Diagnostic Principles and Applications

Robert B. Taylor

Diagnostic Principles and Applications

Avoiding Medical Errors, Passing Board
Exams, and Providing Informed Patient Care

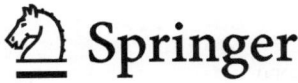 Springer

Robert B. Taylor, MD
Department of Family Medicine
Oregon Health & Science University
Portland
Oregon
USA

ISBN 978-1-4614-1110-9   ISBN 978-1-4614-1111-6 (eBook)
DOI 10.1007/978-1-4614-1111-6
Springer New York Heidelberg Dordrecht London

Library of Congress Control Number: 2013932843

Printed on acid-free paper

Springer is part of Springer Science+Business Media (www.springer.com)

I saw on the sand the footprints of an animal, and easily decided that they were those of a little dog. Long and faintly marked furrows, imprinted where the sand was slightly raised between the footprints, told me that it was a bitch whose dugs were hanging down, and that consequently she must have given birth only a few days before. Other marks of a different character, showing the surface of the sand had been constantly grazed on either side of the front paws, informed me that she had very long ears; and, as I observed that the sand was always less deeply indented by one paw than by the other three, I gathered that the bitch belonging to our august queen was a little lame, if I may venture to so say so.

Voltaire. The history of Zadig; or, the book of fate: an oriental tale. In: Candide and other writings. New York: The Modern Library; 1956. Originally published in France in 1747.

Diagnosis is founded upon the observation of trifles.

Meador CK. A little book of doctors' rules II. Philadelphia: Hanley & Belfus; 1999.

"Never mind," said Holmes, laughing; "It is my business to know things. Perhaps I have trained myself to see what others overlook. If not, why should you come to consult me?"

Arthur Conan Doyle. A case of identity. In: The adventures of Sherlock Holmes. Hertfordshire: Wordsworth Editions; 1992.

Clinical Practice Notice

Everyone involved with the preparation of this book has worked very hard to assure that information presented here is accurate and that it represents accepted clinical practice. These efforts include confirming that diagnostic methods and drug usage discussed in this text are in accordance with current practice at the time of publication. Nevertheless, diagnostic approaches, therapeutic recommendations, and dosage schedules change with reports of ongoing research, technologic advances, updated guideline recommendations, and other new information.

The use of the information in this book in a specific clinical setting or situation is the professional responsibility of the clinician. The authors, editors, or publisher are not responsible for errors, omissions, adverse effects, or any consequences arising from the use of information in this book and make no warranty, expressed or implied, with respect to the completeness, timeliness, or accuracy of the book's contents.

Preface

This book is intended to make you a better clinician, as you learn some unfamiliar, perhaps even forgotten, pathways to important diagnostic destinations. If this book were a road map, it would be about the *blue highways*—the less-traveled roads, the ones that may become vital when the *red line* major highways don't get you where you need to go. Think about the observation by American laryngologist Chevalier Jackson cited above: When presented with a wheezing patient, an experienced clinician would consider asthma to top the list of diagnostic considerations. But, in certain clinical contexts, the astute clinician might also think of foreign body aspiration, Wegener granulomatosis, parasitic infection, or airway constriction by an aortic aneurysm. Considering these other possibilities is the first step in making the correct diagnosis.

Thus, this is not a typical, "comprehensive" differential diagnosis book, with long lists of diseases, most familiar to practicing clinicians, that might explain a symptom, sign, or abnormal laboratory finding. Instead I present selected topics, the uncommon—and sometimes exasperatingly esoteric—disease causes we sometimes fail to consider. As an analogy, I offer the *Lifeguard Paradox*: If aspiring lifeguards were to spend the bulk of training time practicing what they will do most of the day at work, they would focus on learning to apply sunscreen to their own bodies. But in lifeguarding, unanticipated events happen, and the lifeguard must know how to handle them. In medicine, uncommon diseases and unlikely manifestations of common diseases occur with occasionally-surprising frequency, and we need to review them from time to time.

Of course, clinicians also encounter some diseases—whether everyday or rare—that we especially do not want to overlook, such as toxic megacolon and testicular torsion; when one of these appears in the coming pages, it is tagged as a *must-not-miss diagnosis*.

In this book, the emphasis is on the enlightened uses of traditional diagnostic tools—clinical history, physical examination, and basic laboratory tests and imaging. The more esoteric investigative methods—PET scans and genetic testing—seem to evolve constantly and are best studied in journal and web-based sources that are more timely than books. Because the content of this book is selective, rather than attempting to be all-inclusive, I have tilted my choices toward identification of high-impact diseases. And also because this is a diagnosis book, I have included information about therapy only when I believed it would enrich the discussion or when I wanted to emphasize the urgency of reaching a timely, precise diagnostic end point.

What will you find in this book? I have included the following categories of diagnostic facts:

Classical diagnostic pearls: For example, the patient with acute pericarditis often leans forward to relieve the anterior chest pain.

Red flag symptoms and signs of serious illness: A salty taste when kissing an infant may represent the first clue to a diagnosis of cystic fibrosis.

Counterintuitive clinical manifestations: The patient with gout may have a normal or low serum uric acid level during the acute attack, and nocturnal back pain has, in fact, not been found to be a useful indicator for serious spinal pathology.

Bellwether signs and symptoms allowing an occasional early diagnosis: Abdominal distension is a common early manifestation of ovarian cancer, and patients with gastric cancer sometimes lose their appetite for meat early in the course of the disease.

Curious clinical manifestations that may point to specific diagnoses: Here I think of the aquagenic pruritus of polycythemia vera, with itching that is aggravated by a hot shower. And the cutaneous *wake sign*, skin lesions resembling the wake left by a moving ship, has been described as seen only with scabies.

Who needs this book? As medicine has become increasingly specialized, medical books have become correspondingly limited in their scope. This book, on the other hand, casts a very wide net, presenting diagnostic facts related to all ages and body systems. Thus, intended readers include medical students, residents, and practicing physicians, nurse practitioners, physician assistants, nurses, and, in fact, anyone involved in making diagnostic observations and decisions.

Do *you* need this book? Let's see. If you see real, live patients in any specialty setting and cannot answer the following five questions, I suggest that you put *Diagnostic Principles and Applications* high on your reading list:

1. What are the three characteristics of the scenario in which a diagnosis of breast cancer is often missed?
2. Of all the sites of possible lymphadenopathy, which is the most worrisome?
3. Low back pain that improves with forward flexion of the spine suggests what diagnosis?
4. Hyponatremia may be the clue to what psychiatric disorder?
5. Can you describe the Au–Henkind test for acute iritis, the Wartenberg sign in ulnar nerve palsy, and the Tullio phenomenon as a clue to the cause of vertigo?

What are key features of this book? Medical education and clinical experience are remarkably capricious. A newly minted medical graduate may never have seen a patient with Guillain–Barré syndrome or osteomyelitis of the spine. Even the experienced practitioner may never have encountered anyone complaining of pathologically excessive yawning or a patient with suspected cerebrospinal fluid rhinorrhea. Owing to the variability in individual training and experience, each reader will be well acquainted with some of the entities described in this book, considering what I present to be well known and wondering why I included them at all. Others will find this same information to be new knowledge. For the most part, I have attempted to select facts not generally covered in basic physical examination courses or textbooks.

Traditional diagnosis books are organized by symptoms and signs—hemoptysis, chest pain, or bullous eruption of the skin—in contrast to disease-oriented reference books, which are organized by names of various clinical entities: lung cancer, myocardial infarction, or pemphigus. In this book, I present information under both types of headings, manifestations and diseases. When questions arose, I listed items under the body organ or system in which manifestations are most likely to occur. For example, consider the clue that the patient with herpes zoster who develops a vesicle near the tip of the nose is at risk of developing herpes zoster ophthalmicus; this pearl is presented in Chap. 5 rather than Chap. 4.

To save space, and with apologies to all the often-anonymous et al. coauthors of the world, I have used a shorthand reference style, citing the first author only, plus article title, journal, year, volume, and initial page number. Using an abbreviated reference style allows more pages for facts and still provides enough information to find the article on PubMed, BioMedLib, or Google Scholar. Also, readers will find reference citations listed immediately following the stated fact and commentary, rather than at the end of the chapter; in my own reading I find this placement of references to be especially helpful. In the appendix, I have included a list of a glossary of statistical terms used in the book.

This book is literature-based, by which I mean that all facts in this book are found somewhere in the medical literature. Not all assertions, however, are classically evidence-based. We just don't know with precision (or, at least, I could not locate) the sensitivity or specificity of uncommonly occurring clinical manifestations, such as upbeating nystagmus sometimes observed in Wernicke encephalopathy, or the positive predictive value of some uncommon observations, such the *red ear syndrome* that has occurred in some patients with migraine. Some phenomena presented, such as yellow vision with digitalis intoxication, represent examples of often repeated clinical lore, validated by repeated observations of experienced clinicians, and are included because they seem to have weathered the test of time, supported by a few case reports. But most of what is presented here, such as the positive correlation of a high pulse pressure and white coat hypertension, has been subjected to statistical analysis and peer review. I recognize that some of what I describe is controversial and that future clinical studies may lead us to reconsider what we think is true and wise today. I urge the reader to use this book as a series of prompts and then consult the current literature before making clinical decisions if in unfamiliar territory.

In my research for this book, I found that a number of my reference citations for physical findings and diagnostic maneuvers—such as the Lisker tibial tap sign for deep vein thrombophlebitis of the lower extremity, discussed in Chap. 6—are found in literature that some may call *dated*. Today, teaching indicator symptoms and physical biomarkers of disease seems to be out of style in medical school, and as Verghese writes, "Because the echocardiogram, magnetic resonance imaging, and computed tomographic can precisely characterize anatomy, the physical exam is too often viewed as redundant" [2]. I hold that so-called old-fashioned historical clues and physical signs are not only part of our medical heritage; their recognition can often spell the difference between prompt identification of disease and an expensive, time-consuming journey through the clinical laboratory and diagnostic imaging suite. In fact, with the inconsistent quality of medical school teaching regarding the physical examination and the rising costs of high-tech healthcare, I think this book is needed more than ever.

How should you use this book? This is not a classical course text to be studied in a classroom setting. Nor is it a clinical reference book, intended to be *searched* but not really *read*. This is a "topical" book, presenting a somewhat eclectic collection of facts that someday may prove useful in specific puzzling situations. Hence, the book should be *read*, cover to cover. Put it at your bedside; take it to the beach; enjoy it on a plane trip. The goal is both to learn diagnostic principles and applications today and to imprint them deep in your memory for future reference. I continue to like my metaphor of *Post-It* notes used to describe my book: *Essential Medical Facts Every Clinician Should Know* [3]. What you read today may not be clinically pertinent for months or years, but when the time comes, the information is there, *posted* in memory. Then, just to confirm your recollection, you can find it here again using the index provided or perhaps check out the original report on-line.

In addition to my *read, post it, recollect, and confirm* approach, the book's index will be a good place to look when faced with a head-scratching, seemingly unsolvable diagnostic puzzle. Use the index to locate the answers to the five questions posed above.

It is axiomatic that the most common diseases occur most commonly. What clinician has not heard the axiom that when you hear hoofbeats, expect to hear horses, not zebras? But it is also true that we all encounter the uncommon entity occasionally, perhaps when we least expect to do so. Knowing the contents of this book can help you recognize the unlikely disease manifestation of a *horse* disorder or spot the *zebra* diagnosis when it presents itself in the middle of a busy office session or on an exam question.

Finally, this book is intended to be easy to read, with just enough statistical details to support assertions, without becoming excessively burdened with methodologic minutiae. I have attempted to enrich your knowledge of our heritage by including a few historical anecdotes. And most of all, I have done my best to make this book clinically useful in, as the title says:

Preventing medical errors

Passing board examinations
and

Providing informed patient care

1. Jackson C. A new diagnostic sign of foreign body in trachea of bronchi, the "asthmatoid wheeze." Am J Med Sci. 1918;156:626.
2. Verghese A. Culture shock: patient as icon, icon as patient. N Engl J Med. 2008;359:2748.
3. Taylor R. Essential medical facts every clinician should know. New York: Springer; 2011.

Portland, OR, USA   Robert B. Taylor, MD

Acknowledgments

Anyone who has ever written a single-author book such as this soon realizes that the what appears in print is, in no way, the product of a single mind. This book has many contributors; most are probably not aware of the help they were to me.

Some of these otherwise anonymous contributors are: my personal physician for a quarter century, William (Bill) Toffler, MD, one of the great diagnosticians among us; my professional colleagues, also for the past 25+ years, John Saultz, MD, and Scott Fields, MD; Bob Bomengen, MD, good friend and an inspirational frontier doctor; (the late) Peter Goodwin, valued fellow physician and another good friend; and Charles Visokay, MD, who helped me get started in medical writing. In addition, I gratefully acknowledge the guidance and support of my Springer editor, Katharine Cacace.

My most insightful writing colleague is my wife, Anita D. Taylor, MA Ed, an accomplished author and academician, and sometimes painfully honest critic.

Finally, I thank Doctors Osler, Hutchinson, Wilms, Scheuermann, Graves, Kallmann, Waardenburg, and all the others who have recognized the connections between clinical manifestations and disease causes. Many of these physicians have lent their names to clinical signs, maneuvers, tumors, and syndromes. These observations, studied and reported, are the bedrock of today's *Diagnostic Principles and Applications*.

Contents

Chapter 1
Undifferentiated Problems

For most diagnoses, all that is needed is an ounce of knowledge,
an ounce of intelligence, and a pound of thoroughness.

Anonymous [1]

Contents

R.B. Taylor, *Diagnostic Principles and Applications,*
DOI 10.1007/978-1-4614-1111-6_1, © Springer Science+Business Media, LLC 2013

The undifferentiated manifestations of disease can present challenging puzzles, calling for diagnostic acumen, the casting of a wide, yet rational, net, and as the quotation cited above advises, *a pound of thoroughness*. What are the undifferentiated problems? They are those that cannot—at least as first glance—be ascribed to any single organ or body system, thus generally eluding ownership by a specific medical specialty. The undifferentiated problems include fever, fatigue, anorexia, and the others listed above and discussed below.

Because many of these undifferentiated problems can be, well, nonspecific, there will be the temptation to employ the *Casablanca strategy*. This tendency to exhaust all etiologic possibilities in the first round of testing is named for the closing scenes of the movie Casablanca when, following Rick's shooting of Major Strasser, Captain Renault orders: "Round up the usual suspects." Of course, this strategy will not solve the crime, but it will buy some time for Victor and Ilsa to escape [2]. Such a strategy allows the clinician to feel that every possibility is being explored but at considerable expense and at the risk of turning up a host of misleading findings. In just such a setting, recognition of subtle clues or knowledge of statistical probabilities may be more valuable than a comprehensive battery of tests.

1. Anonymous. From: Strauss MB. Familiar medical quotations. Boston: Little and Brown; 1968. p. 99.
2. Memorable quotes for Casablanca 1942. Available at: http://www.imdb.com/title/tt0034583/quotes.

Fever

In most instances, unexplained fever is not caused by a rare or exotic disease, but by an uncommon presentation of a common disease.

Fever of unknown origin (FUO) has been defined as fever greater than 38.3 °C (100.9 °F) on several occasions over at least 3 weeks with no diagnosis after the appropriate initial testing. Bleeker-Rovers reports that infection is the cause in about one-quarter of instances, followed by tumor and noninfectious inflammatory diseases. Yet, in half of all cases, no firm diagnosis could be elucidated [1].

Zenone, in France, reviewed 144 cases of community-acquired FUO. Of these an etiologic diagnosis was determined in 107 patients, with the following distribution: noninfectious inflammatory disorders (35.5 %), infections (30.8 %), miscellaneous causes (20.6 %), and malignancies (13.5 %). No specific cause for the fever could be identified in 37 patients (25.7 % of the total). The author noted the higher frequency of giant cell arteritis and polymyalgia rheumatica in the elderly and Epstein-Barr virus and cytomegalovirus infections in younger patients [2].

From Turkey comes a paper reminding us that the spectrum of causes can vary with geographic location; presenting a study of 71 patients with FUO in which infection was the most common etiology (32 patients, 45.1 %) with tuberculosis the culprit in 40 % of these infections [3].

1. Bleeker-Rovers CP, et al. Fever of unknown origin. Semin Nucl Med. 2009;39:81.
2. Zenone T. Fever of unknown origin in adults: evaluation of 144 cases in a non-university hospital. Scand J Inf Dis. 2006;38:632.
3. Colpan A. Fever of unknown origin: analysis of 71 consecutive cases. Am J Med Sci. 2007;337:92.

Heat stroke—an elevation of core temperature to 40 °C (104 °F) or greater associated with central nervous system disturbances—is a red-flag emergency requiring immediate intervention, with rapid lowering of the core temperature.

Heat stroke, a *must-not-miss diagnosis*, must not be confused with less serious heat-related syndromes such as heat cramps, heat exhaustion, and heat syncope, situations in which movement to a cool environment, hydration, and less drastic cooling measures will suffice [1].

Be aware that in acute heat stroke the presence or absence of sweating lacks diagnostic value: The patient may have anhidrosis or may continue to perspire [2].

1. Sandor RP. Heat illness; on-site diagnosis and cooling. Phys Sportsmed. 1997;25:35.
2. Becker JA. Heat-related illness. Am Fam Physician. 2011;83:1325.

Fever is one of the manifestations of the DRESS syndrome, a potentially lethal reaction to a drug such as a sulfonamide, allopurinol, or an anticonvulsant such as phenobarbital, phenytoin (Dilantin), or carbamazepine (Tegretol).

DRESS is an acronym for *d*rug *r*ash with *e*osinophilia and *s*ystemic *s*ymptoms. To diagnose the DRESS syndrome, the patient must exhibit three of the following manifestations: fever, exanthematous rash, eosinophilia, atypical circulating lymphocytes, and hepatitis. The DRESS syndrome may be confused with sepsis, especially in a patient taking a sulfonamide for an infection, or even thrombotic thrombocytopenic purpura [1].

1. Fleming P, et al. The DRESS syndrome: the great mimicker. Pharmacotherapy. 2011;31:45e.

Fatigue

Although fatigue is a common presenting symptom in office practice, laboratory testing provides results that affect management in only 5 % of patients.

The above statement is the conclusion of Rosenthal et al., who remind us that the differential diagnosis of fatigue must include mental disorders such as depression, lifestyle issues such as sleep deprivation, medication side effects, chronic diseases such as anemia and hypothyroidism, and life-threatening diseases such as cancer [1]. Harvey et al. hold that the most commonly occurring comorbid condition in patients with chronic fatigue syndrome is depression [2]. Depression, of course, will not show up on laboratory testing.

1. Rosenthal C, et al. Fatigue: an overview. Am Fam Physician 2008;78:1173.
2. Harvey SB, et al. Chronic fatigue syndrome: identifying zebras amongst the horses. BMC Med. 2009;7:58.

Fatigue is surprisingly prevalent among adolescents, occurring more commonly in girls than boys.

In a study of 1,718 boys and 1,749 girls, 20.5 % of girls and 6.5 % of boys scored above the clinical cutoff on the Individual Strength Checklist, and of these, 80.0 % of girls and 61.5 % of boys reported severe fatigue for ≥ 1 month [1].

1. ter Wolbeek M, et al. Severe fatigue in adolescents: a common phenomenon? Pediatrics. 2006;117:e1078.

Chronic fatigue syndrome (CFS), a distinct disorder, is generally an exclusion diagnosis made after other physical and psychological causes have been ruled out.

The diagnosis of CFS is based on finding the new onset of fatigue causing 50 % or greater reduction in activity for at least 6 months (the major criterion), accompanied by the presence of various other manifestations such as mild fever, muscle weakness, recurrent headache, migratory joint pain, and sleep disturbance (minor criteria) [1]. Although diagnostic testing is often undertaken to exclude causes such as anemia, hypothyroidism, fibromyalgia, and Lyme disease, CFS patients are typically found to have frustratingly normal laboratory test results. There is, for the record, no test that can conclusively confirm—or refute—the diagnosis of CFS [2]. CFS is one of those clinical presentations in which as McDonald states: "Time is often a better diagnostician than the best anatomic pathologist" [3].

1. Fukuda K, et al. The chronic fatigue syndrome: a comprehensive approach to its definition and study. International Chronic Fatigue Syndrome Study Group. Ann Intern Med. 1994;121:953.
2. Alfredo AF. Chronic fatigue syndrome: etiology, diagnosis and treatment. BMC Psychiatry. 2009;Suppl+1:S1.
3. McDonald EC. Quoted in: Meador CK. A little book of doctors' rules II. Philadelphia: Hanley & Belfus; 1999. p. 220.

Once in a while, a patient with chronic fatigue will have a zebra diagnosis.

Before labeling the patient as having CFS, be sure to consider physical causes. The list of possibilities is long and includes such entities as adrenal insufficiency, valvular heart disease, cardiomyopathy, endocarditis, restrictive lung disease, renal failure, chronic liver disease, tuberculosis, human immunodeficiency virus (HIV) infection, and a variety of malignancies [1].

Just to highlight an uncommon cause of fatigue, in a series of patients with chronic mercury toxicity (think of a diet very high in *large-fish* seafood), 88.8 % of patients had memory loss, 32.3 % reported severe fatigue, and 27.5 % had depression [2].

1. Harvey SB, et al. Chronic fatigue syndrome: identifying zebras amongst the horses. BMC Med. 2009;7:58.
2. Wojcik DP, et al. Mercury toxicity presenting as chronic fatigue, memory impairment and depression. Neuro Endocrinol Lett. 2006;8:415.

Chronic fatigue may be an early symptom of multiple sclerosis (MS).

In MS patients, fatigue occurs commonly and is one of the most disabling manifestations of the disease [1]. MS must be part of the differential diagnosis of CFS, especially in young women. Morrow et al., reviewing a large sample of cases, conclude that "self-reported fatigue, while correlated with self-reported depression, is not significantly related to cognitive capacity in MS" [2].

1. Kos D, et al. Origin of fatigue in multiple sclerosis: review of the literature. Neurorehabil Neural Repair. 2008;22:91.
2. Morrow SA, et al. Subjective fatigue is not associated with cognitive impairment in multiple sclerosis: cross sectional and longitudinal analysis. Mult Scler. 2009;8:998.

Consider Sjögren syndrome in the differential diagnosis of fatigue.

Sjögren syndrome, a systemic disease with diverse manifestations that may include dry eyes, dry mouth, and arthralgia, can also cause fatigue [1]. This connection is likely to be made more often and earlier in the future, owing to the disclosure by tennis star Venus Williams that for 4 years she lacked stamina and was subsequently misdiagnosed as having exercise-induced asthma. Her true diagnosis was Sjögren syndrome.

1. Dass S, et al. Reduction of fatigue in Sjögren syndrome with rituximab; results of a randomized, double blind, placebo-controlled pilot study. Arch Rheum Dis. 2008;67:1541.

Anorexia

Anorexia, with decreased hunger and early satiety, may be more common than generally believed.

Anorexia has been reported in approximately one of three older women and men [1]. Among these individuals, depression is the most common cause identified [2]. Other causes to consider include chronic infections such as viral hepatitis, HIV infection, and tuberculosis; endocrine diseases such as diabetes mellitus and Addison disease; inflammatory causes such as pancreatitis and rheumatoid arthritis; chronic disease such as chronic renal failure and Alzheimer disease; any of a number of drugs such as amphetamines and alcohol; eating disorders; and, of course, a variety of neoplasms such as cancer of the colon or lung.

1. Thoma DR. Anorexia: etiology, epidemiology and management in older people. Drugs Aging. 2009;26:557.
2. Morley JE. Anorexia in older persons: epidemiology and optimal treatment. Drugs Aging. 1996;8:134.

Anorexia may be an early symptom of acute hepatitis of various types.

One manifestation of liver disease may be the loss of appetite. In addition, smokers may describe that cigarettes *taste bad*. In acute viral hepatitis, the pre-icteric phase may be characterized by anorexia, perhaps accompanied by malaise, nausea, vomiting, and pains in muscles and joints [1]. Early recognition of viral hepatitis can be important because, for example, in preschoolers hepatitis A infection sometimes causes liver failure [2].

1. Gujral H, et al. Understanding viral hepatitis: a guide for primary care. Nurse Pract. 2009;34:23.
2. Latifa T. Current issues in the management of pediatric viral hepatitis. Liver Int. 2010;30:5.

Unintentional Weight Loss

Unintentional weight loss (UWL) may herald both morbidity—increased susceptibility to infection, impaired wound healing, and greater susceptibility to bedsores—and increased risk of death. Yet the data for the implications of unintentional and intentional weight loss are not crystal clear.

Unintentional weight loss commands our attention when the patient loses 4.5 kg (10 lb) or more than 5 % of body weight over 6–12 months, especially if the decrement is progressive. Bouras reports that UWL occurs in up to 13 % of elderly individuals and 50–60 % of nursing home residents [1].

Simonsen reviewed a collection of studies on intentional weight loss (IWL), finding three with increased mortality, two with decreased mortality, and four lacking a relationship between IWL and total mortality [2].

Allison et al. may offer some insight into the issue of weight loss and mortality. In a review of two large, population-based cohort studies, they found that among individuals who were not severely obese, weight loss was linked to increased mortality, but loss of body fat (measured by skinfolds) was associated with a decreased mortality rate [3].

1. Bouras EP, et al. Rational approach to patients with unintentional weight loss. Mayo Clin Proc. 2001:76;923.
2. Simonsen MK, et al. Intentional weight loss and mortality among initially healthy men and women. Nutr Rev. 2008;66:375.
3. Allison DB, et al. Weight loss increases and fat loss decreases all-cause mortality rate: rates from two independent cohort studies. Int J Obes Relat Metab Disord. 1999;23:603.

Involuntary weight loss should prompt a search for a treatable cause.

In an early study, Marton et al. evaluated 91 patients with involuntary weight loss, finding physical causes of weight loss in 59 patients (65 %); of these physical causes of weight loss were clinically evident on initial examination in 55 individuals (a number that I find quite high). In 32 (35 %) of the 91 patients, no physical cause of weight loss was detected [1].

In a subsequent study, Rabinowitz et al. reviewed 154 patients with UWL, finding that 36.3 % had neoplasms, notably those of the gastrointestinal (GI) tract. In 23.3 % of patients, no causative disease was found. The other half of the patients studied were found to have assorted disorders, especially GI and psychiatric diseases. Contrary to what might be expected, few instances of UWL were attributed to hyperthyroidism or diabetes mellitus [2].

1. Marton KI, et al. Involuntary weight loss: diagnostic and prognostic significance. Ann Intern Med. 1981;95:568.
2. Rabinowitz M, et al. Unintentional weight loss: a retrospective analysis of 154 cases. Arch Int Med. 1986;146:186.

When unintentional weight loss occurs in a nursing home resident, think of depression or medication effects.

A study of 156 nursing home residents ages 51–105 years with UWL revealed depression as the cause in 36 % of individuals. Other causes included medication effects, psychotropic drug reduction, dementia, and obsessive–compulsive disorder [1]. A report by McMinn et al. highlights the contribution of medication side effects to UWL in older adults. Parenthetically, this same paper points out that when cancer is the cause, the prognosis is often poor because, by the time weight loss is noted, the tumor is likely to be in an advanced stage [2].

1. Morley JE, et al. Causes of weight loss in a community nursing home. J Am Geriatr Soc. 1994;42:583.
2. McMinn J, et al. Investigation and management of unintentional weight loss in older adults. BMJ. 2011;342:d1972.

A patient with cancer, involuntary weight loss and anorexia may have the cancer cachexia syndrome (CCS), found in at least one person in five who dies of cancer.

CCS can lead to poor cancer treatment tolerance and decreased quality of life. The availability of treatment options—including psychosocial interventions and a variety of pharmacologic possibilities, such as progestins, steroids, and the antiemetic metoclopramide (Reglan)—makes efforts at early recognition worthwhile [1].

1. Hopkinson JB. Management of weight loss and anorexia. Ann Oncol. 2008;19:S289.

Involuntary weight loss may be an early sign of Alzheimer disease.

In a study of 449 older persons followed for 6 years, 125 developed dementia of the Alzheimer type (DAT); 324 did not develop dementia. The weight loss of those with DAT was 1.2 lb per year, compared with 0.6 lb per year in the non-dementia group [1].

1. Johnson DK, et al. Accelerated weight loss may precede diagnosis in Alzheimer disease. Arch Neurol. 2006;63:1312.

Sleep Disorders

Insomnia and other sleep disorders can coexist with a host of other conditions, sometimes in a causative role and or as a result of concurrent disease. Elucidating which, if either, can be a diagnostic challenge.

Insomnia may go hand in hand with drug use and abuse; psychiatric disease such as anxiety, depression, and posttraumatic stress disorder; cardiovascular disease such as heart failure with paroxysmal nocturnal dyspnea; chronic obstructive lung disease and asthma; GI diseases such as inflammatory bowel disease; arthritis of various types; and pain from any source. In most cases, the disease causes the insomnia, but not always [1]. And then, in addition, there are the primary sleep disorders such as sleep apnea, restless leg syndrome, and circadian rhythm disturbances.

Bloom et al. remind us of the bidirectional relationship between sleep disorders and health problems of aging, including depression, hypertension, and cardiovascular and cerebrovascular disease [2].

1. Billiard M, et al. Is insomnia best categorized as a symptom or a disease? Sleep Med. 2004;6:S35.
2. Bloom HG, et al. Evidence-based recommendation for the assessment and management of sleep disorders in older persons. J Am Geriatr Soc. 2009;57:761.

The patient who falls asleep in the course of an office visit may have narcolepsy, but don't overlook the possibility of the obesity-hypoventilation syndrome (OHS), aka the *Pickwickian* syndrome.

The eponym comes from Joe, the *fat boy*, described by Charles Dickens in his story, *The Posthumous Papers of the Pickwick Club*. Weitzenblum et al. describe the OHS as chronic alveolar hypoventilation in an obese individual with a body mass index greater than 30 kg/m². Most are not hypercapnic, even in the face of severe obesity. Many Pickwickian patients also have diabetes mellitus, hypertension, and heart failure, and the disease has a high mortality [1].

1. Weitzenblum E, et al. Obesity-hypoventilation syndrome. Rev Mal Respir. 2008;25:391.

The patient, especially an adolescent, who goes to sleep very late and sleeps late in the morning may have delayed sleep phase syndrome (DSPS).

Yes, there may be a reason why your teenager seems to live in a distant time zone. Patients with DSPS turn in and arise much later than what we consider normal. In one review of 33 DSPS patients, the mean bedtime was 4 a.m. and the mean time of arising was 10:38 a.m. [1]. The problem is much more than the household disruption caused by a dyssynchronous sleep cycle. Patients with DSCS tend to have daytime sleepiness and poor function at school or on the job [2]. Of the 33 patients described by Regenstein, 25 had a diagnosis of depression, either currently or in the past [1].

Because the syndrome can seem consistent with a young person's personal choices, the distinction between disease and lifestyle can be murky.

1. Regenstein QR, et al. Delayed sleep phase syndrome: a review of its clinical aspects. Am J Psychiatry. 1995;152:602.
2. Stores G. Sleep disorders in general and adolescence. J Fam Health Care. 2009;19:51.

Rapid eye movement (REM) sleep behavior disorder (RBD) is manifested as abnormal, often violent motor behavior with a loss of electromyographic atonia during REM sleep.

Robust chin and limb muscle activity occurs commonly, with the potential to disrupt sleep and even injure the bed partner [1]. RBD occurs in 0.5 % of the population [2]. For the record, that is 1 in every 200 adults, making this a not uncommon disease. The significance of RBD is this: A number of studies have identified RBD as an early marker for neurodegenerative diseases, such as Parkinson disease, Lewy body dementia, multiple system atrophy, and DAT [1–4].

1. Gagnon JF, et al. Mild cognitive impairment in rapid eye movement sleep behavior disorder and Parkinson's disease. Ann Neurol. 2009;66:39.
2. Zoetmulder M, et al. Rapid eye movement sleep behavior disorder—diagnosis, causes and treatment. Ugeskr Laeger. 2009;171:1849.
3. Postuma RB, et al. Quantifying the risk of neurodegenerative disease in idiopathic REM sleep behavior disorder. Neurology. 2009;72:1294.
4. Iranzo A, et al. Rapid eye movement sleep behavior disorder as an early marker for a neurodegenerative disorder: a descriptive study. Lancet Neurol. 2006;5:572.

Although periodic leg movement disorder is readily apparent electromyographically on nocturnal polysomnography, restless leg syndrome (RLS) is a clinical diagnosis [1].

Periodic leg movement disorder, a common cause of interrupted sleep, may not be considered in the differential of insomnia. Restless leg syndrome, on the other hand, has achieved widespread recognition, owing to television advertisements for dopamine agonists directed at patients.

RLS is especially likely to be found in patients on dialysis, who may also report insomnia and excessive daytime sleepiness [2].

1. Wolkove N, et al. Sleep and aging: sleep disorders commonly found in older people. Can Med Assoc J. 2007;176:1255.
2. Al-Jahdali HH, et al. Restless legs syndrome in patients on dialysis. Saudi J Kidney Dis Transpl. 2009;20:378.

Syncope

The most common causes of syncope are the neurally mediated disorders—generally benign conditions related to vasodilation or vagally mediated changes in heart rate resulting in transient cerebral hypoperfusion.

Syncope—the most common cause of transient loss of consciousness—occurs at some time in the lives of about 40 % of adults [1]. The most common presentation is sudden *collapse*, followed before long by full recovery largely independent of the ministrations of well-meaning bystanders. Most events last about 30 s, and unconsciousness after 5 min has passed must be viewed with suspicion.

Diligent clinical observation and investigation reveal a plausible cause in 50–80 % of patients with syncope, which is important because red-flag causes such as cardiac arrhythmias may warrant hospitalization [2]. Even in the face of some ominous causes, a study of 305,932 patients over 5 years revealed an overall mortality rate in patients with syncope of 0.28 % ($p = 0.07$), with the odds ratio for death increasing with age [3].

Mussi et al. remind us that syncope, especially that related to orthostatic hypotension, can cause falls resulting in injuries, with the risk greatest in the elderly [4].

1. Parry SW, et al. An approach to the evaluation and management of syncope in adults. BMJ. 2010;340:468.
2. Ouyang H, et al. Diagnosis and evaluation of syncope in the emergency department. Emerg Med Clin North Am. 2010;28:471.
3. Alshekhlee A, et al. Incidence and mortality rates of syncope in the United States. Am J Med. 2009;122:181.
4. Mussi C, et al. Orthostatic hypotension as cause of syncope in patients older than 65 years admitted to emergency departments for transient loss of consciousness. J Gerontol A Biol Sci Med Sci. 2009;64:801.

In contrast to the low overall mortality risk attributed to syncope, the risk of dying is high in patients with cardiac syncope.

Up to one-third of patients with cardiac syncope who are untreated may die within a year [1]. Tachy- and bradyarrhythmias are the most common types of cardiac syncope. Other cardiovascular causes of syncope include atrial fibrillation, sick sinus syndrome, myxoma, hypertrophic cardiomyopathy, pulmonary hypertension, and aortic stenosis.

1. Seegers J, et al. Cardiac syncope: diagnosis and therapy. Herzschrittmacherther Electrophysiol. 2011;22:107.

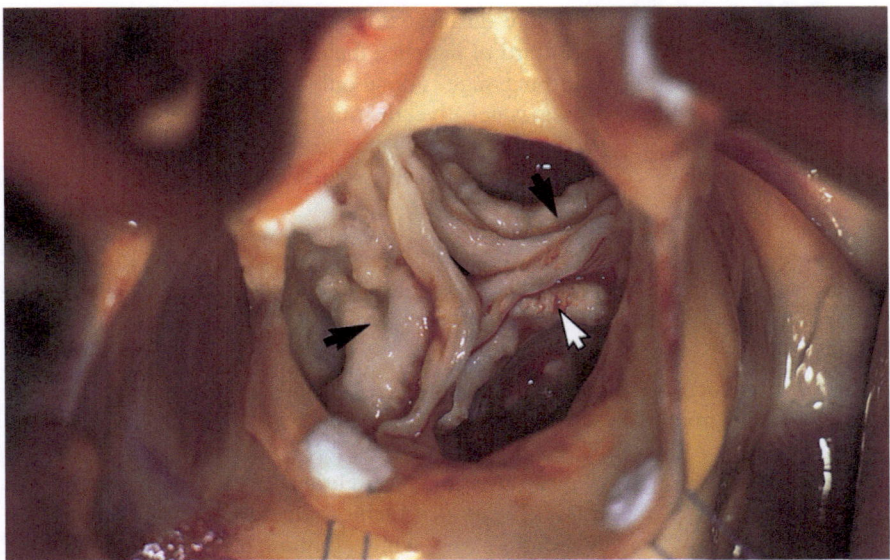

Fig. 1.1 Degenerative aortic stenosis. Stenosis is caused by calcification, which may involve the whole body of the cusps or be localized in the form of lumps or bars of calcium (*arrows*)

Consider aortic stenosis in the older individual who experiences the new onset of syncopal episodes.

Syncope (or near-syncope), along with angina pectoris and heart failure, are the three chief keys to the diagnosis of aortic stenosis in the elderly, although the disease may be diagnosed before these manifestations occur by careful auscultation of a systolic murmur [1] (see Fig. 1.1). Doppler echocardiography can provide diagnostic confirmation and provide an estimate of disease severity [2].

Early detection and intervention in patients with aortic stenosis is vital. Untreated patients with aortic stenosis have been reported to have a survival time after the first occurrence of syncope of 27 ± 15 months [3].

1. Aronow WS. Recognition and management of aortic stenosis in the elderly. Geriatrics; 2007;62:23.
2. Otto CM. Aortic stenosis: clinical evaluation and optimal timing of surgery. Cardiol Clin. 1998;16:353.
3. Horstkotte D, et al. The natural history of aortic valve stenosis. Eur Heart J. 1988;9 Suppl E:57.

The older individual with syncope may have carotid sinus sensitivity.

Often not considered in the differential diagnosis of syncope, carotid sinus sensitivity can be diagnosed by detecting ≥ 3 s of cardioinhibitory asystole or a ≥ 50-mm decrease in systolic blood pressure during carotid massage [1]. Parry et al. have demonstrated that in up to one-third of patients, the diagnosis of carotid sinus sensitivity will be missed if carotid massage is done only in the supine position. They recommend that if the supine test is negative, the massage should be repeated in the head-up tilt position [2]. Detection of carotid sinus sensitivity is important because many patients with this disorder will benefit from cardiac pacing [2].

1. Benditt DG, et al. Syncope: therapeutic approaches. J Am Coll Cardiol. 2009;53:1741.
2. Parry SW, et al. Diagnosis of carotid sinus hypersensitivity in older adults: carotid sinus massage in the upright position is essential. Cardiovasc Med. 2000;83:22.

Syncope associated with intermittent unilateral claudication of an arm may be caused by the subclavian steal syndrome (SSS).

SSS describes the reversal of flow through the vertebral artery which may be caused by stenosis of the proximal subclavian or brachiocephalic artery [1]. Chan-Tack describes an elderly woman with SSS who, while climbing a flight of stairs, turned her head to the left and abruptly passed out. Her left arm had a much-reduced blood pressure and peripheral pulses detectable only by Doppler ultrasonography [2]. I am happy to report that, aside from the risk of falls, the symptoms described rarely lead to permanent neurological damage [1].

1. Smith JM, et al. Subclavian steal syndrome: a review of 59 consecutive cases. J Cardiovasc Surg (Torino). 1994;35:11.
2. Chan-Tack KM. Subclavian steal syndrome: a rare but important cause of syncope. South Med J. 2001;94:445.

Flushing

When a patient complains of cutaneous flushing, think first of drug effects.

Niacin is the drug we first consider when a patient describes flushing. Often pre-scribed for dyslipidemic patients, niacin induces widespread and annoying cutane-ous vasodilation, an action of the drug that, when the extended-release formulation is used, can sometimes be reduced by premedication with aspirin [1].

A type of niacin-induced flushing may be experienced by patients using so-called abuse-resistant oxycodone, to which niacin has been added to prevent ingestion of large quantities of tablets by causing flushing and itching [2].

Other drugs that may cause flushing include:

- Aminophylline
- Amyl nitrite
- Dipyridamole
- Nitroglycerine
- Papaverine
- Hydralazine
- Isoproterenol
- Reserpine
- Theophylline
- Tolazoline

In addition, alcohol can cause flushing, a situation which should not present a diag-nostic dilemma. What may be more puzzling is the Antabuse-like flushing that occurs when a diabetic person treated with chlorpropamide (Diabinese) ingests alcohol [3].

1. Kamanna VS, et al. The mechanism and mitigation of niacin-induced flushing. Int J Clin Pract. 2009;63:1369.
2. Pharmacology watch. 2011;9:2.
3. Groop L, et al. Roles of chlorpropamide, alcohol and acetaldehyde in determining the chlorpro-pamide-alcohol flush. Diabetologia; 1984;26:34.

The patient with cutaneous flushing unresponsive to usual therapy—such as estro-gen use in menopausal women—may have metastatic carcinoid syndrome (CS).

The most common type of endocrine tumor, CS, classically causes flushing, diar-rhea, breathlessness, and wheezing (see Fig. 1.2). The hallmark manifestation of flushing is found in 85 % of CS patients. Symptoms may be precipitated by inges-tion of alcohol or chocolate [1, 2].

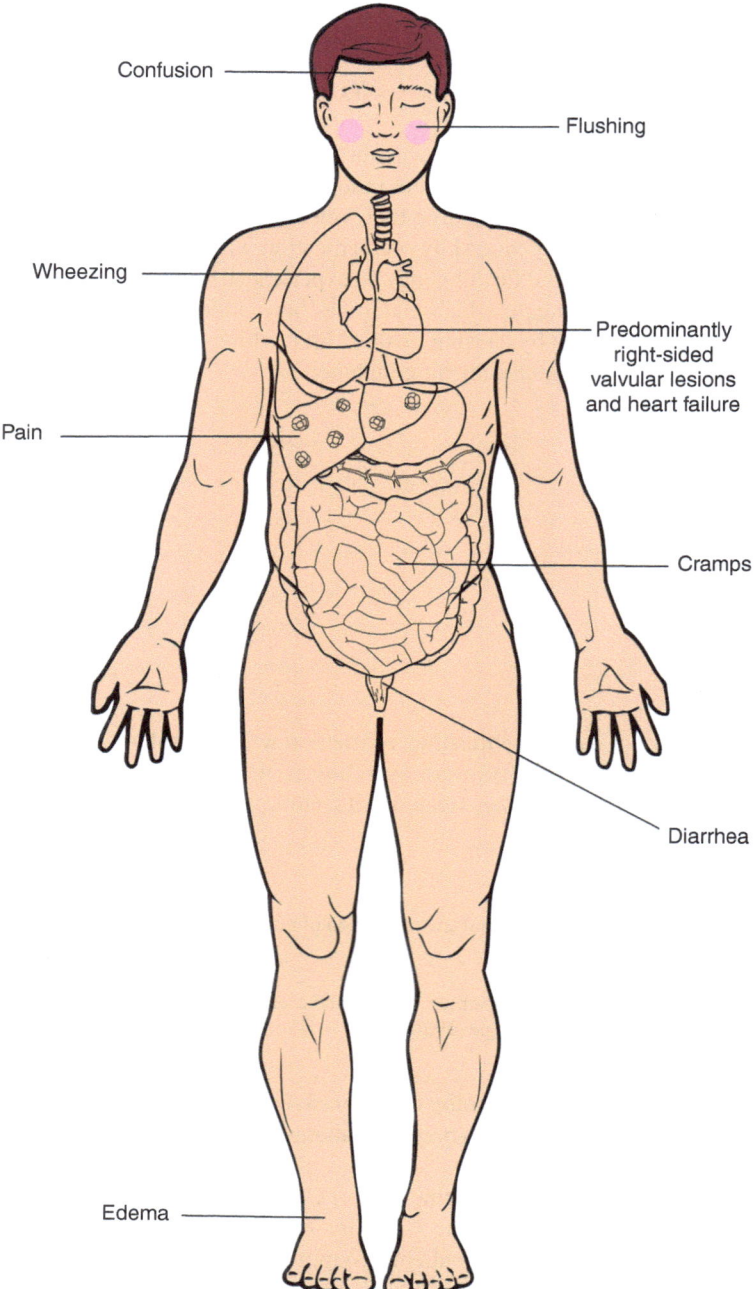

Fig. 1.2 Manifestations of carcinoid tumor

Most tumors begin in the intestine; the syndrome is typically noted when metastasis has occurred, generally to the liver. Heart valve involvement, an ominous sign, occurs in half of all patients [3].

Testing beginning with detection of increased urinary excretion 5-hydroxy indole acetic acid (5-HIAA) will help differentiate CS from systemic mastocytosis, medullary thyroid carcinoma, pheochromocytoma, and idiopathic flushing [4].

1. Jayasena CN, et al. Carcinoid syndrome. Medicine. 2009;37:454.
2. Brendelow J, et al. Carcinoid syndrome. Eur J Surg Oncol. 2008;34:289.
3. Weinreich C, et al. Carcinoid heart disease: two clinical cases and a review. J Endocrinol Metab Diabetes S Afr. 2011;16:96.
4. Aldrich LB, et al. Distinguishing features of idiopathic flushing and carcinoid syndrome. Arch Intern Med. 1988;148:2614.

Asymmetrical facial flushing describes the Harlequin syndrome, named for a humorous, distinctively masked character found in the Italian *Commedia Dell'arte* and later plays.

This rare syndrome involves diminished unilateral facial flushing and sweating in response to exercise or heat; it is caused by a localized autonomic dysfunction on the involved side. These patients often also have Horner syndrome, with ptosis and meiosis on the non-flushing side of the face [1]. Willaert describes two new cases and 85 patients previously reported in the literature [2].

1. Bremner F, et al. Pupillographic findings in 39 consecutive cases of harlequin syndrome. J Neuroophthalmol. 2008;28:171.
2. Willaert WI, et al. Harlequin syndrome: two new cases and a management proposal. Acta Neurol Belg. 2009;109:214.

Night Sweats

Night sweats, a common occurrence, are underreported, and thus many causes—both benign and ominous—are clinically undetected.

Night sweats, conveniently defined as episodes of drenching diaphoresis requiring that the person change bedclothes, occurred in 41 % of 2,267 adult patients interviewed in one study [1].

Some patients will also describe daytime sweats.

According to Sir William Osler, in endocarditis "sweating is a very frequent symptom, and is worthy of special notice, from the peculiarly drenching character, which is … usually far beyond the average mark of phthisis (tuberculosis, TB) or pyaemia" [2]. In my medical school classes ca 1960, my teachers emphasized that the first diagnosis to consider in a patient with night sweats should be TB. Lymphoma is also on the list of diseases in which night sweating is a dominant symptom. Other diseases to consider are malignancy (other than lymphoma), infection (other than tuberculosis), hyperthyroidism, human immunodeficiency virus infection, obstructive sleep apnea, menopausal hot flashes, carcinoid syndrome, alcohol abuse, and gastroesophageal reflux disease (GERD) [3].

1. Mold JW, et al. Prevalence of night sweats in primary care patients. J Fam Pract. 2002;51:452.
2. Osler W. Gulstonian lectures on malignant endocarditis. Lancet. 1885;1:459.
3. Viera AJ, et al. Diagnosing night sweats. Am Fam Physician. 2003;67:1019.

When a pregnant woman describes the new onset of night sweats, think first of gastroesophageal reflux disease.

Based on the study of two patients and a deep literature review, Young et al. report that profuse night sweats affect approximately 60 % of pregnant women and that anti-reflux treatment may bring relief to those with GERD [1].

1. Young P, et al. Gastroesophageal reflux as a cause of night sweating. An Med Interna (Spanish). 2007;24:285.

Consider panic attacks in the differential diagnosis of night sweats.

Following their study of 2,267 patients, Mold et al. emphasize the importance of investigating both panic attacks and sleep disorders in patients with night sweats, citing these as causative entities that need further investigation [1].

1. Mold JW, et al. Prevalence of night sweats in primary care patients. J Fam Pract. 2002;51:452.

In addition to disease causes, drugs can be the source of night sweats.

The list of drugs that might cause episodic sweating is long. Here are some of the "usual suspects" [1]:

Drug class	Examples
Antidiabetic agents	Insulin, oral agents
Antipyretics	Nonsteroidal anti-inflammatory agents
Antidepressants	Tricyclics, selective serotonin receptor antagonists
Sympathomimetics	Phenylephrine
Gonadotropin-releasing hormone (GnRH) agonists	Leuprolide
Cholinergic agonists	Bethanechol
Other drugs	Bromocriptine, cyclosporine, omeprazole, sildenafil, tamoxifen, theophylline

1. Su CW, et al. What's the best diagnostic evaluation of night sweats? J Fam Pract. 2007;56:493.

In children, night sweats may accompany atopic and respiratory disease.

In a study involving 6,381 children ages 7.7–10.7 years, So et al. found night sweats "to be significantly associated with male gender, younger age, allergic rhinitis, tonsillitis and symptoms suggestive of sleep apnea, insomnia, and parasomnia" [1].

1. So HK, et al. Night sweats in children: prevalence and associated factors. Arch Dis Child. doi:10.1136/ADC.2010.199638.

Selected Undifferentiated Problems

In a book presenting chosen topics—in our case, observations and insights related to diagnosis—there are some items that just don't fit convenient headings and yet are too good to leave out. So, I have clustered them at the end of each chapter under the rubric *selected problems*. The following are some of these.

The initial appearance of frostbite may be deceptively benign [1].

The sentence above, taken directly from the paper by Imray et al., should be remembered when examining a patient with any degree of cold injury. Initial symptoms, which might be misleading, are a sense of cold numbness and impaired sensation, with the patient experiencing a sense of clumsiness [1] (see Fig. 1.3).

Cold injuries have played pivotal roles in history. In his journey to Rome over the Alps in 218 BCE, Hannibal lost half his army to cold injuries. And during the Russian campaign in World War II, more than 15,000 German soldiers required

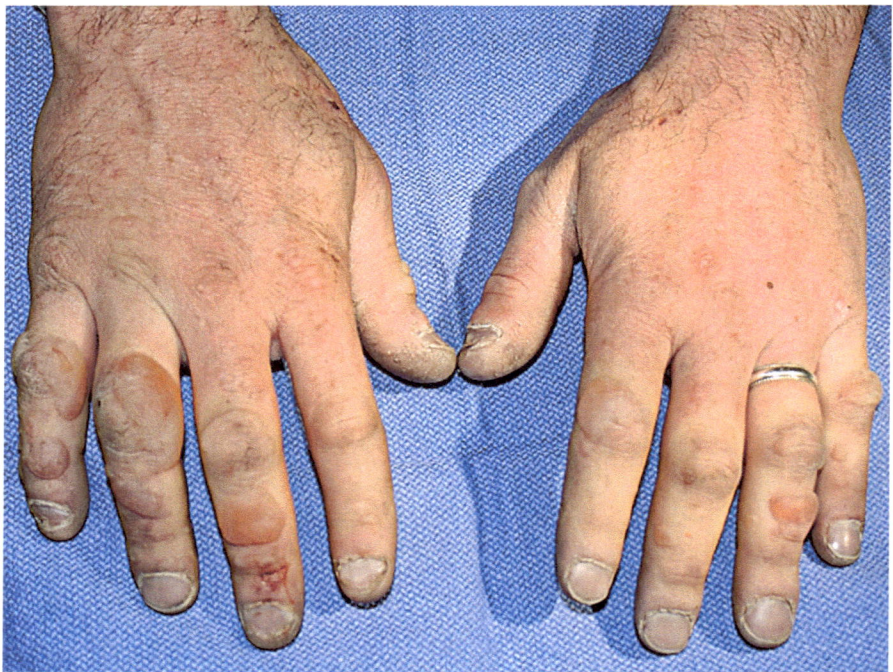

Fig. 1.3 A 37-year-old male with bilateral second- and third-degree frostbite of the hands, with multiple blisters on the fingers which ranged from clear to hemorrhagic

amputations due to frostbite [1]. The patient with cold injury may not be a skier or mountaineer. He or she might also be an elderly individual or perhaps a homeless person exposed to a cold environment. Risk factors for frostbite include inadequate clothing, constrictive clothing, smoking, diabetes, atherosclerosis, dehydration, psychiatric illness, and alcohol use. In a review of 79 frostbite cases in a Northern Canadian hospital, 53 % of patients had consumed alcohol and 16 % had psychiatric illness [2].

1. Imray C, et al. Cold damage to the extremities: frostbite and nonfreezing injuries. Postgrad Med J. 2009;85:481.
2. Urschel JD. Frostbite: predisposing factors and predictors of poor outcome. J Trauma. 1990;30:340.

When an elderly patient falls, think about medication use as a possible contributing factor.

Following a systematic review of 22 studies involving 79,081 individuals, Woolcott et al. concluded, "The use of sedatives and hypnotics, antidepressants, and benzodiazepines demonstrated a significant association with falls in elderly individuals" [1]. Bartlett et al. emphasize the increased risk of a new benzodiazepine prescription [2]. Other risk factors include a history of prior falls, the use of scatter rugs, and, as seen recently in our practice, the recent installation of blackout curtains in a bedroom.

1. Woolcott JC, et al. Meta-analysis of the impact of 9 medication classes on falls in elderly persons. Arch Int Med. 2009;169:1952.
2. Bartlett G. Association between risk factors for injurious falls and new benzodiazepine prescribing in elderly persons. BMC Fam Pract. 2009;10:1.

Frontal bossing can be caused by a variety of diseases.

Hydrocephalus in infancy is the most common cause of frontal bossing. In the elderly, think of Paget disease [1] (see Fig. 1.4). Other causes include rickets (not altogether absent in the developed world), craniosynostosis, congenital heart disease, and, today seen less commonly in advanced stages, syphilis [1–3].

1. Orient JM, editor. Sapira's art and science of diagnosis. 3rd ed. Philadelphia: Lippincott, Williams & Wilkins; 2005. p. 172.
2. Weisberg P, et al. Nutritional rickets among children in the United States; review of cases reported between 1986 and 2003. Am J Clin Nutr. 2004;80:16975.
3. Boop FA. Synostectomy versus complex cranioplasty for the treatment of sagittal synostosis. Childs Nerv Sys. 1996;12:371.

Fig. 1.4 This patient displays many of the classic features of Paget's disease, including severe bowing of the right lower leg, frontal bossing, and deafness as manifested by her hearing aid

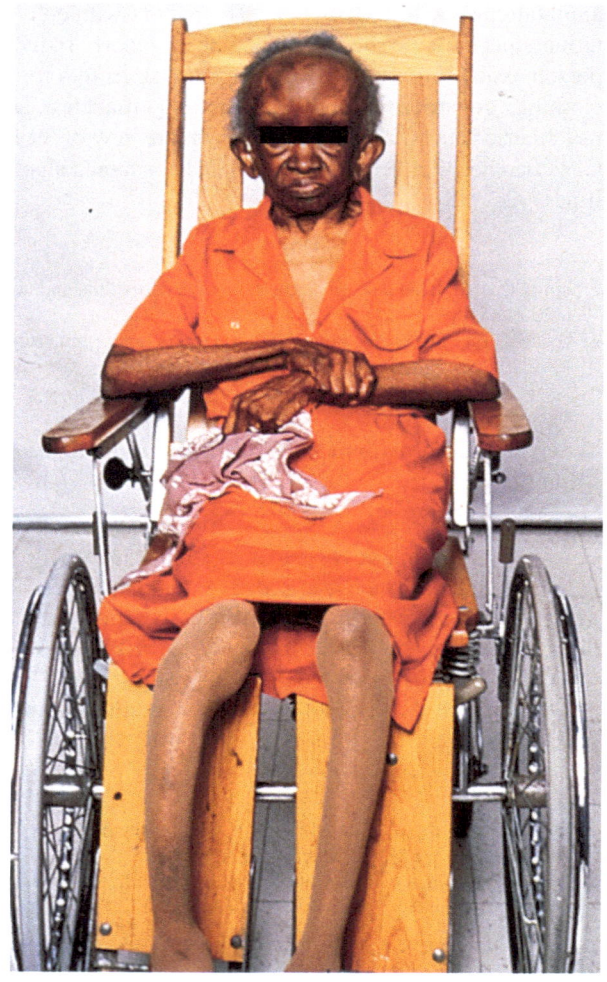

The man with post-ejaculatory allergy-type and flu-like symptoms may have postorgasmic illness syndrome (POIS).

In a study of 45 men with suspected POIS, ejaculation was followed by flu-like syndrome in 78 % and local allergic reactions involving the eyes (44 %) and nose (33 %) of subjects. Many also described concentration difficulties and exhaustion [1]. The diagnosis is confirmed by finding a positive skin-prick test using autologous semen. Successful treatment using hyposensitization with autologous semen has been reported [2].

1. Waldinger MD, et al. Postorgasmic illness syndrome (POIS) in 45 Dutch Caucasian males: clinical characteristics and evidence for an immunogenic pathogenesis, part 1. J Sex Med. 2011;8:1164.
2. Waldinger MD, et al. Postorgasmic illness syndrome (POIS) in 45 Dutch Caucasian males: clinical characteristics and evidence for an immunogenic pathogenesis, part 2. J Sex Med. 2011:8:1743.

Chapter 2
Infants and Children

Children are not simply micro-adults, but have their own specific problems.

Pediatrician Béla Schick, MD (1877–1967) [1]

Contents

R.B. Taylor, *Diagnostic Principles and Applications*,
DOI 10.1007/978-1-4614-1111-6_2, © Springer Science+Business Media, LLC 2013

When compared to adults, children have more sensitive thermostats, thinner skin, narrower airways, more sensitive gastrointestinal tracts, and a limited repertoire of ways to communicate their symptoms. Add to this the panoply of congenital diseases—both hereditary and environmentally caused—and we can appreciate the special diagnostic challenges often presented when disease occurs in the infant or child.

1. Schick B. Quoted in: Wolf IJ. Aphorisms and facetiae of Béla Schick, the early years. New York: Waverly Press; 1965.

Congenital Disorders

When a parent reports that a child's skin tastes salty when kissed, think of cystic fibrosis (CF).

The concern for a child that tastes salty—*a child that tastes salty when kissed will die soon*—has been known for more than 400 years, first described by a Spanish observer in the early seventeenth century [1]. Today an elevated sweat chloride test is considered "almost pathognomonic" for cystic fibrosis, the most common severe inherited recessive disease in white children and adults [2, 3].

Because early detection and intervention provides improved outcomes, newborn screening for CF is increasingly available in the USA [4].

1. de Fonteca J, et al. Diez privilegios pare mugeres prenadas. Spain: Henares; 1606.
2. Quinton PM. Cystic fibrosis: lessons from the sweat gland. Physiology. 2007;22:212.
3. de Aguero MI, et al. Protocol for the diagnosis and follow up of patients with cystic fibrosis. Ann Pediatr. 2009;71:250.
4. Farrell PM, et al. Guidelines for the diagnosis of cystic fibrosis in newborns through older adults: Cystic Fibrosis Foundation Consensus Report. J Pediatr. 2008;2:S4.

A child with craniofacial abnormalities that resemble *elfin facies* may have Williams syndrome.

Williams syndrome, named after the physician who first described the disorder in 1961, seems to be one of the few diseases that have managed to retain their eponymic descriptor [1]. Caused by a genetic abnormality, the disorder presents with the characteristic facies and impaired development and mental function. In one study 53 % of affected children were found to have cardiovascular defects, notably supravalvular aortic stenosis [2].

Bennett describes these patients as often having "an unusual, outgoing personality" and "an unusual command of language, often resulting in a superficial overestimation of cognitive abilities" [3].

1. Williams JD, et al. Supravalvular aortic stenosis. Circulation. 1961;24:1311.
2. Eronen M, et al. Cardiovascular manifestations in 75 patients with Williams syndrome. J Med Genet. 2002;39:554.
3. Bennett FC, et al. The Williams elfin facies syndrome: the psychological profile as an aid in syndrome identification. Pediatrics. 1978;61:303.

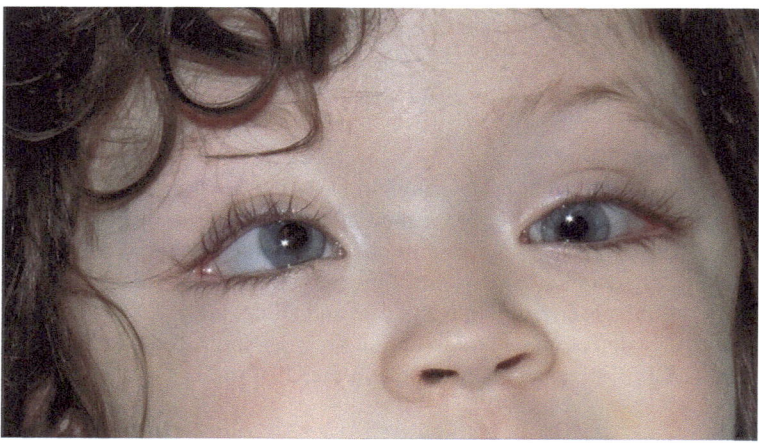

Fig. 2.1 Characteristic facies of the child with Kabuki syndrome. Note the elongated palpebral fissures, eversion of the lower lateral eyelids, arched eyebrows with the lateral one-third particularly sparse, and depressed nasal tip

The child whose facial appearance resembles the makeup of actors in traditional Japanese Kabuki theater—notably eversion of the lower eyelid—may have Kabuki syndrome.

Described first in 1981, Kabuki syndrome is a congenital and probably genetic neurodevelopmental disorder (see Fig. 2.1). Physical manifestations may include postnatal growth impairment, heart abnormalities, joint laxity, and hearing loss [1, 2]. These children tend to exhibit poor communication skills, clumsy social interaction, and restricted interests and repetitive behaviors; some have frank autism or autistic-like behavior [2].

Based on their reported case and several like cases in the literature, Casanova et al. suggest that there may be an association between Kabuki syndrome and neoplastic disease [3].

1. Niikawa N, et al. Kabuki make-up syndrome of mental retardation, unusual facies, large and protruding ears, and postnatal growth deficiency. J Pediatr. 1981;99:565.
2. Sari BA, et al. Case report: autistic disorder in Kabuki syndrome. J Autism Dev Disord. 2008;38:198.
3. Casanova M, et al. Cancer predisposition in children with Kabuki syndrome. Am J Med Gen. 2010;155:1504.

A triad of facial characteristics characterizes the fetal alcohol syndrome: smooth philtrum, thin vermillion border, and small palpebral fissures (see Fig. 2.2).

These features are easier to identify in children and may be more difficult to detect after puberty [1]. Behavioral manifestations may include cognitive and executive

Discriminating
features

Associated
features

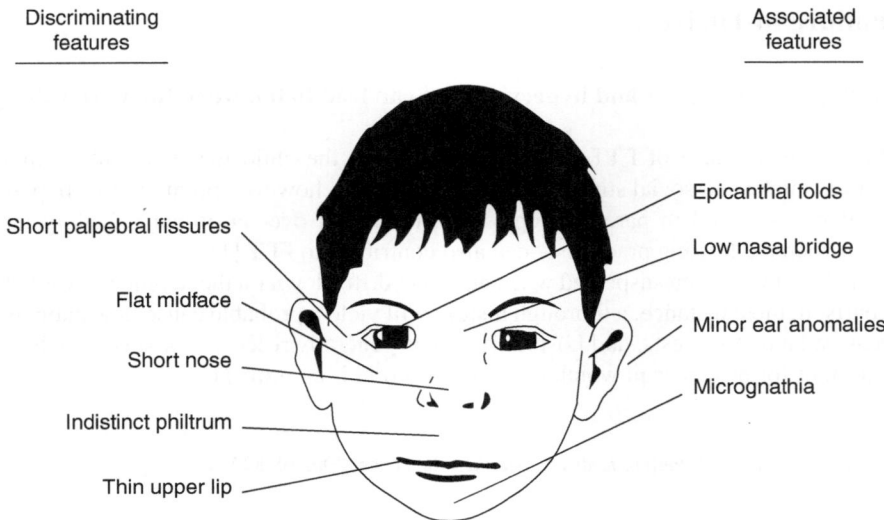

Epicanthal folds

Short palpebral fissures

Low nasal bridge

Flat midface

Minor ear anomalies

Short nose

Micrognathia

Indistinct philtrum

Thin upper lip

Fig. 2.2 Facial features particularly characteristic of a child with fetal alcohol syndrome

function deficits; impaired motor function, such as tremors or clumsiness; attention and hyperactivity problems; and poor communication abilities.

Considering that one in 25 women report binge drinking (five or more drinks of alcoholic beverages on any single occasion) while pregnant, it seems likely that the fetal alcohol syndrome is underdetected.

1. Paton SJ, et al. An overview of fetal alcohol spectrum disorders for physicians. Prim Care Rep. 2010;16:5.
2. Floyd RL, et al. Recognition and prevention of fetal alcohol syndrome. Obstet Gynecol. 2005;106:1059.

Failure to Thrive

Both parental neglect and hypervigilance can lead to failure to thrive (FTT).

Neglect as a cause of FTT is quite logical, with the child receiving suboptimal caloric intake and social stimulation. Krugman et al., however, point out that hypervigilance—related to parental depression, obsession over an infant's feeding, or even coercive feeding practices—can also contribute to FFT [1].

FFT is most often suspected when an infant drifts down on the height and weight charts. In most instance, a thorough history will yield a probable cause, few patients require laboratory tests, and hospitalization is generally reserved for severe malnutrition or for instances in which safety of the child is an issue [1].

1. Krugman SD, et al. Failure to thrive. Am Fam Physician. 2003;68:879.

Not all instances of failure to thrive will have psychosocial causes; some patients will have organic disease, including some zebras.

FTT is so often associated with cystic fibrosis that growth monitoring has been suggested as a screening tool for this genetic disorder [1]. Gastrointestinal abnormalities, including celiac disease and duodenal stenosis or webs, can cause FFT [2]. Cuevas reports puzzling infant weight loss in a patient found to have idiopathic hypercalcemia [3]. Other causes of FTT include chronic infection, cow's milk allergy, liver disease, genetic abnormalities, and metabolic disorders [4].

1. van Dommelen P, et al. Growth monitoring to detect children with cystic fibrosis. Horm Res. 2009; 72:218.
2. Sarkar S, et al. Vomiting and food refusal causing failure to thrive in a 2 year old: an unusual and late manifestation of congenital duodenal web. BMJ Case Rep. 2011. doi:10.1136/bcr.01.2011;3779.
3. Cuevas M. Infant with failure to thrive. Clin Pract. 2011;4:364.
4. Krugman SD, et al. Failure to thrive. Am Fam Physician. 2003;68:879.

Fever

Fever in an infant younger than 28 days should receive a full evaluation for sepsis and the infant should be admitted to the hospital for antibiotic therapy.

The above statement is the recommendation found in Emergency Medicine Clinics of North America in 2010, making fever during the first 4 weeks of life a red-flag finding. In this report, fever is defined as a rectal temperature greater than 38.0 °C (100.4 °F), whether recorded in the clinical setting or at home [1].

1. Claudius I, et al. Pediatric emergencies associated with fever. Emerg Med. 2010;28:67.

Bacterial markers may help detect serious bacterial causes in young febrile children.

Although most childhood fever has a benign cause, some febrile children will have a serious bacterial infection such as meningitis, pneumonia, urinary tract infection, or bacteremia. Following a study of the use of white blood cell count, absolute neutrophil count, and C-reactive protein in 119 patients, Pratt et al. concluded that these biomarkers were useful but were more predictive of serious bacterial infection if the fever duration exceeded 12 h. Of the three markers, C-reactive protein proved to be superior—better sensitivity and specificity—when compared to the other two bacterial markers in predicting serious bacterial infection [1].

1. Pratt A, et al. Duration of fever and markers of serious bacterial infection in young febrile children. Pediatr Int. 2007;49:31.

Clinicians should pay special attention to the febrile child with a skin infection, which may represent methicillin-resistant Staphylococcus aureus (MRSA); sickle cell disease, which puts the patient at special risk; or mental status changes, which may point to herpes simplex virus infection of the central nervous system.

Also at high risk for serious cause of childhood fever are those who have not received timely immunization against bacterial meningitis [1].

1. Claudius I, et al. Pediatric emergencies associated with fever. Emerg Med. 2010;28:67.

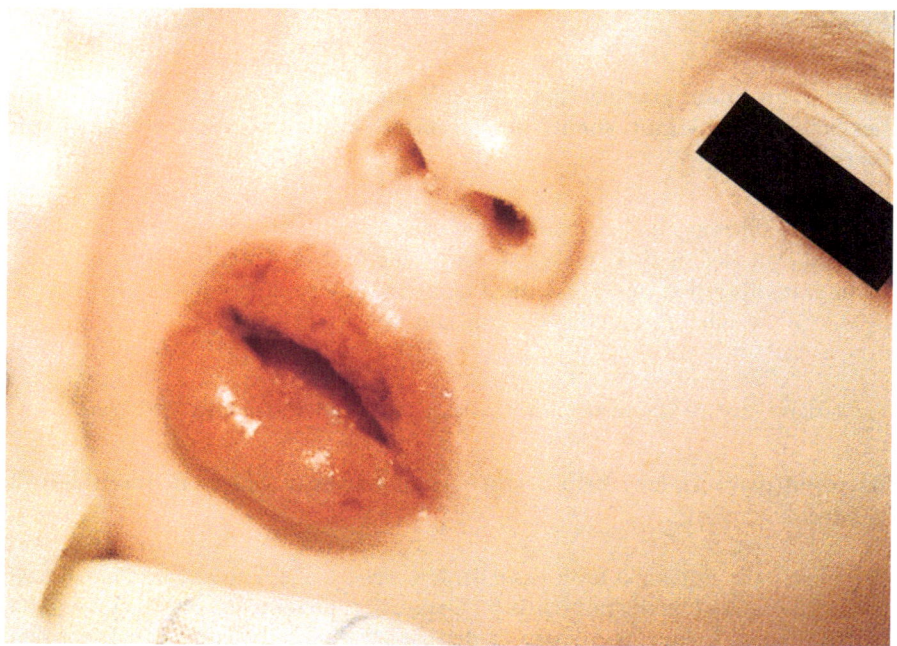

Fig. 2.3 Mucous membrane changes in Kawasaki disease

Kawasaki disease (KD) should be considered in any child with a fever of five or more day's duration.

Many, perhaps most, clinicians have never seen a case of Kawasaki disease, aka mucocutaneous lymph node syndrome. KD, one of the spectrum of vasculitides of childhood, is characterized by fever, rash, erythema of the oral mucosa and lips, and cervical lymphadenopathy [1] (see Fig. 2.3). Of all the manifestations of KD, fever occurs most commonly, and rarely are all features present at the onset of the disease [2].

Prompt diagnosis, within 5–10 days of onset, followed by use of aspirin and intravenous immunoglobulin can reduce the 20–30 % risk of coronary artery lesions seen in untreated cases [2].

1. Newburger JW, et al. Diagnosis, treatment, and long-term management of Kawasaki disease: a statement for health professionals from the Committee on Rheumatic Fever, Endocarditis and Kawasaki disease, Council on Cardiovascular Disease in the Young, American Heart Association. Circulation. 2004;110:2747.
2. Harnden A, et al. Kawasaki disease. BMJ. 2009;338:1514.

The febrile child with other manifestations may have PFAPA (periodic fever, aphthous lesions, pharyngitis, and cervical adenitis).

There indeed seems to be such a syndrome, although it was unknown to me before I began my research for this book. Feder et al. studied 105 children with PFAPA, noting that the mean duration of fever was 4.1 days and the mean interval between febrile episodes was 29.8 days. In addition to the manifestations mentioned above, patients reported headache (44 %), mild abdominal pain (41 %), and vomiting with fever spikes (27 %) [1].

I include this curious syndrome because of the various therapies reported useful. Individual episodes of fever were treated successfully with prednisone; cimetidine therapy was followed by resolution of fever in 7 of 26 patients, and in 11 of 11 patients, fever resolved following tonsillectomy [1].

1. Feder HM, et al. A clinical review of 105 patients with PFAPA (a periodic fever syndrome). Acta Paediatr. 2010;99:178.

Crying Infant

We should cast a wide diagnostic net when the patient is a crying afebrile child.

Freedman et al. studied 237 crying afebrile infants age less than 1 year. Of these, only 12 (5.1 %) had serious underlying disease, with three of these infants having urinary tract infections. History and physical examination yielded a cause in 66.3 % of instances, and in only two children did laboratory or other testing in the absence of a suggestive clinical picture contribute to the diagnosis.

With that said, you don't want to miss a treatable cause of the uncontrolled crying. Some etiologies to consider include post-vaccine reaction, corneal abrasion (commonly caused by an infant's fingernail), open diaper pin, cellulitis, pneumonia, incarcerated hernia, intussusception, and appendicitis.

1. Freedman SB. The crying infant: diagnostic testing and frequency of serious underlying disease. Pediatrics. 2009;123:841.

Hip Pain

The most likely cause of acute hip pain in a child ages 3–10 years of age is transient synovitis of the hip (TSH) [1].

However, transient synovitis for the hip must be differentiated from septic arthritis, a *must-not-miss diagnosis* [1]. In many instances of TSH, there will be a preceding history of a nonspecific upper respiratory infection.

Helpful tests to distinguish self-limited and benign TSH from potentially devastating septic arthritis include the following: Septic arthritis of the hip classically causes inability to bear weight, fever, elevated white blood count, elevated erythrocyte sedimentation rate (ESR), and elevated C-reactive protein. Yet in a study of clinical prediction algorithms, Sultan concluded that even with all five variables meeting threshold values, the predicted probability of septic arthritis was only 59.9 % [2]. Ultrasound may reveal hip effusion in both disorders, and joint aspiration is recommended if septic arthritis is suspected [1].

Here I will offer another diagnostic pearl: When evaluating a limping child, examine all joints in the extremity, not just the one reported to hurt. The patient may, for example, be experiencing pain referred from the knee to the hip.

1. Hart JJ. Transient synovitis of the hip in children. Am Fam Physician. 1996;54:1596.
2. Sultan J, et al. Septic arthritis or transient synovitis of the hip in children: the value of clinical prediction algorithms. J Bone Joint Surg. 2010;92B:1289.

The child with TSH may develop Perthes disease a few months later.

In one series of 275 children with TSH, 10 individuals (3.4 %) developed Perthes disease, aka Legg–Calvé–Perthes disease, 1–5 months later [1] (see Fig. 2.4).

1. Landin LA, et al. Transient synovitis of the hip: incidence, epidemiology and relation to Perthes disease. J Bone Joint Surg. 1987;69B:238.

Fig. 2.4 Legg–Calvé–
Perthes disease of the hip
with whole head involvement
in the fragmentation stage

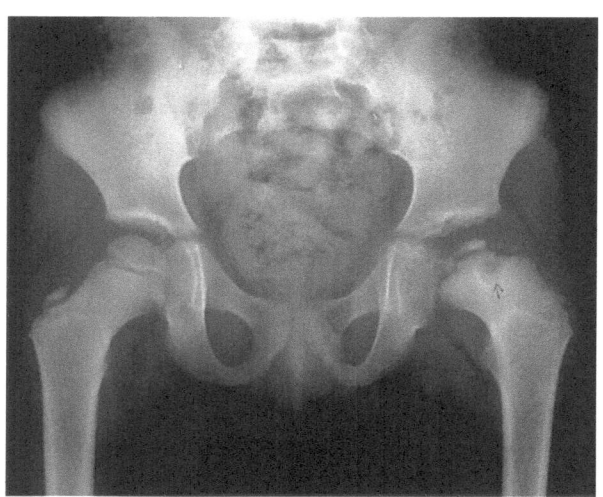

Cough and Stridor

Stridor at rest in a croupy child indicates the presence of severe airway obstruction.

Croup is a bit of a wastebasket term, including spasmodic croup, laryngotracheitis, laryngotracheobronchitis, and laryngotracheobronchopneumonia. The hallmark of all of this, in addition to fever and coryza, is the high-pitched barking cough, reminiscent of a seal at the zoo. Stridor is a more ominous sign, signaling some degree of airway blockage, especially when accompanied by a rapid respiratory rate and by subcostal and intercostal retractions. All this describes a setting in which death could occur [1, 2].

1. Cherry JD. Clinical practice: croup. N Engl J Med. 2008;24:384.
2. Zoorob R, et al. Croup: an overview. Am Fam Physician. 2011;83:1067.

The child with a respiratory tract infection who assumes the *tripod* position—sitting leaning forward with the chin thrust forward and neck hyperextended—may have acute epiglottitis.

Listen for stridor, a distinctive type of wheeze described as a "loud musical sound of constant pitch" [1]. Stridor is found in four of every five children with acute epiglottitis, a *must-not-miss diagnosis* [2]. Classically, children with acute epiglottitis are described as having the *three Ds*: dyspnea, dysphagia, and drooling. In many instances, the child will be reluctant to lie down and, instead, assume the tripod position [3] (see Fig. 2.5). For the record, the tripod position is, or perhaps was, also

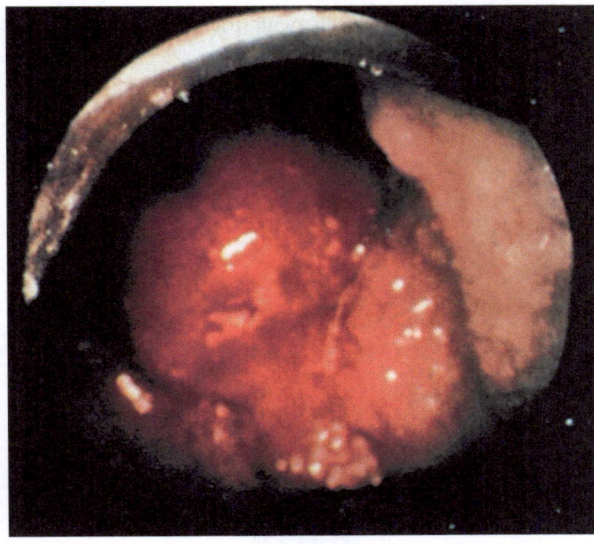

Fig. 2.5 Epiglottitis, as seen by direct laryngoscopy, with a beefy red appearance of the epiglottis characteristic of acute epiglottitis in children

a classic sign of paralytic polio, as weakened lower body muscles could not support the child's body weight when seated on a flat surface, that is, a bed.

In this setting, a lateral neck roentgenogram may be helpful in diagnosis, although in one study, predictions of severity based on roentgenographic readings did not correlate well with clinical severity [4].

1. Hollingsworth HM. Wheezing and stridor. Clin Chest Med. 1987;8:231.
2. Mayo-Smith MF, et al. Acute epiglottitis: an 18-year experience in Rhode Island. Chest. 1995;108:1640.
3. Stroud RH, et al. An update on inflammatory disorders of the pediatric airway: epiglottitis, croup, and tracheitis. Am J Otolaryngol. 2001;22:268.
4. Mills JL. The usefulness of lateral neck roentgenograms in laryngotracheobronchitis. Am J Dis Child. 1979;133:1140.

On rare occasions, what seems to be croup or epiglottitis will turn out to be laryngeal diphtheria.

Think about this in the setting of patient unlikely to have had routine immunizations. Then look for a membranous pharyngitis [1].

1. Cherry JD. Croup. N Engl J Med. 2008;358:384.

The child with chronic stridor may have laryngomalacia.

Laryngomalacia is the most common cause of chronic stridor in young children [1].

1. Lachman DC, et al. A toddler with stridor. Clin Pediatr. 2009;48:878.

Cardiovascular Disease

Circulatory manifestations—cyanosis and poor peripheral perfusion—are red flags in the recognition of serious infection in children.

In a systematic review, Van den Bruel et al. analyzed 30 studies, finding that cyanosis (positive likelihood ratio range 2.66–52.20) and poor peripheral perfusion (LR 2.39–38.80) were red flags in identifying serious illness in children. Other useful indicators identified in the study were rapid breathing (positive likelihood ratio range 1.26–9.78) and petechial rash (LR 6.18–83.70) [1].

1. Van den Bruel A, et al. Diagnostic value of clinical features at presentation to identify serious infection in children in developed countries: a systematic review. Lancet. 2010;375:834.

Critical congenital heart disease (CCHD) in newborn infants is often unrecognized.

A population-based retrospective study in California of 898 infants who died of CCHD before 1 year of age led to the estimate that up to 30 infants per year died in the state of a missed or possibly late diagnosis of CCHD. The median age at death was less than 2 weeks. The most common missed diagnoses were hypoplastic left heart syndrome and coarctation of the aorta [1].

1. Chang RK, et al. Missed diagnosis of critical congenital heart disease. Arch Pediatr Adolesc Med. 2008;162:969.

Exertional syncope in childhood may be the tip-off to the diagnosis of hypertrophic cardiomyopathy (HCM), the most common cause of death in young athletes.

In a study of 467 cases of pediatric cardiomyopathy, hypertrophic cardiomyopathy was present in 42 % of subjects, and dilated cardiomyopathy in 51 %, with restrictive, other types and unspecified types making up the balance [1]. HCM, an asymmetric enlargement of the left ventricle, is an autosomal dominant disease that affects about 1 in 500 persons. A lower threshold for use of electrocardiography and echocardiography in screening of young athletes may reduce the risk of sudden death during sports [2, 3].

1. Lipshultz SE, et al. The incidence of pediatric cardiomyopathy in two regions of the United States. N Engl J Med. 2003;348:1647.
2. Maron BJ. Sudden death in young athletes. N Engl J Med. 2003;349:1064.
3. Maron BJ. Hypertrophic cardiomyopathy and other causes of sudden cardiac death in young competitive athletes, with considerations for preparticipation screening and criteria for disqualification. Cardiol Clin. 2007;25:399.

Abdominal Pain

The child who attempts to relieve severe, intermittent abdominal pain by drawing the legs up to the abdomen may have intussusception.

Intussusception, obstruction occurring when a segment of intestine invaginates into itself, generally occurs during the first 2 years of life (see Fig. 2.6). Episodes of inconsolable crying, with the legs drawn up, may alternate with pain-free periods. Finding occult or gross blood in the stool helps support the diagnosis [1, 2].

1. Watson NA, et al. Case report: intussusception—a cause of chronic abdominal symptoms and weight loss. Clin Radiol. 1994;49:723.
2. Isbister WH. Enteric intussusception after acute trauma. Am J Surg. 1970;120:101.

In a child with acute abdominal pain, think of constipation as a cause.

Loening-Baucke et al. reviewed the charts of 962 children age 4 years or less seen over a 6-month period. Of these, 9 % had a visit for acute abdominal pain. The cause of the abdominal pain in 48 % of these children was constipation, making this the

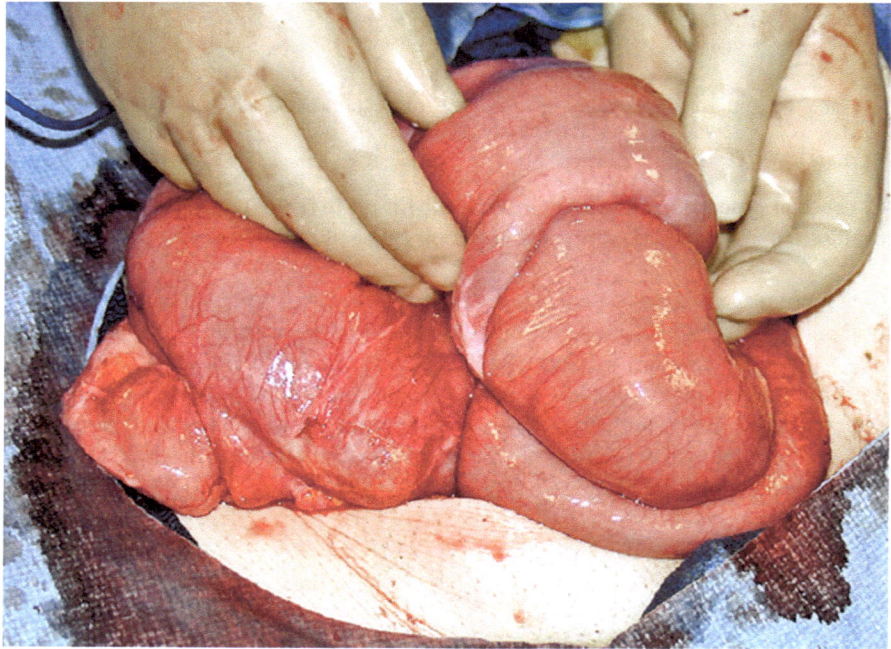

Fig. 2.6 Large obstructing intussusception

most common cause identified in this series [1]. In a retrospective chart review of the causes of constipation, 85 % of 137 children evaluated for constipation had functional constipation, while the remaining 15 % had organic disorders such as Hirschsprung disease [2].

1. Loening-Baucke V, et al. Constipation as a cause of acute abdominal pain in children. J Pediatr. 2007;151:666.
2. Khanna V, et al. Etiology and clinical spectrum of constipation in Indian children. Indian Pediatr. 2010;47:1025.

When you are evaluating a child with chronic, recurrent abdominal pain, think of the possibility of abdominal migraine (AM).

This is the conclusion of Carson et al. following a retrospective chart review of 458 children evaluated with recurrent abdominal pain. According to the International Classification of Headache Disorders, AM is an idiopathic disorder characterized by attacks of midline, moderate to severe abdominal pain lasting 1–72 h with vaso-motor symptoms, nausea and vomiting. In the study described, 20 patients (4.4 %) met formal criteria for AM and another 50 patients (11 %) met all but one criterion. Yet no patient in the cohort received a diagnosis of AM. The investigators conclude: "Among children with chronic, idiopathic, recurrent abdominal pain, AM represents about 4–15 %" [1].

1. Carson L, et al. Abdominal migraine: an under-diagnosed cause of recurrent abdominal pain in children. Headache. 2011;51:707.

Child Abuse and Neglect

Be suspicious when a child's fracture is attributed to falling from a piece of furniture.

Falling out of bed is generally a low-impact, benign event. Lyons et al. studied records involving 124 falls from cribs and 83 from beds by children younger than 6 years. The heights of these falls ranged from 25 to 54 in., the highest being those instances in which the child climbed over crib rails. The result: minor bumps and scratches, one simple skull fracture noted on x-ray, and one fractured clavicle. There were no serious injuries in this study [1].

The benignity of falling from bed is significant because, for example, one report tells that half of all child abuse victims have fractures and 17 % of abused children in a series reported had fracture as the first indication of abuse [2].

On a personal note, I have seen a few clavicular and wrist fractures in children, often boys older than 6 years, who fall from the top level of a double bunk bed, a height which may be up to 70 in., landing on an uncarpeted floor.

Other causes of suspicion in the setting of a childhood fracture would be an injury that seems excessive for the mechanism described, an injury attributed to a sibling, or an unwitnessed injury. We must consider child abuse a *must-not-miss diagnosis*.

1. Lyons TJ, et al. Falling out of bed: a relatively benign occurrence. Pediatrics. 1993;92:125.
2. Sinal SH, et al. Physical abuse of children: a review for orthopedic surgeons. J South Orthop Assoc. 1998;7:264.

The child with unexplained fractures may have osteogenesis imperfecta (OI) and not be a victim of child abuse at all.

In both settings—osteogenesis and physical abuse—there may be multiple fractures in various stages of healing. Because OI, a genetic disorder of increased bone fragility, occurs rarely, it sometimes will not be considered in the diagnosis of unexplained or multiple fractures. Other manifestations of osteogenesis imperfecta include hearing loss, blue sclera, and short stature [1, 2] (see Fig. 2.7).

1. Pandya NK, et al. Unexplained fractures: child abuse or bone disease? Clin Orthop Relat Res. 2011;469:805.
2. Rauch F, et al. Osteogenesis imperfecta. Lancet. 2004;363:1377.

The unusually docile child may be an abused child.

Several papers have reported the overly placid and docile affect of some abused children, reflecting acceptance of their status as chronic victims [1, 2].

Fig. 2.7 Five-year-old child with osteogenesis imperfecta. Note osteopenia and healing fracture of proximal tibia pretreatment (**a**) and metaphyseal bands, healed midtibial fracture, and acute distal tibial fracture post treatment (**b**)

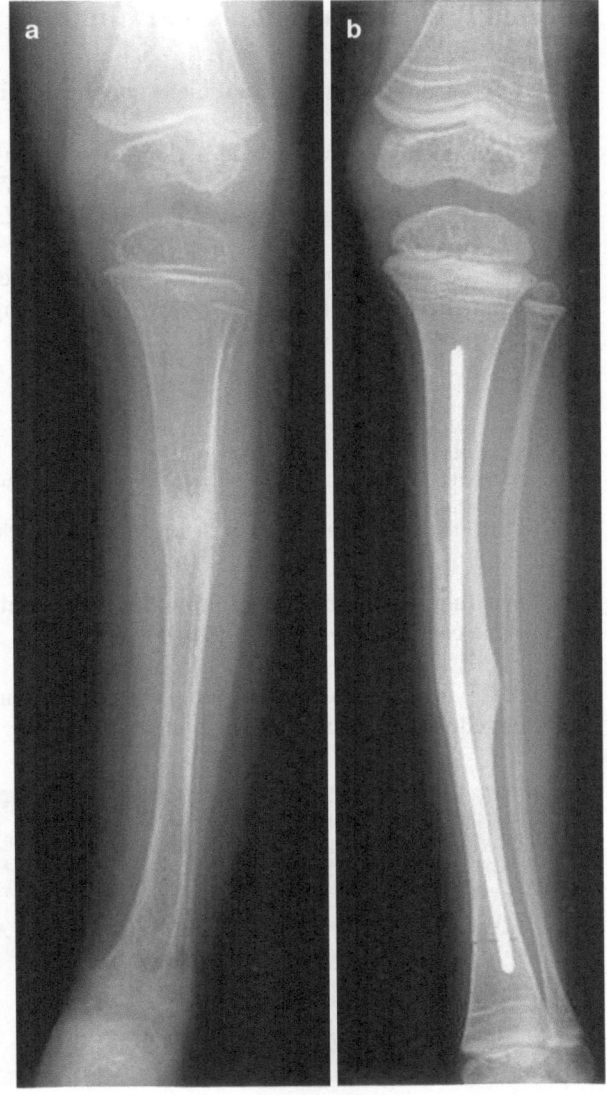

1. Vizard E. Child sexual abuse—the child's experience. Br J Psychother. 1988;5:77.
2. Kinard EM. The psychological consequences of abuse for the child. J Soc Issues. 1979;35:82.

Selected Problems of Infants and Children

A child with a solitary abdominal mass may have Wilms tumor.

Other manifestations may include abdominal pain, hypertension, or hematuria. There is an increased risk in children with Beckwith–Wiedemann syndrome and in children in families with a history of Wilms tumor [1]. Early detection and intervention has helped achieve a cure rate over 85 % [2].

In the teaching setting, this is not a time when the attending should invite a troupe of medical students to examine the mass (see Fig. 2.8). Vigorous palpation can cause spread of the tumor [3].

1. Scott RH, et al. Surveillance for Wilms tumor in at-risk children: pragmatic recommendations for best practice. Arch Dis Child. 2006;91:995.
2. Speafico F, et al. Wilms tumor: past, present and (possibly) future. Expert Rev Anticancer Ther. 2006;6:249.
3. Taylor RB. Essential medical facts every clinician should know. New York: Springer; 2011. p. 139.

Facial swelling in an infant, beginning before 6 months of age, may be caused by infantile cortical hyperostosis (Caffey disease).

The disease, named after American pediatrician John Caffey (1895–1978), is characterized by periosteal inflammation and thickening, with soft-tissue swelling.

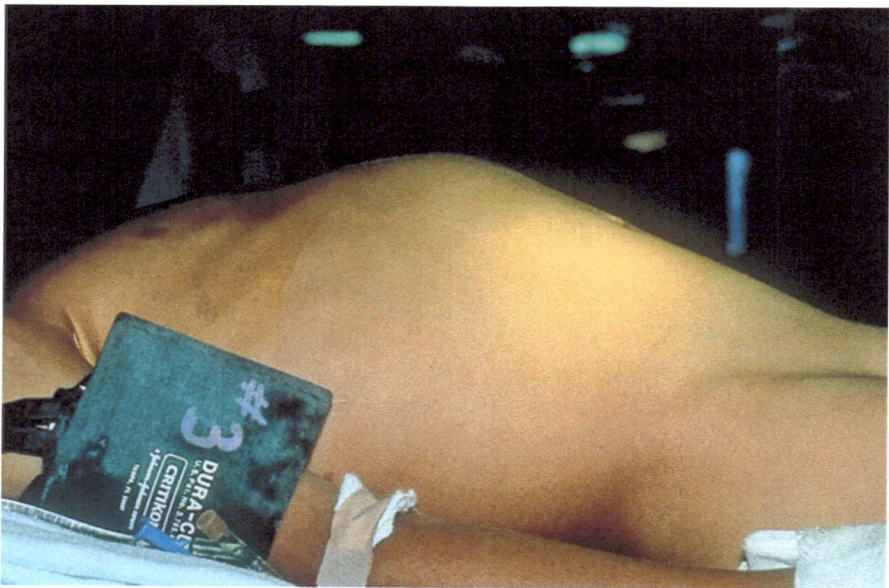

Fig. 2.8 A palpable mass is the most common presentation of Wilms tumor

Various bones may be involved: mandible, scapula, clavicle, and long bones. Other manifestations include persistent fever as high as 40 °C (104 °F), tenderness over involved bones, leukocytosis, and an elevated ESR. Most changes resolve spontaneously by 2 years of age [1, 2].

1. Kamoun-Goldrat A, et al. Infantile cortical hyperostosis (Caffey disease): a review. J Oral Maxillofac Surg. 2008;66:2145.
2. Staheli LT, et al. Infantile cortical hyperostosis (Caffey disease): sixteen cases with a late follow-up of eight. JAMA. 1968;203:384.

When you see a child with palpable purpura in the absence of thrombocytopenia, think of Henoch–Schonlein purpura (HSP).

The most common systemic vasculitis of childhood, HSP, typically (but not always) occurs before 10 years of age. Often the disease is preceded by an upper respiratory infection. HSP patients also typically have abdominal pain and arthritis. Up to half of HSP patients will develop renal involvement, which may be treated with corticosteroids [1, 2].

1. McCarthy HJ, et al. Clinical practice: diagnosis and management of Henoch-Schonlein purpura. Eur J Pediatr. 2009;169:643.
2. Reamy BV, et al. Henoch-Schonlein purpura. Am Fam Physician. 2009;80:697.

A child with abnormal liver function tests may have Wilson disease (WD).

In a study of 57 consecutive cases of children with WD, 19 were referred because of abnormal liver function tests, notably elevated transaminase levels. This was more than the 18 patients identified by family screening [1]. Other manifestations may include the characteristic yellow-gold ring at the periphery of the iris of the eye (Kayser–Fleischer ring), movement disorders such as ataxia or tremor, decreased serum ceruloplasmin levels, and elevated urinary copper excretion [1].

1. Manolaki N, et al. Wilson disease in children: analysis of 57 cases. J Pediatr Gastroenterol Nutr. 2009;48:72.

A child who seems to have cognitive problems may actually have suboptimal sleep caused by enuresis.

Enuresis affects 5–10 % of children in the early grades of school and up to 1 % of adults. The worst outlook is for those children who wet the beds most nights and not just from time to time [1].

In one study of 88 patients with enuresis, coexistent constipation was found in 62 % of patients with primary enuresis ($n=79$) and 67 % of those with secondary enuresis ($n=9$). The authors suggest that these patients are not monosymptomatic and should be considered to have elimination dysfunction [2].

1. Nevsue T. Diagnosis and management of nocturnal enuresis. Curr Opin Pediatr. 2009;21:199.
2. Akvol I. An overlooked issue in children presenting with enuresis: constipation. J Pediatr Urol. 2010;6:S66.

Food allergy in children is probably overdiagnosed.

Noimark et al. report that while 6–8 % of children may have some sort of food allergy at some time during childhood, an estimated 20 % of children have eliminated one or more foods from their diet because of perceived allergy. They cite the dangers of poor nutrition that can result from an unsupervised elimination diet [1].

There is hope for these children. In a retrospective chart review of 125 children aged 1–19 years on elimination diets based primarily on positive serum immunoglobulin E (IgE) results, the outcome of oral food challenges allowed 84–93 % of foods being avoided to be returned to the diet [2].

1. Noimark L, et al. Nutritional problems related to food allergy in childhood. Pediatr Allergy Immunol. 2008;19:188.
2. Fleischer DM, et al. Oral food challenges in children with a diagnosis of food allergy. J Pediatr. 2011;158:578.

Beta-lactam allergy is also overdiagnosed.

Once an entry such as *penicillin allergy* appears on a clinical record, it seems to linger forever. Yet several studies question this practice. One study involved testing 166 history-positive children were tested for penicillin and, in a few instances, cephalosporins. Negative skin tests were followed by oral challenge. Then the testing was repeated a few months later, looking for possible resensitization. In the initial testing, four children tested positive by skin test and six by oral challenge. Subsequent testing of 98 subjects with initial negative tests revealed only two children who were resensitized. In a later survey of 71 of these 96 children, 59 had received beta-lactam antibiotics and only one had developed a minor rash [1]. In another study of 85 children with suspected beta-lactam allergy, oral challenge tests with the culprit antibiotic yielded skin rashes in only 6.8 %, with no rash more severe than the original event [2].

1. Hershkovich J, et al. Beta lactam allergy and resensitization in children with suspected beta lactam allergy. Clin Exp Allergy. 2009;39:726.
2. Caubet JC, et al. The role of penicillin in benign skin rashes in childhood: a prospective study based on drug rechallenge. J Allergy Clin Immunol. 2011;127:218.

Chapter 3
The Nervous System

From the brain, and from the brain only, arise our pleasures, joys,
laughter and jests, as well as our sorrow, pains, grief and tears.
Hippocrates (460–377 BCE) [1]

Contents

R.B. Taylor, *Diagnostic Principles and Applications*,
DOI 10.1007/978-1-4614-1111-6_3, © Springer Science+Business Media, LLC 2013

Of course, the nervous system is much more than the brain only. Consider the complexity of the peripheral nervous system, with motor, sensory, and autonomic nerves. Taken together, the human nervous system offers abundant opportunity for pleasure and joy, but also for malfunction causing paralysis, pain, and tears. In this chapter, I will discuss diagnostic insights into some of these maladies, beginning with the seemingly universal symptom of headache.

1. Hippocrates. The sacred disease. Sect. XVII.

Headache

Evidence-based red-flag symptoms in headache patients are (1) paralysis, (2) papilledema, and (3) drowsiness, confusion, memory impairment, and loss of consciousness.

Headache, and especially migraine headache, is a common complaint faced by clinicians. One study of 120,000 US households led to the assertion that 40 % of women and 20 % of men will experience migraine during their lifetimes, with most of these problems beginning before age 35 years [1]. This is the highest estimate I have seen.

Although most headaches have benign causes—that is, not life-threatening—some patients will have serious disease such as intracranial bleeding or cancer. Over the years, guidelines have been promulgated to help guide clinicians as to when to use expensive imaging to look for these ominous causes of headache. These guidelines generally have described red flags as onset of headache after age 50, new-onset headache, worst-ever headache, rapidly increasing headache frequency, abnormal neurologic findings, and other manifestations such as stiff neck and fever [2, 3]. As tends to be the case with guidelines, the studies reviewed in compiling indications sometimes lacked robust statistical support.

Sobri et al. provide some statistically grounded guidance, studying 111 headache patients of whom 39 had abnormal neuroimaging. Sensitivity and specificity of red flags were analyzed to determine the cutoff point to predict abnormal neuroimaging. Three manifestations—paralysis, papilledema, and drowsiness, confusion, memory impairment, and loss of consciousness were each found to be statistically significant (p values < 0.05) on both univariate and multivariate analysis [4]. This is not to say that other manifestations, considered in context, might not suggest the need for diagnostic imaging.

1. Stewart WF, et al. AMPP Advisory Group. Cumulative lifetime migraine incidence in women and men. Cephalgia. 2008;28(11):1170.
2. Solomon GD, et al. Standards of care for treating headache in primary care. National Headache Foundation. Cleve Clin J Med. 1997;64(7):373.
3. Silberstein SD for the US Headache Consortium. Practice parameter: evidence-based guidelines for migraine headache. Report of the Quality Standards Subcommittee of the American Academy of Neurology. Neurology. 2000;55(6):754.
4. Sobri M, et al. Red flags in patients presenting with headache: clinical indications for neuroimaging. Br J Radiol. 2003;76:532.

Migraine associated with transient monocular visual loss—retinal migraine—carries a risk of permanent visual impairment.

Retinal migraine, sometimes called ocular migraine, is the diagnosis when a patient describes transient episodes of reversible monocular scotomata or blindness occurring in connection with a headache. Careful inquiry will be needed to distinguish this phenomenon from the lesser scotomata sometimes occurring as part of the migraine aura [1]. Although sometimes challenging, the distinction is important because of the prognosis. Grosberg et al. described six cases of retinal migraine and reviewed an additional 40 patients reported in the literature. They found that 43 % of these patients eventually suffered some degree of irreversible visual loss [2].

1. Russell MB, et al. A nosographic analysis of the migraine aura in a general population. Brain. 1996;119(2):355.
2. Grosberg B, et al. Retinal migraine reappraised. Cephalgia. 2006;26(11):1275.

Middle-aged migraineurs with aura have an increased risk of late-life brain infarcts on magnetic resonance imaging (MRI).

Scher et al. conducted a population-based study of 4,689 persons, 57 % women, followed for more than 25 years. They found a 40 % greater incidence of late-life brain infarcts when compared with headache-free patients, with the noteworthy finding of a nearly twofold increase in the prevalence of cerebral infarcts in women [1].

Perhaps migraine with aura is not as "benign" as we have assumed and is, in fact, a key risk factor for cerebrovascular disease, especially in women.

1. Scher AI, et al. Migraine headache in middle age and late-life brain infarcts. JAMA. 2009;301:2594.

Eleven percent of migraineurs have restless legs syndrome (RLS).

In a study of 1,041 patients, the 11.4 % frequency of RLS in migraineurs was higher than in tension-type headache patients (4.6 %) and cluster headache patients (2.0 %) ($p = 0.002$) [1]. Understanding this correlation will help you recognize the comorbidity and understand the interrupted sleep in affected patients.

1. Chen PK, et al. Association between restless legs syndrome and migraine. J Neurol Neurosurg Psychiatry. 2010;81:524.

Brain Ischemia

A transient ischemic attack (TIA) typically lasts less than 1 h [1].

Thus, a brain ischemia syndrome lasting more than 60 min may be a manifestation of a cerebral infarction [2, 3].

1. Caplan LR. Transient ischemic attack: definition and natural history. Curr Atheroscler Rep. 2006;8:276.
2. Albers GW, et al. Transient ischemic attack – proposal for a new definition. N Engl J Med. 2002;347:1713.
3. Caplan LR. Transient ischemic attack with abnormal diffusion-weighted imaging results: what's in a name? Arch Neurol. 2007;64:1080.

There is a constellation of bedside findings that can help distinguish a hemorrhagic stroke from an ischemic stroke.

The differentiation of hemorrhagic and ischemic strokes is vital because the therapies differ. Here, from a review by Runchey and McGee of studies published in 1966–2010, are six findings significantly increasing the likelihood that a stroke is hemorrhagic [1]:

- Coma (likelihood ratio [LR] 6.2)
- Neck stiffness (LR 5.0)
- Seizures accompanying the neurologic deficit (LR 4.7)
- Diastolic blood pressure >110 mm/Hg (LR 4.3)
- Vomiting (LR 3.0)
- Headache (LR 2.9)

1. Runchey S, et al. Does this patient have a hemorrhagic stroke? Clinical findings distinguishing hemorrhagic stroke from ischemic stroke. JAMA. 2010;303:2280.

Associated symptoms and signs can help identify specific types of stroke.

Here are a few clues that may prove helpful:

Altered consciousness: Impaired alertness suggests that a stroke is hemorrhagic. If there are focal signs, think of intracerebral bleeding, but if there are no localizing signs, consider subarachnoid hemorrhage. Sudden onset of headache also suggests that a stroke is hemorrhagic [1].

Fever: A patient with fever accompanying a stroke may have an embolism from bacterial endocarditis. Finding a heart murmur helps confirm this diagnosis [2].

Atherosclerosis: The presence of a carotid bruit and other signs of atherosclerosis increases the likelihood that a stroke is occlusive [3].

Seizure: If the patient has a seizure associated with a stroke, the cause may be hemorrhagic or ischemic, but probably not thrombotic [4].

1. Arboix A, et al. Hemorrhagic sensorimotor stroke: spectrum of disease. J Neurol Res. 2011;1:90.
2. Cooper HA, et al. Subclinical brain embolization in left-sided infective endocarditis. Circulation. 2009;120:585.
3. Pickett CA, et al. Carotid bruits and cerebrovascular disease risk: a meta-analysis. Stroke. 2010;41:2295.
4. Szaflarski JP, et al. Incidence of seizures in the acute phase of stroke: a population-based study. Epilepsia. 2008;49:974.

In detection of all types of stroke syndromes, magnetic resonance imaging is much more sensitive than non-contrast computed tomography (CT).

A study of 356 patients with suspected acute stroke revealed that MRI had a sensitivity of 83 % (95 % CI, 78–88 %) and a specificity of 97 % (95 % CI, 92–99 %). All patients were tested with both methods, and in comparison, non-contrast CT had a sensitivity of only 26 % (95 % CI, 20–32 %) and a specificity of 98 % (95 % CI, 93–99 %) [1]. CT is, however, quite sensitive in the identification of hemorrhagic stroke [2].

1. Chalela JA, et al. Magnetic resonance imaging and computed tomography in emergency assessment of patients with suspected acute stroke: a prospective comparison. Lancet. 2007;369:293.
2. Caplan LR. Imaging and laboratory diagnosis. In: Caplan's stroke: a clinical approach. ed 4. Philadelphia: Saunders; 2009. p. 87.

Dementia and Delirium

Frontotemporal dementia (FTD), more common than generally believed, is characterized by manifestations that can help differentiate this disease from Alzheimer disease (AD).

A victim of the campaign to purge eponyms from the medical lexicon, what was once called Pick disease, to honor Dr. Arnold Pick, a psychiatrist from Prague who described the syndrome in 1892, is now termed frontotemporal dementia. Although considered uncommon until recently, we now estimate that 20–50 % of persons under age 65 with dementia have FTD [1]. The pathologic hallmark of the disease is atrophy in the frontal and temporal lobes of the brain [2]. See Fig. 3.1.

The features that might help distinguish FTD from AD are onset before age 65; disinhibition, with muting of the little voice that warns that something really shouldn't be said or done; personality change; hyperorality; and roaming behavior. In a study of 21 FTD patients and 42 AD patients, all FTD patients and none of the AD patients exhibited three of the five manifestations described [3]. Also, memory seems to be less affected than in AD [1]. Making the correct diagnosis is important because there are some differences in management of the two diseases, including

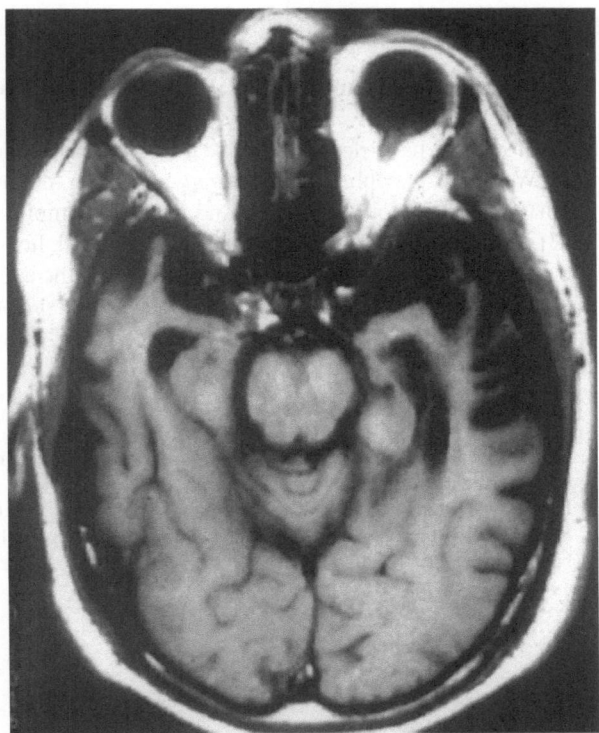

Fig. 3.1 Frontotemporal lobar degeneration

the fact the FTD often affects younger, working individuals who can benefit from advance planning [2].

1. Cardarelli R, et al. Frontotemporal dementia; a review for primary care physicians. Am Fam Physician. 2010;82:1372.
2. Lantz MS, Buchalter EN. Pick's disease. Available at: http://www.clinicalgeriatrics.com/article/4261?page=0,1.
3. Mendez MF, et al. Pick's disease versus Alzheimer's disease: a comparison of clinical characteristics. Neurology. 1993;43(2):289.

An Alzheimer-signature MRI biomarker that predicts AD in cognitively normal adults has been described.

Dickerson et al. propose that focusing on cortical thinning in regions known to be affected in AD can identify atrophy in asymptomatic individuals up to a decade before dementia [1].

The questions then arise: Do you or I really want to know this information? And is there anything we could do to change the outcome?

1. Dickerson RC, et al. Alzheimer-signature MRI biomarker predicts AD dementia in cognitively normal adults. Neurology. 2011;76:1395.

Vertical nystagmus can indicate Wernicke encephalopathy.

Several reports have described upbeating and downbeating nystagmus in patients with Wernicke encephalopathy, a *must-not-miss* neurologic emergency that can result in death if not recognized and treated promptly with intravenous thiamine [1–3]. The disease is typically related to prolonged, heavy alcohol use. However, in one case reported, there was no such history, and the encephalopathy was attributed to sequelae of anorexia nervosa [3]. The classic description of Wernicke encephalopathy tells of confusion, ataxia, and oculomotor dysfunction, although this trio is seen together in a minority of cases.

1. Shin BS, et al. Upbeat nystagmus changes to downbeat nystagmus with upward gaze in a patient with Wernicke's encephalopathy. J Neurol Sci. 2010;298:145.
2. Koontz DW, et al. Wernicke encephalopathy. Neurology. 2004;63:394.
3. Sharma S, et al. Wernicke's encephalopathy presenting with upbeating nystagmus. J Clin Neurosci. 2002;9:476.

The demented patient in the hospital or nursing home who suddenly becomes delirious may have acute urinary retention.

This scenario, especially likely to occur in elderly men with enlarged prostates, is a urologic emergency calling for prompt bladder decompression—rather than the administration of sedative drugs [1, 2].

1. Van Rompaey BV, et al. Risk factors for delirium in intensive care patients: a prospective cohort study. Crit Care. 2009;13:R77.
2. Thorne MB, et al. Acute urinary retention in elderly men. Am J Med. 2009;122:815.

Choreoathetosis, Tremors, and Tics

The onset of choreiform movements in a Hispanic child may be the beginning of Huntington disease (HD).

Huntington disease is a progressive, incurable disease characterized by chorea and cognitive impairment that typically appear during the fourth or fifth decade of life. The presence of this autosomal dominant disease can be confirmed by genetic testing.

The world's largest concentration of HD patients is in Venezuela, many found in the area near Lake Maracaibo, and study of these patients led to discovery of the HD gene in 1993. The original progenitor of the family lived in the early 1800s and has had some 14,000 descendants, many with the disease. Among these families, many children suffer from the disease and may experience seizures in addition to the chorea and cognitive changes [1].

The disease in not confined to Venezuelans. Alonso et al. studied 691 Mexican HD patients in 401 families. When compared to HD populations in other countries, the Mexican patients had a higher frequency of infantile cases, shorter disease duration, and a lower suicide rate [2].

1. Hereditary Disease Foundation. The Venezuela Huntington's disease project. Available at: http://www.hdfoundation.org/html/venezuela_huntington.php.
2. Alonso ME, et al. Clinical and genetic characteristics of Mexican Huntington's disease. Mov Disord. 2009;24:2012.

Asterixis is found in more than hepatic encephalopathy.

Asterixis, the so-called flapping tremor, was first described in 1949 in patients with advanced liver failure and encephalopathy [1]. The word derives from "a-" combined with *sterixis*, a Greek word referring to a fixed position. In addition to hepatic encephalopathy, asterixis has been described in patients with renal failure, carbon dioxide poisoning, and stroke [2]. Drugs can also cause asterixis; two examples from the literature are carbamazepine (Tegretol) and gabapentin (Neurontin) [3, 4].

1. Adams RD, et al. The neurological changes in the more common types of severe liver disease. Trans Am Neurol Assoc. 1949;74:217.
2. Kim JS. Asterixis after unilateral stroke: lesion location of 30 patients. Neurology. 2001; 56:533.
3. Naoko S, et al. A case of symptomatic epilepsy associated with carbamazepine-induced asterixis. Neurol Med. 2006;64:183.
4. Sechi GP, et al. Asterixis and toxic encephalopathy induced by gabapentin. Prog Neuropsychopharmacol Biol Psychiatry. 2004;26:195.

Although various types of tics occur commonly in school children, vocal tics suggest one of three diagnoses: Tourette syndrome (TS), Huntington disease, or Sydenham chorea (SC).

A study of 4,479 Swedish schoolchildren revealed that 6.6 % of subjects ages 7–15 years had or had experienced a tic disorder during the previous 12 months [1]. Vocal tics are sudden, recurrent, involuntary vocalizations, often loud, and sometimes complex, such as repeating certain phrases out of context (palilalia) or echoing the words of others (echolalia).

Swain et al. report, "The diagnosis of TS should be in doubt in the absence of simple tics. Vocal tics can be helpful in ruling out other diagnoses because they are rare in other neurologic conditions. Exceptions include Huntington's disease and SC" [2].

The diagnosis of TS is suspect in the absence of throat clearing and grunting [3].

1. Khalifa N, et al. Prevalence of tic disorders and Tourette syndrome in a Swedish school. Dev Med Child Neurol. 2003;45:315.
2. Swain JE, et al. Tourette syndrome and tic disorders: a decade of progress. J Am Acad Child Adolesc Psychiatry. 2007;46:947.
3. Robertson MM, Trimble MR, Lees AJ. The psychopathology of the Gilles de la Tourette syndrome. A phenomenological analysis. Br J Psychiatry. 1988;152:383.

Essential tremor (ET), the most common of all pathologic tremors, may be associated with cognitive impairment and an increased risk of Parkinson disease (PD).

We no longer call the disease "benign" essential tremor. This common disorder, which can be transmitted in an autosomal dominant fashion in about half of instances, affects 0.4–6 % of the population and, owing to motor impairment and perhaps to reduced cognitive function, leads up to a quarter of affected persons to modify their careers or end them early [1]. Several studies have found cognitive impairment in ET patients, in a pattern described by Lacritz et al. as "not unlike that seen in Parkinson's disease" [2, 3].

But wait; there's more. Patients with ET are four times more likely to develop PD than individuals without ET. In the study by Benito-León et al., 12 (5.8 %) of 207 ET patients developed PD after a median time of 3.3 years [4]. Conversely, first-degree relatives of patients with PD have an increased risk of ET, most noteworthy in families of patients with younger-onset PD and with the tremor-predominant (or mixed) form of PD [5].

A generous serving of alcohol often suppresses the tremor of ET, a phenomenon which some might consider a diagnostic feature of the disease [1].

1. Crawford P, Zimmerman EE. Differentiation and diagnosis of tremor. Am Fam Physician. 2011;83:697.
2. Lacritz LH, et al. Cognitive functioning in individuals with "benign" essential tremor. J Int Neuropsychol Soc. 2002;8:124.

3. Frisina PG, et al. An explanatory-comparative study with Parkinson's and Alzheimer's disease patients. J Am Med Dir Assoc. 2009;10:238.
4. Benito-León J, et al. Risk of Parkinson's disease and Parkinsonism in essential tremor: a population based study. J Neurol Neurosurg Psychiatry. 2009;80:423.
5. Rocca WA, et al. Increased risk of essential tremor in first-degree relatives of patients with Parkinson's disease. Mov Disord. 2007;22:1607.

Parkinson Disease

Tremor is present in most idiopathic Parkinson disease patients but is uncommon in drug-induced Parkinsonism.

Parkinson's early description, published in 1817, describes the typical onset of disease: The first symptoms perceived are a slight sense of weakness (not paralysis,) with a proneness to trembling in some particular part: sometimes in the head but most commonly in one of the hands (especially the nondominant hand, i.e., the left in most persons) [1].

In recent years we have seen an increasing number of patients with drug-induced Parkinsonism: Culprits include metoclopramide, perphenazine, chlorpromazine, haloperidol, flupenthixol, zuclopenthixol, and occasionally even antidepressants. Blount et al. report that, in contradistinction to idiopathic Parkinsonism, tremor is uncommon in these patients [2].

Describing the phenomenon as "musicophilia," Sacks tells that rhythmic music can have a beneficial effect in relieving PD patients' movement restrictions [3].

1. Parkinson J. An essay on the shaking palsy. London: Whittingham and Rowland; 1817.
2. Blount BW, et al. Parkinson disease. CME bulletin. 2010;2:1. Available at: http://www.aafp. org/online/etc./medialib/aafp_org/documents/cme/selfstudy/bulletins/parkinsonpdf.Par.0001. File.dat/Parkinson.pdf.
3. Sacks O. Musicophilia. London: Picador; 2007. p. 248.

Micrographia can be the earliest sign of Parkinsonism.

McLennan et al. report that micrographia—small handwriting—is a sentinel manifestation in about 5 % of PD patients, occurring before any other signs of the disease are noted. They also note that micrographia is generally unresponsive to the various treatment methods used for PD [1]. Described by Gangadhar et al. as showing both smaller letters and greater velocity fluctuation compared to normal handwriting [2], the progressive development of micrographia can sometimes be demonstrated in the office by reviewing medical history forms and signatures written by the patient over the years. Having the patient draw a spiral may help differentiate Parkinson disease from essential tremor. See Fig. 3.2.

There are other, albeit less specific, early signs of PD. These include constipation, depression, impaired sense of smell, and disordered sleep [3].

1. McLennan JE, et al. Micrographia in Parkinson's disease. J Neurol Sci. 1972;15:141.
2. Gangadhar G, et al. A computational model of Parkinsonism handwriting that highlights the role of the indirect pathway in the basal ganglia. Hum Mov Sci. 2009;28:602.
3. Grossett DG, et al. Guideline Development Group. Diagnosis and pharmacological management of Parkinson's disease: summary of SIGN guidelines. BMJ. 2010;340:b5614.

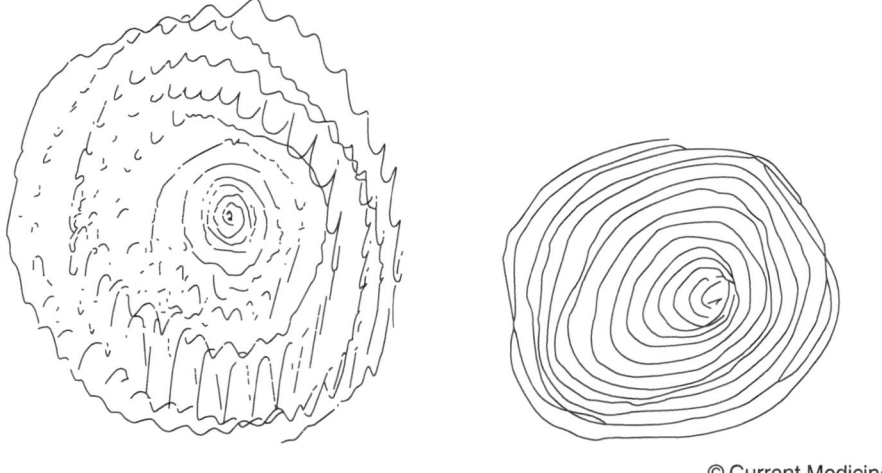

© Current Medicine

Fig. 3.2 Spirals drawn by patients with essential tremor (*left*) and Parkinson disease tremor (*right*). Essential tremor can interfere with drawing a smooth spiral, as seen in the *left* panel. The patient with Parkinson disease typically has a tremor at rest that decreases upon action or writing; however, the spiral may be micrographic and eccentric, as in the *right* panel (*Courtesy of* Seth Pullman, MD, Columbia University Medical Center, New York, NY)

The "bicycle" sign can help identify patients with atypical Parkinsonism.

Atypical Parkinsonism is characterized by "more extensive extranigral pathology," resulting in problems with coordination and balance. Aerts et al. studied 156 consecutive patients with PD, asking each, "Can you still ride a bicycle?" Before the onset of disease, 111 patients reported being bicyclists. Of the group, 34 of 64 atypical Parkinsonism patients had ceased cycling, compared with only 2 of the 45 patients with typical PD (sensitivity 52 %; specificity 96 %; CI 0.64–0.83) [1].

1. Aerts MB, et al. The "bicycle sign" for atypical Parkinsonism. Lancet. 2011;377(9760):125.

Parkinson disease patients who report visual hallucinations often experience progressive cognitive decline.

In a study of 20 non-demented hallucinating PD patients, 45 % developed dementia over the following 12 months, and nearly 70 % showed some sort of cognitive impairment [1]. In light of this study, visual hallucination in a PD patient should be considered a risk factor for the development of dementia.

1. Ramirez-Ruiz B, et al. Cognitive changes in Parkinson's disease patients with visual hallucinations. Dement Geriatr Cogn Disord. 2007;23:282.

The Neuropathies

The type 2 diabetic patient with polyneuropathy may not report "numbness of the feet."

There are many causes of chronic polyneuropathy, including vitamin B12 deficiency; alcohol; inherited disorders such as Charcot–Marie–Tooth disease, amyloidosis, syphilis, acquired immunodeficiency disorder (AIDS) or its treatment; toxins such as mercury and lead; and drugs such as vincristine, isoniazid, metronidazole, and statins. The most commonly encountered form, however, is diabetic peripheral neuropathy.

Up to half of older type 2 diabetic patients have peripheral neuropathy, and many of these are asymptomatic [1]. Franse et al. studied 588 type 2 diabetic patients with a mean age of 66.8 years, finding polyneuropathy in 32 % of subjects. The strongest association of polyneuropathy was with age, and the sensitivity and specificity of "numbness of the feet" were 28 and 93 %, respectively [2].

1. Boulton AJM. Management of diabetic peripheral neuropathy. Clin Diab. 2005;23:9.
2. Franse LV, et al. 'Numbness of the feet' is a poor indicator for polyneuropathy in Type 2 diabetic patients. Diab Med. 2000;17:105.

In daily practice, the 128-Hz tuning fork is the best way to test for diabetic polyneuropathy.

Meijer et al. tested the 128-Hz tuning fork against two well-regarded international (International Consensus on the Diabetic Foot) and national (Dutch *Nederlandse Diabetes Federatie-Centraal Beleids Orgaan*) test instruments. The single use of the tuning fork yielded predictive results similar to the extended test scores and much better results when compared to monofilament testing [1].

Going further, Oyer et al. tested the clanging 128-Hz tuning fork on the toes of diabetic patient and also evaluated the monofilament test. They found the tuning fork test to be reproducible and accurate, with a mean duration of vibration sensation of 10.2 s, with a standard deviation of ±1.3 s. This study also found the tuning fork test to be superior to the monofilament test in detecting neuropathy [2].

1. Meijer JW, et al. Back to basics in diagnosing polyneuropathy with the tuning fork! Diabetes Care. 2005;28:2201.
2. Oyer DS, et al. Quantitative assessment of diabetic peripheral neuropathy with use of the clanging tuning fork test. Endocr Pract. 2007;13:5.

The earliest manifestation of Guillain–Barré syndrome (GBS) may be pain.

Although we think of this immune-mediated disease as an ascending motor paralysis, a prospective cohort study of 156 GBS patients revealed that 36 % of subjects experienced pain in the 2 weeks preceding the onset of weakness, and 66 % had pain during the first 3 weeks of the disease [1]. Moulin et al.'s report found the most common pain syndromes to be deep aching back and leg pain and dysesthetic pain in the extremities. They reported poor correlation of pain intensity with neurologic disability [2].

When pondering a cause of GBS, think first of a recent *Campylobacter jejuni* infection, found in about one quarter of GBS patients [3].

As a historical note, Goldman et al. propose, based on Bayesian analysis of probabilities, that US President Franklin D. Roosevelt's paralytic illness was not poliomyelitis, but GBS [4].

1. Ruts L, et al. Pain in Guillain-Barré syndrome: a long-term follow up study. Neurology. 2010;75:1439.
2. Moulin DE, et al. Pain in Guillain-Barré syndrome. Neurology. 1997;48:328.
3. Hughes RAC, et al. Guillain-Barré syndrome. Lancet. 2005;366(9497):1653.
4. Goldman AS, et al. What was the cause of Franklin Delano Roosevelt's paralytic illness? J Med Biogr. 2003;11:232.

Bell palsy (BP) may herald the onset of diabetes mellitus or Parkinson disease.

A study of 148 BP patients versus 128 control subjects found the prevalence of abnormal glucose metabolism significantly higher in BP subjects ($p < 0.001$) than in controls [1]. And Savica et al. conducted a population-based case–control study of the relationship of PD and prior BP, finding a history of prior BP in 6 of 196 PD patients and no similar occurrence in 196 control subjects [2].

Figure 3.3 depicts the typical findings of Bell palsy.

1. Bosco D, et al. Bell's palsy: a manifestation of prediabetes? Acta Neurol Scand. 2011;123:68.
2. Savica R, et al. Bell's palsy preceding Parkinson's disease: a case–control study. Mov Disord. 2009;24:1530.

Not all cases of Bell palsy are idiopathic.

Although Herpes simplex virus type 1 is thought to be the leading suspect in Bell palsy, we still consider the disease idiopathic because firm evidence is lacking [1]. Other causes of facial nerve paralysis include Guillain–Barré syndrome, Lyme disease, otitis media, Ramsay Hunt syndrome, sarcoidosis, tumor, stroke, and multiple sclerosis. There is even one report of a facial palsy following use of cervical traction [2]. The point here is that assuming all patients with Bell palsy to have idiopathic disease will result in failure to diagnose some important—possibly even life-threatening—causes of facial nerve paralysis.

To present another instance of medical detective work, Maloney speculates that the wry smile of the Mona Lisa portrait is "Leonardo da Vinci's anatomically precise representation of a new mother affected by Bell's palsy subsequent to her recent pregnancy" [3].

Fig. 3.3 Bell palsy (left seventh nerve weakness)

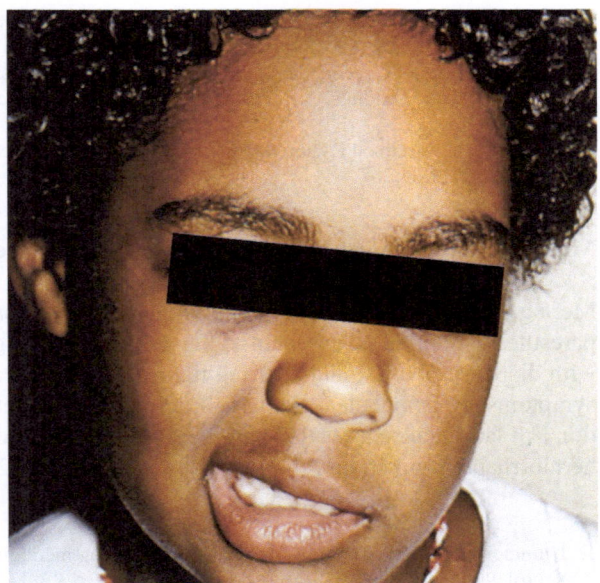

1. Tiemstra JD, et al. Bell's palsy: diagnosis and management. Am Fam Physician. 2007;76:997.
2. So EC. Facial nerve paralysis after cervical traction. Am J Phys Med Rehabil. 2010;89:849.
3. Maloney WJ. Bell's palsy: the answer to the riddle of Leonardo da Vinci's Mona Lisa. J Dent Res. Available at: http://scholar.google.com/scholar?hl=en&q=Bell%E2%80%99s+palsy%3A +the+answer+to+the+riddle+of+Leonardo+da+Vinci%E2%80%99s+Mona+Lisa&btnG=Sear ch&lr=lang_en&as_sdt=1%2C38&as_ylo=2007&as_vis=0.

The time-honored tests for carpal tunnel syndrome (CTS)—Tinel, Phalen, reverse Phalen, and carpal compression tests—are more sensitive for tenosynovitis than for carpal tunnel syndrome.

CTS is the most commonly encountered peripheral nerve entrapment syndrome. In a study of 232 individuals with CTS matched with 182 controls, Miedany et al. found the sensitivity of the commonly used clinical tests to be higher for tenosynovitis than for carpal tunnel syndrome: Tinel sign, 46 % versus 30 %; Phalen test, 92 % versus 47 %; reverse Phalen test, 75 % versus 42 %; and carpal tunnel compression test, 95 % versus 42 %. In addition all four tests showed higher specificity for tenosynovitis than for CTS [1].

The diagnosis of CTS rests on the triad of symptoms, physical findings, and electrodiagnostic studies. Yet, Homan et al. report "poor overlap" among these three findings. Among 449 subjects with CTS, only 23 (5 %) with one of the three findings met all three criteria for the dominant hand [2].

In 2012 Bilkis et al. describe a modified Phalen test (MPT), using sensory testing in the Phalen position. Following a study of 66 hands by a blinded examiner, they concluded that the "MPT demonstrates greater accuracy than the traditional Phalen test for predicting CTS" [3].

1. Miedany EL, et al. Clinical diagnosis of carpal tunnel syndrome: old tests—new concepts. Joint Bone Spine. 2008;75:451.
2. Homan MM, et al. Agreement between symptom surveys, physical examination procedures and electrodiagnostic findings for carpal tunnel syndrome. Scand J Work Environ Health. 1999;25:115.
3. Bilkis S, et al. Modified Phalen's test as an aid in diagnosing carpal tunnel syndrome. Arthritis Care Res. 2012;64:287.

Meralgia paresthetica (MP) can be an iatrogenic disease.

Meralgia paresthetica, an entrapment of the lateral femoral cutaneous nerve causing paresthesia, numbness, and pain in the anterolateral thigh, is classically associated with diabetes, obesity, and wearing tight belts. Other causes of anterolateral thigh symptoms are spinal stenosis, large uterine leiomyomata, and lumbar disc herniation [1]. Iatrogenic causes that have been reported include hip surgery, laparoscopic herniorrhaphy, and antipsychotic-induced weight loss [2, 3].

1. Trummer M, et al. Lumbar disc herniation mimicking meralgia paresthetica: case report. Surg Neurol. 2000;54:80.
2. Eubanks S, et al. Meralgia paresthetica: a complication of laparoscopic herniorrhaphy. Surg Laparosc Endosc. 1993;3:381.
3. Chlebowski S, et al. Meralgia paresthetica: another complication of antipsychotic-induced weight loss. Obes Rev. 2009;10:700.

The tip-off to the diagnosis of Charcot–Marie–Tooth (CMT) disease may be the finding of pes cavus.

Charcot–Marie–Tooth disease, a hereditary demyelinating peripheral neuropathy and the most common genetic nerve disorder, usually involves the legs before the arms. Pes cavus is a common early sign, found in 12 of 22 CMT patients studied by Sabir et al. [1] See Fig. 3.4. Patients typically develop atrophy of the peroneal muscle groups, manifested as thin lower legs.

1. Sabir MB, et al. Pathogenesis of pes cavus in Charcot-Marie-Tooth disease. Clin Orthop Relat Res. 1984;184:223.

The diabetic patient with peripheral neuropathy may, in fact, have a metformin-induced vitamin B12 deficiency.

There have been a number of recent reports of metformin-induced vitamin B12 deficiency, including a number of instances involving symptoms of peripheral neuropathy [1–3]. In one report, 10 (6.2 %) of 162 patients with cobalamin deficiency were considered to have metformin-associated deficiencies [4].

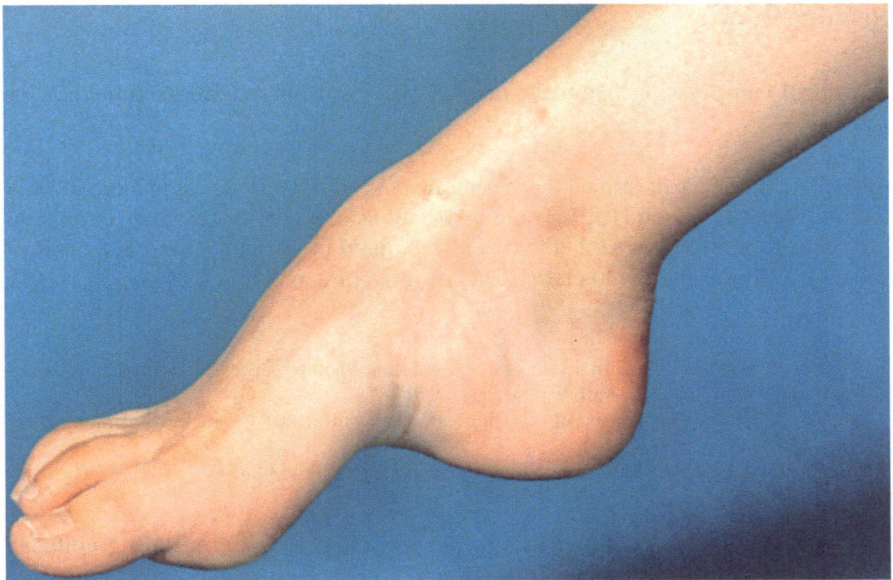

Fig. 3.4 Talipes cavus in Charcot–Marie–Tooth disease

Although straying beyond the realm of diagnosis, I wonder if patients using metformin might benefit from routine supplementation with oral vitamin B12.

1. Liu KW, et al. Metformin-related vitamin B12 deficiency. Age Ageing. 2006;35:200.
2. Bell DS. Metformin-induced vitamin B12 deficiency presenting as a peripheral neuropathy. South Med J. 2010;103:265.
3. Nervo M, et al. Vitamin B12 in metformin-treated diabetic patients: a cross-sectional study in Brazil. Rev Assoc Med Bras. 2011;57:46.
4. Andres E, et al. Metformin-associated vitamin B12 deficiency. Arch Intern Med. 2002;162:2251.

Wartenberg sign, the phenomenon of the fifth finger being caught on the edge of the pants pocket when a patient attempts to put the hand into the trouser side pocket, is sometimes seen in patients with ulnar palsy.

The patient has persistent abduction of the fifth digit owing to weakness of the interosseous muscles and of the joint flexors innervated by the ulnar nerve [1].

1. Wartenberg R. Kleine Hilfsmittel der neurologichen diagnostik. Nervenarzt. 1930;3:594.

Seizures

Vertebral compression fractures may be the result of unwitnessed convulsive seizures.

Several reports have described these occurrences, with the fractures tending to be in the mid-thoracic region [1, 2]. These associations must, however, be taken in context: Finelli et al. reviewed 2,800 patients admitted to hospital with a diagnosis of seizure, finding that only 30 (1.1 %) had sustained fractures [3].

1. Aboukasm AG, et al. Nocturnal vertebral compression fracture: a presenting feature of unrecognized epileptic seizures. Arch Fam Med. 1997;6:185.
2. Napier RJ, et al. Diagnosis of vertebral fractures in post-ictal patients. Emerg Med. 2011;28:169.
3. Finelli PF, et al. Seizure as a cause of fracture. Neurology. 1989;39:858.

The patient's history can provide important clues in differentiating epilepsy versus psychogenic nonepileptic seizures (PNES).

There is a relatively high prevalence of PNES in patients referred to epilepsy centers, estimated to be 15–30 % by Bodde et al. These authors go on to state that the time lag between the first symptom and the eventual diagnosis of PNES is 7 years [1].

Why is the distinction important? The definitive diagnosis guides treatment decisions, with epileptic seizures treated with anticonvulsant drugs and PNES treated with psychotherapy [2].

History may be the most useful tool. Schwabe tells that epileptic patients tend to describe seizures in a coherent manner, while PNES patients more often present accounts that are difficult to fathom [2]. Plut et al. find that epileptic patients often offer metaphors describing the seizure as an "agent/force or event/situation," while PNES patients use metaphors of "space/place" [3].

In a study of 30 patients with epilepsy, 30 patients with PNES, and 30 control subjects, depression and dissociative mechanisms had a higher prevalence as precursors in the PNES group than in epileptics ($p < 0.001$) and controls ($p < 0.001$) [4]. And a study by Walczak et al. found weeping during 14 % of psychogenic nonepileptic seizures in PNES patients, but none during observed epileptic seizures [5].

1. Bodde NM, et al. Psychogenic non-epileptic seizures—diagnostic issues. Clin Neurol Neurosurg. 2009;111(1):1.
2. Schwabe M, et al. Listening to people with seizures: how can linguistic analysis help in the differential diagnosis of seizure disorders? Commun Med. 2008;5:59.
3. Plut L, et al. Seizure metaphors differ in patients' accounts of epileptic and psychogenic non-epileptic seizures. Epilepsia. 2009;50:994.
4. Mazza M, et al. Non-epileptic seizures are predicted by depressive and dissociative symptoms. Epilepsy Res. 2009;84:91.
5. Walczak TS, et al. Weeping during psychogenic non-epileptic seizures. Epilepsia. 1996;37:208.

Multiple Sclerosis

Elation and inappropriate laughing, taken in context with other symptoms, can help in recognition of the patient with multiple sclerosis (MS).

In his description of the disease in 1877, Charcot described "foolish laughter with no cause" [1]. Some have used the term "pathological laughter" [2]. One writer has described this as a "happy state of mind," with mild elation and denial of disability [3]. You may also think of this as a morbid optimism.

O'Connor estimates the prevalence of euphoria in MS as 10–60 %, which seems to me to be a wide range. Other common manifestations of MS include fatigue, sensory loss (especially in the legs), cognitive changes, depression, optic neuritis, optic atrophy, nystagmus, vertigo, ataxia, spasticity, and bladder dysfunction [3].

About a third of patients will have a positive Lhermitte sign—a sense of electrical shock when the neck is flexed—although this sign lacks specificity for MS [5].

1. Pratt RTC. An investigation of the psychiatric aspects of disseminated sclerosis. J Neurol Neurosurg Psychiatry. 1951;14:326.
2. Hoegerl C, et al. Pathological laughter in a patient with multiple sclerosis. J Am Osteopath Assoc. 2008;108:409.
3. Finger S. A happy state of mind: a history of mild elation, denial of disability, optimism, and laughing in multiple sclerosis. Arch Neurol. 1998;55:241.
4. O'Connor P. The Canadian Multiple Sclerosis Working Group. Key issues in the diagnosis and treatment of multiple sclerosis. Neurology. 2002;59:S1.
5. Kanchandani R, et al. Lhermitte's sign in multiple sclerosis: a clinical survey and review of the literature. J Neurol Neurosurg Psychiatry. 1982;45:308.

The onset of multiple sclerosis after age 50 is uncommon, but not rare.

Noseworthy et al. found that of 838 patients in a large MS clinic, the disease began late in life (after age 50) in 9.4 % of individuals. In these older subjects, disability progressed more rapidly than in younger persons [1].

1. Noseworthy J, et al. Multiple sclerosis after age 50. Neurology. 1983;33:1537.

Spinal Cord Disorders

When evaluating one of the legions of patients with acute low back pain, there are four red flags for spinal fracture: being female, age greater than 70 years, prolonged steroid use, and significant trauma.

A group in Australia studied 1,172 patients with a chief complaint of acute low back pain, asking them to respond to 25 red-flag questions. There were 11 cases of serious pathology, including 8 vertebral fractures. The investigators propose a diagnostic prediction rule based on four items—female sex, age above 70 years, significant trauma, and prolonged steroid use. This diagnostic prediction rule was "moderately associated with the presence of fracture" (CI, 0.654–1.014; $p = 0.001$) [1].

1. Henschke N, et al. Prevalence of and screening for serious spinal pathology in patients presenting to primary care settings with acute low back pain. Arthritis Rheum. 2009;60:3072.

Urinary retention in a patient with back and leg pain is characteristic of the cauda equina syndrome (CES), especially in the setting of bilateral sciatica.

An uncommon condition associated with spinal cord compression, the CES is typically caused by a large midline disc herniation, although tumor can also be a cause. Other symptoms are overflow incontinence, saddle anesthesia, and bilateral sciatic pain, leg numbness, and weakness. See Fig. 3.5. CES is a surgical emergency calling for prompt decompression of the spinal canal [1, 2]. The disease may be first noted during the postoperative period, with manifestations incorrectly attributed to postoperative findings [1].

Although clinically rare, CES is described by the Medical Protection Society (MPS, London) as having a "disproportionally high medicolegal profile." Their 2009 report describes 63 likely claims worldwide over a 5-year interval [3]. If for no other reason than the disorder's medicolegal profile, CES must be considered a *must-not-miss diagnosis*.

1. Spector LR, et al. Cauda equina syndrome. Am Acad Orthop Surg. 2008;16:471.
2. Ma B, et al. Cauda equina syndrome: a review of clinical progress. 2009;122:1214.
3. Cauda equina syndrome. MPS Casebook. London; 2009. Available at: http://www.medicalprotection.org/uk/casebook-september-2009/cauda-equina-syndrome.

A neck injury followed by complaints of numb, clumsy hands may signal a central cord syndrome (CCS).

Described as the most common incomplete spinal cord injury, CCS is a problem shared by two disparate groups: the elderly and athletes involved in contact sports,

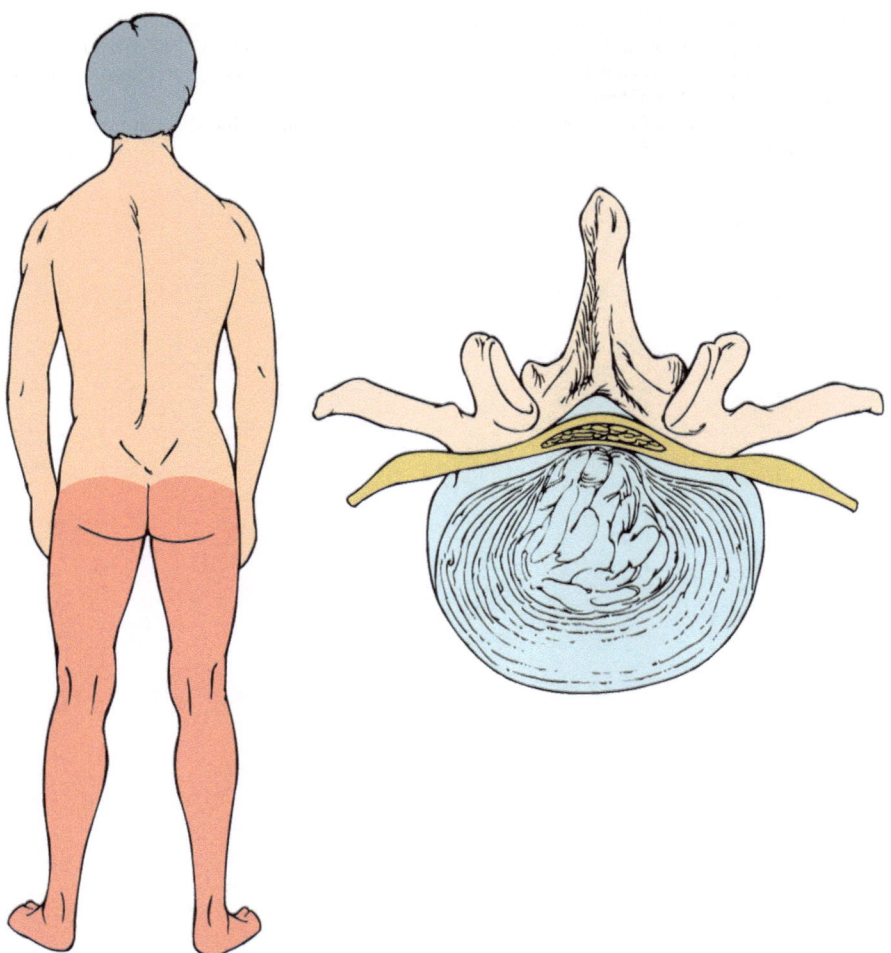

Fig. 3.5 Cauda equina compressed by disc and area affected with weakness and numbness

such as football. Elderly individuals often have predisposing factors, such as degenerative spinal disease, spinal stenosis, or cervical spondylosis. Athletic injuries such as helmet-to-helmet impact or falls can cause cervical hyperextension with damage to the ligamentum flavum [1–3].

The classic pathology is ischemia or bleeding into the central spinal cord, yielding the symmetry of the findings and, owing to the arrangement of nerves in the spinal cord, the apparent paradox of greater weakness in the upper extremities than in the lower. Other, often later, manifestations of CCS include spasticity, gait disturbance, bladder dysfunction, and neuropathic pain [1–3].

1. Nakajima M, et al. Midcervical central cord syndrome: numb and clumsy hands due to midline cervical disc protrusion at the C3-4 level. J Neurol Neurosurg Psychiatry. 1995;58:607.
2. Aarabi B, et al. Hyperextension cervical spine injuries and traumatic central cord syndrome. Neurosurg Focus. 2008;25:9.
3. McKinley W, et al. Incidence and outcomes of spinal cord injury clinical syndromes. J Spinal Cord Med. 2007;30:215.

Trauma

Any alteration in mental status following trauma is a concussion.

This definition covers everything from the athlete's self-report of a "slight ding" to lying unconscious on the ground [1]. The importance of this broad definition of concussion lies in the epidemiology of the problem. A prospective cohort study of 100 nationally representative US high schools elicited injury reports in various sports where head trauma might occur. There were 1,308 concussions reported during more than five million athlete exposures, yielding an estimated 395,000 concussions sustained nationally. They also found that, using various guidelines, 15–40 % of athletes returned to play prematurely. Remarkably, 15.8 % of high school football players suffering a concussion with loss of consciousness returned to play within 24 h [2].

When the mental status and neurologic examinations are normal, imaging is generally unnecessary. There are, however, three evidence-based indications for imaging: prolonged unconsciousness, focal neurologic deficits, and worsening symptoms [1].

1. McConnell A, et al. Concussion care: simple strategies, big payoffs. J Fam Pract. 2009;58:410.
2. Yard EE, et al. Compliance with return to play guidelines following concussion in US high school athletes, 2005–2008. Brain Inj. 2009;23:888.

In seeking laboratory confirmation of a cerebrospinal fluid (CSF) rhinorrhea, the gold standard is beta-2-transferrin.

CSF rhinorrhea was recognized as early as Roman times as a consequence of head trauma, and over the years the diagnosis of suspected CSF rhinorrhea has generated a rich treasury of lore. The use of glucose oxidase test strips lacks specificity [1, 2]. Such use was labeled a "plastic pearl" by Hull and Morrow [1].

Decherd and Bailey suggest the halo sign, present as a halo on bed linens as blood forms a dark ring around the clear CSF. The authors, however, describe this test as "not very accurate." These same authors also suggest that when the rhinorrhea is collected on a linen handkerchief, a dry, stiff residue suggests nasal secretions and a soft cloth indicates CSF. I would also not bet my diagnostic reputation on these tests [3]. Other authors suggest that CSF is probably present in the nasal discharge if the glucose test is positive, no blood is noted, the blood glucose is <6 mmol/L^{-1}, and the patient has no evidence of an upper respiratory infection [4].

The best laboratory test for a CSF fistula is beta-2-transferrin, a protein present only in three body fluids: perilymph, vitreous humor, and CSF. The test is both sensitive and specific. One milliliter of secretions is needed, and the fluid can sometimes be collected by the patient at home. Unfortunately the test result may not be known for a few days [5].

1. Hull HF, et al. Glucorrhea revisited: prolonged promulgation of another plastic pearl. JAMA. 1975;234:1052.
2. Katz RT, et al. Glucose oxidase stick and cerebrospinal fluid rhinorrhea. Emerg Med J. 2005;22:556.
3. Decherd ME, et al. Cerebrospinal fluid leaks. Available at: http://74.125.155.132/scholar?q=ca che:vKUCTI7sfAMJ:scholar.google.com/+Decherd+ME,+Bailey+BJ.+Cerebrospinal+fluid+l eaks.+&hl=en&as_sdt=0,38.
4. Baker EH, et al. New insights into the glucose oxidase stick test for cerebrospinal fluid rhinor-rhea. Emerg Med. 2005;22:556.
5. Bleier BS, et al. Preliminary study on the stability of beta-2 transferrin in extracorporeal cere-brospinal fluid. Otolaryngol Head Neck Surg. 2010;144:101.

Selected Problems of the Nervous System

Gait and balance problems are typically the presenting findings in idiopathic normal pressure hydrocephalus.

This treatable neurologic disorder is a type of hydrocephalus occurring in adults, usually in individuals over 60 years of age. See Fig. 3.6. The classic triad of manifestations is gait disturbance, urinary incontinence, and dementia [1]. The symptoms can overlap with Alzheimer disease and even, in the setting of gait dysfunction, with Parkinson disease. Making the correct diagnosis is vital because many patients experience improvement in their symptoms following placement of a ventricular shunt [2].

1. Thynne K. Normal pressure hydrocephalus. J Neurosci Nurs. 2007;39:27.
2. Tsakanikas, et al. Normal pressure hydrocephalus. Semin Neurol. 2007;27:58.

Tinnitus can be a symptom of idiopathic intracranial hypertension (IIH).

In one study of 23 patients with IIH, 4 (23.5 %) complained of a pulsatile intracranial noise [1]. Others have estimated the occurrence of pulsatile tinnitus in IIH as

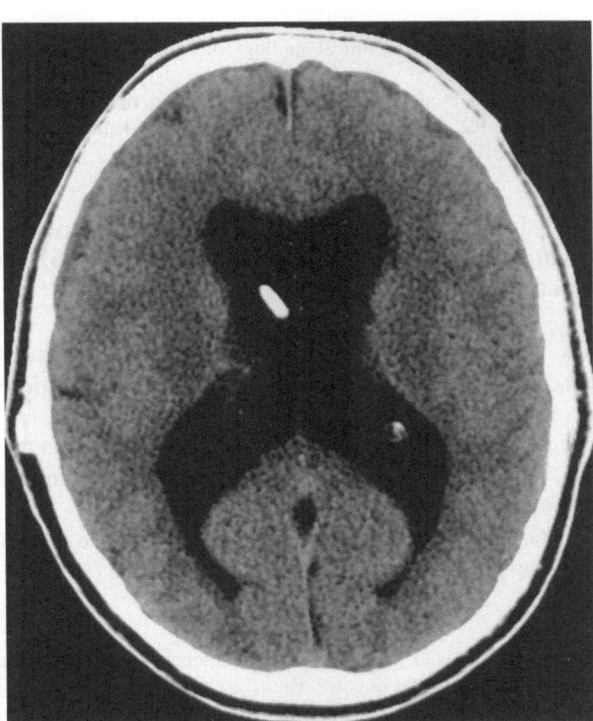

Fig. 3.6 Computed tomography scan of a patient with normal-pressure hydrocephalus, showing dilated ventricles

high as 50 % [2]. Of course, in IIH the most common presenting symptoms are visual, notably blurred vision and transient visual obscuration, found in 88 % of patients, with symptoms attributed to increased intracranial pressure in the study by Aavirt-Soudry et al. and headache, present in 65 % of subjects [1].

1. Aavirt-Soudry S, et al. Idiopathic intracranial hypertension after 40 years of age: clinical features in 23 patients. Eur J Ophthalmol. 2008;18:989.
2. Standridge SM. Idiopathic intracranial hypertension in children: a review and algorithm. Pediatr Neurol. 2010;43:337.

Acoustic neuroma can cause a decreased corneal reflex and nystagmus.

Granted, the most common signs of an acoustic neuroma are unilateral hearing impairment (97 % of patients) and tinnitus and disequilibrium (70 % of patients). A report of difficulty with balance in the dark may be a helpful clue [1, 2]. Facial numbness and weakness may occur. The eye signs described above, although uncommon, might be a source of diagnostic confusion if their occurrence with acoustic neuroma is not recognized.

And here is a zebra you may encounter some day: The patient with bilateral acoustic neuroma might have neurofibromatosis—type 2 [3].

1. Harner SG, et al. Clinical findings in patients with acoustic neurinoma. Mayo Clin Proc. 1983;58:721.
2. Harner SG, et al. Diagnosis of acoustic neurinoma. Neurosurgery. 1981;9:373.
3. Karnes PS. Neurofibromatosis: a common neurocutaneous disorder. Mayo Clin Proc. 1998;73:1071.

Transient global amnesia (TGA) in men is more likely to follow some physical event, when compared to women in which TGA more often is linked to an emotional event.

The above is the conclusion of Quinette et al., who reviewed the literature and also described 142 personal cases [1]. In TGA a short-lived episode of alarming and disorienting antegrade amnesia is coupled with a retrograde amnesia for recent events. A link to migraine is debated [2]. The suspected link to migraine is intriguing, because both conditions are associated with an increased frequency of patent foramen ovale [3].

TGA has been reported in connection with use of prescribed medications, including phosphodiesterase-5 inhibitors and statins [4, 5].

1. Quinette PL, et al. What does transient global amnesia really mean? Review of the literature and thorough study of 142 cases. Brain. 2006;129:1640.
2. Schmidtke K, et al. Transient global amnesia and migraine. Eur Neurol. 1998;40:9.

3. Klötzsch C, et al. An increased frequency of patent foramen ovale in patients with transient global amnesia: analysis of 53 consecutive patients. Arch Neurol. 1996;53:504.
4. Machado A, et al. Tadalafil-induced transient global amnesia. J Neuropsychiatry Clin Neurosci. 2010;22:E28.
5. Healy D, et al. Transient global amnesia associated with statin intake. BMJ Case Rep. 2009. doi:10.1136/bcr.06.2008.0033.

A few reports have been published describing degeneration of the central and peripheral nervous system caused by excessive use of denture cream.

The chain of events goes like this: A patient with loose-fitting dentures, a very heavy user of denture cream, is found to have sensory disturbance, difficulty walking, and limb weakness. There may be bone marrow depression with pancytopenia. Laboratory studies ordered by the astute clinician reveal two key results: elevated zinc levels (hyperzincemia) and low copper levels, the latter leading to the neurologic and hematologic abnormalities [1, 2].

They physiologic clue is that excessive zinc ingestion interferes with the absorption of dietary copper, leading to hypocupremia and its resultant pathologic manifestations [2]. These and other reports were validated in a "Dear Doctor" letter from GlaxoSmithKline describing the zinc content of various dental products [3].

1. Hedera PL, et al. Myelopolyneuropathy and pancytopenia due to copper deficiency and high zinc levels of unknown origin II. The denture cream as a primary source of excessive zinc. Neurotoxicology. 2009;30:996.
2. Tezvergil-Mutluay A, et al. Hyperzincemia from ingestion of denture adhesives. J Prosthet Dent. 2010;103:380.
3. Letter from Dr. Howard Marsh, Chief Medical Officer GlaxoSmithKline, Direct communication from pharmaceutical company. 18 Feb 2010.

The person who suddenly develops what seems a foreign accent may have— you guessed it—the foreign accent syndrome (FAS).

Also called (inappropriately, I believe) the foreign language syndrome, FAS can develop suddenly following an event such as a stroke or traumatic brain injury [1]. Last year, my local newspaper recently described a woman from Madras, Oregon, who awoke from oral surgery sedation speaking with what seemed a British accent, a speech pattern that has persisted [2]. A report from Spain describes a case of FAS as a first sign of multiple sclerosis [3].

1. Naidoo R, et al. A case of foreign accent syndrome resulting in regional dialect. Can J Neurol Sci. 2008;35:360.
2. Oregon woman woke with an accent. The Sunday Oregonian. 1 May 2011. p. 1.
3. Villaverde-González R, et al. Foreign language syndrome as a first sign of multiple sclerosis. Rev Neurol. 2003;36:1035.

Chapter 4
The Eye

*Who would believe that so small a space could contain the images
of all the universe? Italian Renaissance painter and writer.*
Leonardo da Vinci (1452–1519) [1]

Contents

R.B. Taylor, *Diagnostic Principles and Applications*,
DOI 10.1007/978-1-4614-1111-6_4, © Springer Science+Business Media, LLC 2013

The *small space* to which da Vinci alludes is, of course, the eye, a brilliantly engineered apparatus that can capture the images of the universe and whisk them along via the optic nerve to be interpreted in the visual cortex.

1. da Vinci L. Codice Antlatico, 345. In: The notebooks of Leonardo da Vinci, vol 1. London: Dover Publications; 1970, Chap. IX.

Red Eye

Some simple maneuvers can help distinguish between conjunctivitis and more severe eye disorders.

Most patients with a red eye will have conjunctivitis, a common and generally benign condition. But some will have uveitis, whether involving the anterior uveal tract (iritis) or the structures posterior to the lens (chorioretinitis or vitreitis). Uveitis threatens vision and calls for ophthalmologic referral. Other causes of red eye are acute glaucoma, trauma, foreign body, and corneal abrasion. Lyme disease is a rare cause of uveitis [1]. How can one differentiate conjunctivitis from more serious entities [2–4]?

> *Visual acuity*: Begin with a question about vision. The patient experiencing some degree of visual loss in the red eye may have uveitis. Then visual acuity should be confirmed with a Snellen chart.
> *Photophobia*: Check for significant photophobia, uncommon with conjunctivitis and suggestive of more severe disease. Be concerned about the patient sitting in the waiting room with the affected eye closed.
> *Irritation*: Ask about a scratchy, gritty sensation in the eye, often reported by patients with conjunctivitis, but not typically seen with uveitis or glaucoma.
> *Fixed pupil*: A fixed pupil that does not react to light suggests the presence of acute angle-closure glaucoma, as does the presence of severe eye pain and/or vomiting.
> *Small pupil*: A very small pupil suggests the cause may be iritis or keratitis.

1. Bodaghi B. Ocular manifestations of Lyme disease. Med Mal Infect. 2007;37:518.
2. Cronau H, et al. Diagnosis and management of red eye in primary care. Am Fam Physician. 2010;81:137.
3. Wirbelauer C. Management of the red eye for the primary care physician. Am J Med. 2006;119:302.
4. Schaller UC, et al. From conjunctivitis to glaucoma. When is a red eye an alarm signal? MMW Fortschr Med. 2002;144:30.

The Au–Henkind test can help differentiate between conjunctivitis and iritis.

The Au–Henkind test is performed as follows: Have the patient close the *red* eye and then further occlude vision in that eye with a paddle or the patient's hand. Then shine a bright light into the uninvolved eye. If the patient reports pain in the occluded, *red* eye, the test indicates the presence of iritis. The Au–Henkind test, which assumes that the consensual light response is intact, is considered to be highly sensitive and specific for acute iritis [1, 2].

1. Au YK. Pain elicited by the consensual pupillary reflex: a diagnostic test for acute iritis. Lancet. 1981;2:1254.
2. Orient JM. Sapira's art and science of diagnosis. 3rd ed. Philadelphia: Lippincott, Williams & Wilkins; 2005. p. 196.

In examination of the red eye, the pattern of conjunctival injection matters.

Diffuse injection of the bulbar and palpebral conjunctiva suggests a primary conjunctival problem, for example, conjunctivitis. The presence of perikeratic injection, especially prominent at the limbus and less pronounced peripherally, suggests more serious disease such as iritis, keratitis, or acute glaucoma [1].

1. Sauer A, et al. Red eye in children. Rev Pract. 2008;58:353.

Eye Pain

Eye pain may signal an ocular emergency, although this is not always the case in children.

Causes of eye pain include acute angle-closure glaucoma, uveitis, optic neuritis, chemical burns, and intraocular foreign bodies [1]. Yet, in children, the cause may be functional eye pain, found to be the case in 73 of 80 children (91 %) ages 2–6 years with a complaint of eye pain but without a red eye or history of an obvious cause of the pain [2].

1. Dargin JM, et al. The painful eye. Emerg Med Clin North Am. 2008;26:199.
2. Richards AL, et al. Eye pain in preschool children: diagnostic and prognostic significance. J AAPOS. 2010;14:383.

The patient who is "sick" with eye pain may have acute angle-closure glaucoma.

Although encountered uncommonly in generalist practice, acute angle-closure glaucoma, a *must-not-miss diagnosis*, has been described as the leading cause of blindness in East Asia [1]. The classic presentation is an older individual who appears in general distress, often describing nausea and severe headache, and covering the eye with the hand. Vomiting may occur as intraocular pressure rises. The affected eye may have a fixed pupil and a ciliary flush and may feel hard to the touch [2, 3]. Sapira describes anecdotes in which patients have gone blind from acute angle-closure glaucoma while undergoing diagnostic imaging for their headaches [4].

In a susceptible patient, acute angle-closure glaucoma can be precipitated by drugs. Examples include epinephrine injections; tri- and tetracyclic antidepressants; pilocarpine; sulfa-based drugs such as hydrochlorothiazide, co-trimoxazole, or topiramate; phenylephrine drops; and nebulized salbutamol [5].

Patients with suspected acute angle-closure glaucoma need emergency ophthalmologic referral—without pupillary dilation, which may make things worse (see Fig. 4.1).

1. Amerasinghe N, et al. Angle-closure: risk factors, diagnosis and treatment. Progress Brain Res. 2008;173:31.
2. Quigley HA. Angle-closure glaucoma—simple answers to complex mechanisms: LXVI Edward Jackson Memorial Lecture. Am J Ophthmol. 2009;148:657.
3. Hiroshi S, et al. Acute angle-closure glaucoma. Ophthalmology. 2005;47:1673.
4. Orient JM, editor. Sapira's art and science of diagnosis, 3rd ed. Philadelphia: Lippincott, Williams & Wilkins; 2005. p. 200.
5. Lachkar Y, et al. Drug-induced acute angle closure glaucoma. Curr Opin Ophthmol. 2007; 18:129.

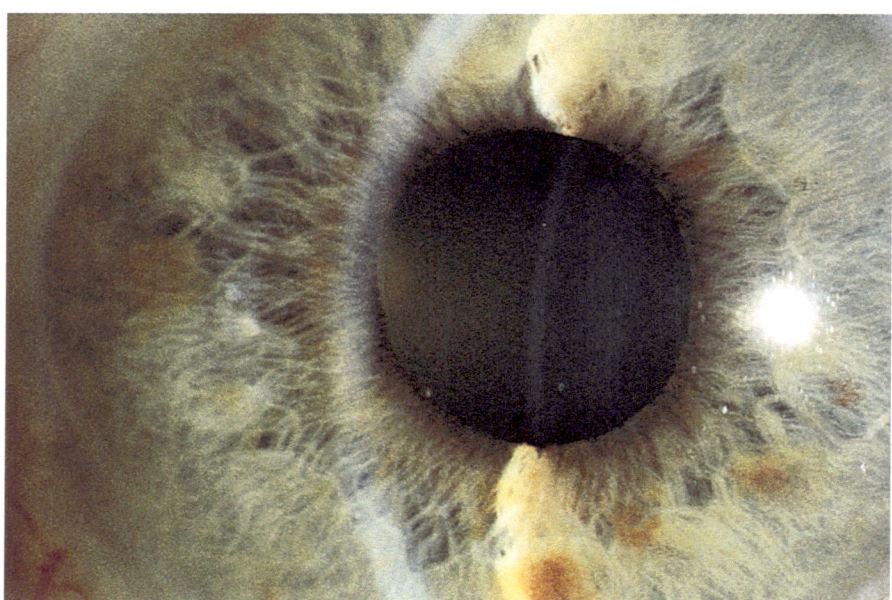

Fig. 4.1 An eye with chronic angle closure glaucoma in which intraocular pressure increased after pupillary dilatation. Note the presence of iris bombé, characterized by marked convexity in the iris configuration

Dry Eye

When a patient begins using artificial tears for dry eyes, consider the diagnosis of Sjögren syndrome.

Akpek et al. have concluded that primary Sjögren syndrome (PSS) is underdiagnosed. They studied medical records of 220 patients with dry eye syndrome. Of these, 24 were found to have PSS, although only eight of these patients (33.3 %) carried the diagnosis at the time of presentation [1]. Because PSS is a progressive autoimmune exocrinopathy that may be manifested as glomerulonephritis, peripheral neuropathy, or skin vasculitis, early diagnosis is important [2]. Witte advises confirmation of PPS as a cause of dry eyes by detection of autoantibodies against Ro(SS-A) and La(SS-B) and/or salivary gland biopsy [3].

1. Akpek EK, et al. Evaluation of patients with dry eye for presence of underlying Sjögren syndrome. Cornea. 2009;28:493.
2. Mavragani CP, et al. The geoepidemiology of Sjögren syndrome. Autoimmune Rev. 2010;9:A305.
3. Witte T. Pathogenesis and diagnosis of Sjögren's syndrome. J Rheumatol. 2010;69:50.

Anisocoria

The first step in the evaluation of anisocoria (pupillary inequality) is determining which eye is abnormal.

If the pupillary abnormality is greater in bright light, there is poor constriction on the abnormal side; that is, the larger pupil is the abnormal one. In contrast, if the anisocoria is greater in relative darkness, there is poor dilation on the affected side, indicating that the abnormality is in the smaller pupil [1].

1. Younge BR. What is the evaluation for anisocoria? In: Lee AG, et al., editors. Curbside consultation in neuro-ophthalmology. New York: Slack; 2008. p. 86.

Adie pupil, generally a benign finding, describes a tonically dilated pupil that reacts poorly or not at all to light (see Fig. 4.2).

Adie pupil must not be confused with the Argyll Robertson (AR) pupil, which has also been called "prostitute's pupil". The AR pupil constricts with accommodation but not with exposure to light. A whimsical mnemonic is that the prostitute *accommodates*, but does not *react*. The AR pupil can be seen with central nervous system syphilis, it's classic cause, as well as various other disorders such as multiple sclerosis, cerebral aneurysm, herpes zoster, Lyme disease, craniopharyngioma, diabetes, and alcoholism [1].

1. Timoney PJ, et al. Douglas Argyll Robertson (1837–1909) and his pupil. Ir J Med Sci. 2010;179:119.

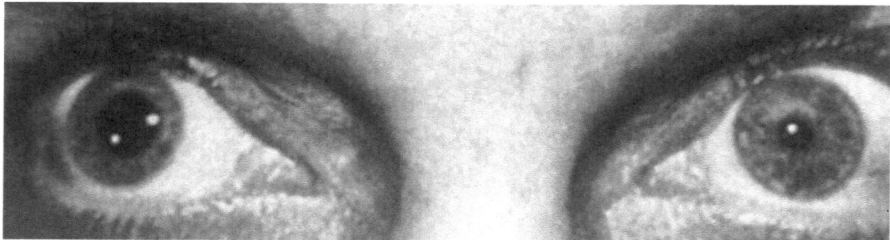

Fig. 4.2 Light-near dissociation in Adie's tonic pupil syndrome in a 38-year-old man with a 4-month history of anisocoria. With bright light, the right pupil fails to constrict, producing noticeable anisocoria. During near viewing, both pupils constrict well

If you encounter a patient with a new onset, unilateral dilated pupil and a sudden, severe headache, the first diagnosis to consider is a *must-not-miss* cerebral aneurysm.

In this setting, the pupillary abnormality can be the tip-off to an impending, potentially devastating intracranial bleed [1].

1. Younge BR. What is the evaluation for anisocoria? In: Lee AG, et al., editors. Curbside consultation in neuro-ophthalmology. New York: Slack; 2008. p. 86.

Diplopia and Ptosis

Binocular diplopia and asymmetric ptosis are found in the majority of patients with myasthenia gravis (MG).

These extraocular muscle weakness manifestations will be the initial manifestation in half of all MG patients, and in about 20 % the disease will continue to be noted only in the extraocular muscles [1, 2]. The diagnosis of this acquired autoimmune disorder can be confirmed using the Tensilon test, detecting elevated titers of acetylcholine receptor or muscle-specific receptor tyrosine kinase (MuSK) antibodies, finding a decremental response on slow repetitive nerve stimulation, and/or noting abnormal jitter on single-fiber electromyography [3].

1. Sommer N, et al. Ocular myasthenia gravis: a critical review of clinical and pathophysiological aspects. Doc Ophthalmol. 1993;84:309.
2. Juel VC, et al. Myasthenia gravis. Orphanet J Rare Dis. 2007;6:44.
3. Benatar M. Pearls: myasthenia. Semin Neurol. 2010;30:35.

Diplopia is the symptom most likely to be reported by patients with Graves ophthalmopathy.

Law et al. report a case of a 71-year-old male with this inflammatory disorder of the orbit typically associated with hyperthyroidism. Treatment of this patient's diplopia involved use of a prism on the left spectacle [1].

1. Law KM, et al. Thyroid disease induced diplopia. Clin Exp Optom. 2009;92:30.

Botulinum toxin injections near the eye can cause diplopia or ptosis.

Aristdemou et al. report three instances of diplopia caused by periorbital botulinum toxin injection, noting that the diplopia was bilateral in two cases. The defect caused by the injection was paresis of the inferior oblique muscle [1]. I found several other reports of ptosis following botulinum toxin injections, including a paper by Racette et al. [2].

1. Aristdemou P, et al. Diplopia associated with the cosmetic use of botulinum toxin for a facial rejuvenation. Ophthal Plast Reconstr Surg. 2006;22:134.
2. Racette BA, et al. Ptosis as a remote effect of therapeutic botulinum toxin B injection. Neurology. 2002;12:1445.

Some cases of diplopia just might be drug related.

In one series, 256 cases of ptosis, diplopia, and ophthalmoplegia following statin therapy are reported [1]. Another paper reports 171 instances of diplopia following the use of fluoroquinolones [2]. In both these associations, the World Health Organization considers the relationship to be *possible*. Stay tuned.

1. Fraunfelder FW, et al. Diplopia, blepharoptosis, and ophthalmoplegia and 3-hydroxy-3-methyl-glutaryl-CoA reductase inhibitor use. Ophthalmology. 2008;115:2282.
2. Fraunfelder FW, et al. Diplopia and fluoroquinolones. Ophthalmology. 2009;116:1814.

Floaters, Night Blindness, and Other Visual Defects

Suspect a retinal detachment in a patient who describes a shower of unilateral vitreous floaters.

Sometimes described as resembling a housefly darting about the visual field, a floater arises as the vitreous gel separates from the retinal surface. The presence of floaters is especially worrisome in individuals older than age 45, as concluded following a prospective study of 350 patients with posterior vitreous detachment. Of the 163 of these subjects who had one to two floaters, with or without light flashes, as the initial symptom, 12 (7.3 %) developed a retinal tear [1]. A family history of retinal detachment increases the risk [2].

1. Byer NE. Natural history of posterior vitreous detachment with early management as the premier line of defense against retinal detachment. Ophthalmology. 1994;101:1503.
2. Go SL, et al. Genetic risk of rhegmatogenous retinal detachment: a familial aggregation study. Arch Ophthalmol. 2005;123:1237.

A *shade being drawn over the eye* is a red-flag symptom suggesting retinal detachment.

Hatten et al. describe a 62-year-old patient with retinal detachment who presented with the "shade drawn over the eye" complaint [1]. Retinal detachment, a *must-never-miss diagnosis*, is especially prominent in boxers and prompted the early retirement of Sugar Ray Leonard in 1982 [2].

1. Hatten B, et al. Retinal detachment. Emerg Med J. 2011;28:83.
2. Maguire JI, et al. Retinal injury and detachment in boxers. JAMA. 1986;255:2451.

Impaired night vision is generally the initial manifestation of retinitis pigmentosa (RP).

RP is described as a group of genetic retinal disorders affecting 1 in 3,500 persons worldwide. There is an increased prevalence in northern Sweden, owing to a *founder* effect on a stable (read nonmigratory) population [1]. The disease often begins in adolescence with the loss of night vision, followed with impaired side vision (so-called tunnel vision) in young adulthood, and, eventually, central vision loss later in life (see Fig. 4.3). Noting black spots peripherally on the retina aids in diagnosis, as does a family history of the disease [2].

1. Golovleva I, et al. Mutation spectra in autosomal dominant and recessive retinitis pigmentosa in northern Sweden. Adv Exp Med Biol. 2010;664:255.
2. Hartong DT, et al. Retinitis pigmentosa. Lancet. 2006;368:1795.

Fig. 4.3 Tunnel vision in retinitis pigmentosa

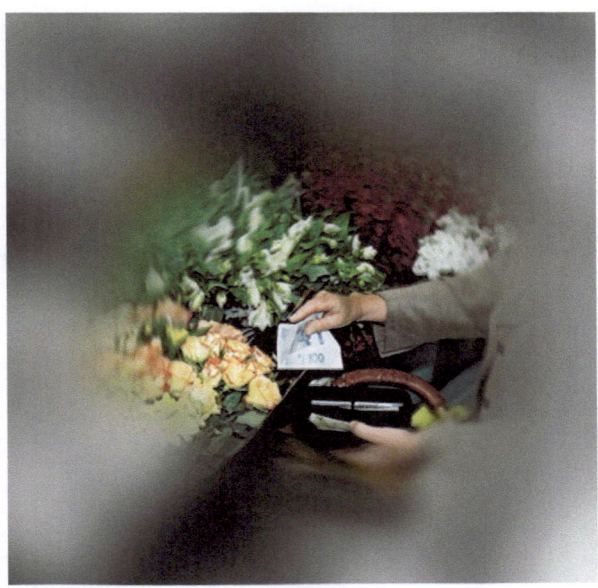

Think of vitamin A deficiency in the undernourished person who describes impaired night vision.

Considered by Dowling et al. to be one of the oldest diseases known to man, nutritional night blindness was described in ancient Egyptian medical writings, along with the recommendation to treat the disease by eating liver [1]. A study of night-blind pregnant women in Nepal found low levels of serum retinol, indicating a poor vitamin A status. In this study, night blindness was associated with low consumption of milk products, fish, meat, and green vegetables [2].

1. Dowling JE, et al. Vitamin A deficiency and night blindness. Proc Natl Acad Sci USA. 1958;44:648.
2. Christian P, et al. Night blindness of pregnancy in rural Nepal: nutritional and health risks. Int J Epidemiol. 1997;27:231.

A sudden monocular visual defect associated with eye pain is an alarm symptom complex strongly suggesting optic neuritis.

In about 10 % of patients, symptoms may be bilateral, and not all patients have eye pain. Optic neuritis may be seen in younger patients and is a common early manifestation of multiple sclerosis [1, 2]. Prompt recognition of this *must-not-miss disease* allows early consideration of therapy with high-dose steroids [2].

Optic neuritis has also been reported following influenza and anthrax immunizations [3, 4].

1. Osborne BJ, et al. Optic neuritis and risk of MS: differential diagnosis and management. Cleveland Clinic J Med. 2010;76:181.
2. Clark D, et al. Optic neuritis. Neurol Clin. 2010;28:573.
3. Hull TP, et al. Optic neuritis after influenza vaccination. Am J Ophthalmol. 1997;124:703.
4. Kerrison JB, et al. Optic neuritis after anthrax vaccination. Ophthalmology. 2002;109:99.

Exophthalmos

The exophthalmos (aka proptosis) of Graves disease can be unilateral or bilateral.

The most common cause of exophthalmos, whether unilateral or bilateral, is Graves disease (see Fig. 4.4). But not all exophthalmos is Graves disease. In one report, Graves disease accounted for more than 15 % of patients with evidence of expanding orbital lesions [1]. Other causes of unilateral exophthalmos include metastatic carcinoma, hemangioma and lymphangioma, idiopathic orbital inflammation, lymphoma, and primary neural tumor. The list of positive causes is shorter when the patient has bilateral exophthalmos: In this setting, think of Graves disease, lymphoma, or Wegener granulomatosis.

One report describes a pulsating unilateral exophthalmos due to a traumatic aneurysm of the intraorbital ophthalmic artery [3].

1. Moss HM. Expanding lesions of the orbit: a clinical study of 230 consecutive cases. Am J Ophthalmol. 1962;54:761.
2. Grove AS Jr, et al. Evaluation of exophthalmos. N Engl J Med. 1975;292:1005.
3. Rahmat H, et al. Pulsating unilateral exophthalmos due to a traumatic aneurysm of the intraorbital ophthalmic artery. J Neurol. 1984;60:102.

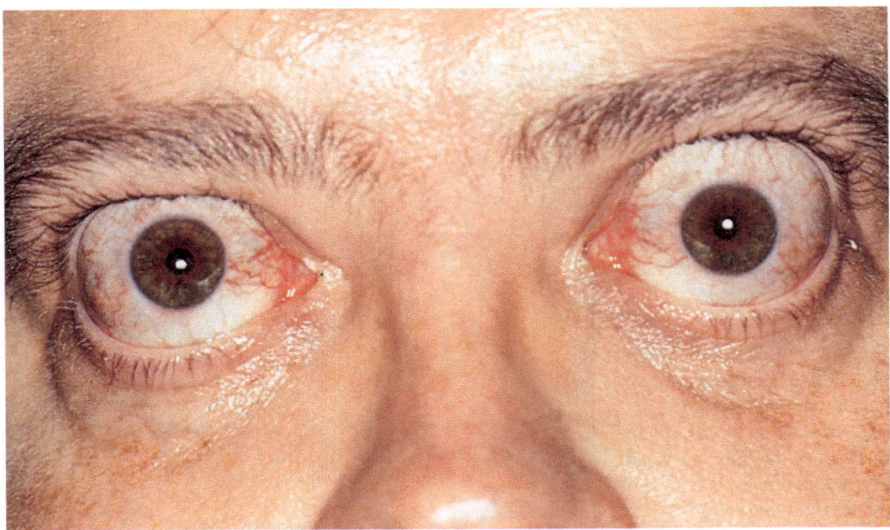

Fig. 4.4 Graves disease with exophthalmos and profound bilateral upper and lower eyelid retraction

Optic Disc Swelling

Papilledema is just one type of optic disc swelling.

Papilledema describes optic disc swelling caused by elevated intracranial pressure, which is often accompanied by other manifestations of increased intracranial pressure, such as headache, nausea and vomiting, visual manifestations, and even altered consciousness (see Fig. 4.5). When you see papilledema, think of idiopathic intracranial hypertension (aka pseudotumor cerebri), intracranial bleeding or inflammation, and tumor. Causes of optic disc swelling other than papilledema include optic neuritis and occlusion of the central retinal artery or vein [1, 2].

In a series of 49 patients with optic disc swelling, the cause was ischemic optic neuropathy in 17 subjects (34.7 %) and optic neuritis in 15 (30.6 %). Seven subjects (14.3 %) had intracranial disease such as papilledema or compressive optic neuropathy [3].

Some patients have congenitally anomalous optic discs that appear swollen, putting these patients at risk of unnecessary clinical tests [1].

1. Van Stavern GP. Optic disc edema. Semin Neurol. 2007;27:233.
2. Whiting AS, et al. Papilledema: clinical clues and differential diagnosis. Am Fam Physician. 1992;45:1125.
3. Jung JJ. Analysis of the causes of optic disc swelling. Korean J Ophthalmol. 2011;25:33.

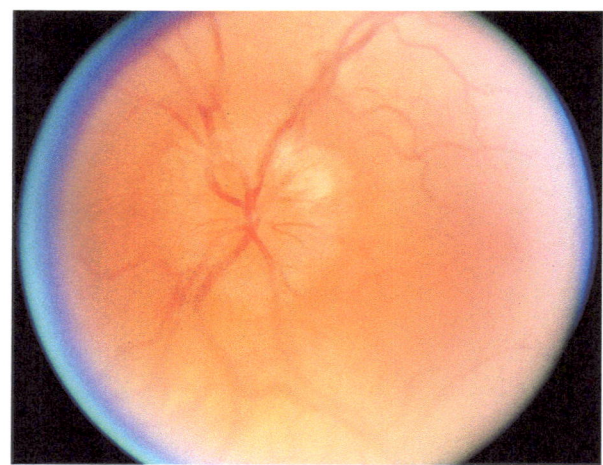

Fig. 4.5 Papilledema. This patient had acute elevation of her intracranial pressure secondary to an abscess. The margins of the optic nerve are blurred, and there is edema of the surrounding retina

Selected Problems of the Eye

Strabismus is the second most frequent manifestation of retinoblastoma in infants.

Leukocoria, an alarming white reflection from the retina of the eye, is well known as the cardinal sign of retinoblastoma, but the fact is that the second most common sign noted in infants with the malignant retina tumor is strabismus [1]. In children over age five, leukocoria remains the most common sign, followed by decreased vision and then strabismus [2].

As an aside: A report by Draper et al. notes an increased incidence of second neoplasms, notably osteosarcoma, in survivors of genetic retinoblastoma, leading to the suggestion that these persons are sensitive to the carcinogenic effects of radiation used to treat the retinal tumor [3].

1. Balmer A, et al. Differential diagnosis of leukocoria and strabismus, first presenting signs of retinoblastoma. Clin Ophthalmol. 2007;1:431.
2. Shields CL, et al. Retinoblastoma in older children. Ophthalmology. 1991;98:395.
3. Draper GJ, et al. Second primary neoplasms in patients with retinoblastoma. Br J Cancer. 1986;53:661.

Xanthopsia, yellow vision, is a classic sign of digitalis intoxication.

In fact, medical historians postulate that the vivid yellow hues in the paintings of Vincent van Gogh from 1886 to 1890 may reflect digitalis effect. The use of absinthe by the artist may have played a role, but another hypothesis has been suggested. Van Gogh had seizures and a popular antiepileptic medication of the time was digitalis [1, 2]. To continue our retrospective speculation, Lanthony suggests that van Gogh's colored haloes may be attributed to glaucoma.

Yellow vision can also be caused by hallucinogens and thiazides and by a number of integrative medicine remedies, including baneberry, oleander, monkshood, hellebore, lily of the valley, and the red squill plant [4, 5].

1. Taylor RB. White coat tales: medicine's heroes, heritage and misadventures. New York: Springer; 2008. p. 171.
2. Lee TC. Van Gogh's vision: digitalis intoxication? JAMA. 1981;245:727.
3. Lanthony P. Van Gogh's xanthopsia. Bull Soc Ophthalmol Fr. 1989;89:1133.
4. Post J. Yellow vision in a patient taking chlorothiazide. N Engl J Med. 1960;263:398.
5. Differential diagnosis for yellow vision perception. DiagnosisPro. Available at: http://en.diagnosispro.com/differential_diagnosis-for/yellow-vision-perception/25352-154.html.

The child with blue sclerae may have osteogenesis imperfecta—or something else.

Blue sclerae represent one of the well-known, multiple-choice-exam-favorite manifestations of osteogenesis imperfecta, an inherited disorder with fragile bones susceptible to multiple fractures. In addition, patients often have short stature, kyphoscoliosis, and hearing defects [1].

Blue sclera, however, can be seen in as many as 87 % of patients with iron deficiency anemia [2]. It may also be noted in patients with Marfan syndrome, Ehlers–Danlos syndrome, and homocystinuria. A rare disease that may include blue sclerae among its manifestations is Kabuki syndrome, a congenital disorder taking its name from the appearance of the patient's face, with eversion of the lower lateral eyelid and other features resembling the makeup of actors in traditional Japanese Kabuki theater [3].

1. Cheung MS, et al. Osteogenesis imperfecta: update on presentation and management. Rev Endocr Disord. 2008;9:153.
2. Kalra L, et al. Blue sclerae: a common sign of iron deficiency? Lancet. 1986;328:1267.
3. Matsumoto N, et al. Kabuki make-up syndrome: a review. Am J Med Gen. 2003;117C:57.

A green-brown ring at the periphery of the cornea is characteristic of Wilson disease.

The Kayser–Fleischer ring represents copper deposition in the Descemet membrane and can typically be seen with the naked eye (see Fig. 4.6). But not all limbal rings represent Wilson disease. High levels of bilirubin can stain a preexisting arcus senilis [1]. Addison disease can also cause a pigmented limbal ring.

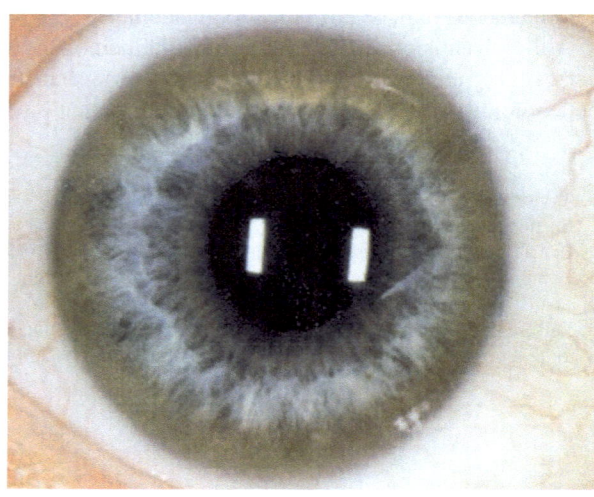

Fig. 4.6 Kayser–Fleischer ring in Wilson disease

Another ocular manifestation sometimes seen in Wilson disease is the sunflower cataract, caused by copper deposits in the lens [2]. Other features of Wilson disease are liver disease, neurologic disorders, and low serum ceruloplasmin levels.

1. Weinberg LM, et al. Fluctuating Kayser-Fleischer-like rings in a jaundiced patient. Arch Intern Med. 1981;141:267.
2. Goyal V, et al. Sunflower cataract in Wilson's disease. J Neurol Neurosurg Psychiatry. 2000;69:163.

Chapter 5
The Ear, Nose, and Throat

*Nature hath given men one tongue but two ears, that we may
hear from others twice as much as we speak.*
Greek philosopher Epictetus (c. 50–c. 138 BCE) [1]

Contents

R.B. Taylor, *Diagnostic Principles and Applications*,
DOI 10.1007/978-1-4614-1111-6_5, © Springer Science+Business Media, LLC 2013

The ear, nose, and throat, together classically abbreviated as ENT before adoption of the more scholarly word *otorhinolaryngology*, are a cluster of structures geographically proximal to one another and, more or less, functionally connected in regard to breathing, swallowing, phonation, and hearing. In considering how to present my collection of ENT facts and pearls, I have chosen to order them as they are traditionally mentioned: *ear* first, then *nose*, and then *throat* (including the lips, tongue, teeth, and other oropharyngeal structures).

1. Epictetus. The golden sayings of Epictetus. Appendix A. Fragments attributed to Epictetus. Boston: Harvard Classics; 1909.

Earache

Symptoms cannot predict acute otitis media (AOM) in young children.

Laine et al. studied 469 children ages 6–35 months, of whom 237 had AOM and 232 had respiratory tract infection without AOM. Restless sleep, the most common cause for parental concern regarding ear infection, was not predictive of AOM (RR 1.0; 95 % CI 0.8–1.2). Also not predictive were ear rubbing, fever, and duration or severity of symptoms. The authors conclude that otologic examination of the tympanic membrane is vital in the clinical diagnosis of acute otitis media, the most common disease for which US children are prescribed antibiotics [1, 2].

1. Laine MK, et al. Symptoms or symptom-based scores cannot predict acute otitis media at otitis-prone age. Pediatrics. 2010;125:e1154.
2. Coker TR, et al. Diagnosis, microbial epidemiology, and the antibiotic treatment of acute otitis media in children: a systematic review. JAMA. 2010;304:2161.

Severe ear pain with unremarkable otoscopic findings may be caused by herpes zoster oticus (HZO), aka Ramsay Hunt syndrome.

First described by American neurologist James Ramsay Hunt (1872–1937) in 1907, HZO describes a reactivation of varicella zoster virus involving the facial nerve. Facial paralysis accompanied by otalgia with auricular vesicles is the classic picture of the disease (see Fig. 5.1). HZO typically occurs in adults and is considered to be rare in children, helping to distinguish this uncommon disease from AOM, which is typically considered a childhood disease [1, 2].

1. Neilan RE, et al. Otalgia. Med Clin North Am. 2010;94:961.
2. Kim D, et al. Ramsay Hunt syndrome presenting as simple otitis externa. CJEM. 2008;10:247.

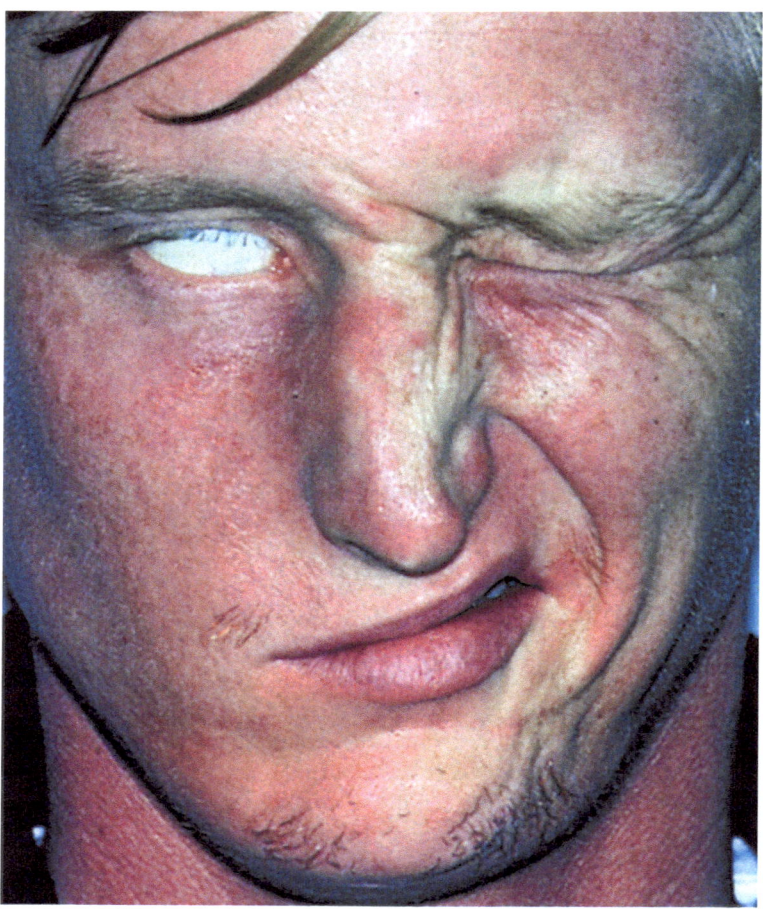

Fig. 5.1 Facial palsy in Ramsay Hunt syndrome. Herpes zoster oticus may involve the seventh and eighth cranial nerves, resulting in ipsilateral facial paralysis, usually transitory, hearing loss, and vertigo. Herpetic vesicles on the external ear or tympanic membrane may be an early and transient finding that is easily overlooked. The syndrome is frequently characterized by severe aural pain

Hearing Loss

Sudden sensorineural hearing loss (SSNHL) sometimes has an identifiable cause but is more likely to be idiopathic.

Sometimes associated with tinnitus or vertigo, SSHL is typically unilateral. About half of all patients with the disorder recover spontaneously, generally within a few weeks [1]. In most instances, the cause is presumed to be viral, but careful diagnostic investigation reveals a specific cause in about 10 % of cases. Among the entities implicated are mitral valve prolapse [3], syphilis [4], and phosphodiesterase-5 inhibitors [5].

Lin et al. describe a study showing that SSNHL increases the chance of stroke, with a 1.64 times greater risk during the next 5 years [6].

1. Schreiber BE, et al. Sudden sensorineural hearing loss. Lancet. 2010;375:1203.
2. Greco A. Sudden sensorineural hearing loss: an autoimmune disease? Autoimmun Rev. 2011; 10:756.
3. Vazquez R, et al. Mitral valve prolapse and sudden deafness (letter). Int J Cardiol. 2008; 124:370.
4. Ibrahim FW, et al. Sudden deafness in a patient with secondary syphilis. J Laryngol Otol. 2009;123:1262.
5. Khan AS, et al. Viagra deafness—sensorineural hearing loss and phosphodiesterase-5 inhibitors. Laryngoscope. 2011;121:1049.
6. Lin HC, et al. Sudden sensorineural hearing loss increases the risk of stroke: a 5-year follow-up study. Stroke. 2008;39:2744.

Unilateral sensorineural hearing loss may point to the diagnosis of acoustic neuroma (AN), aka vestibular schwannoma.

In a retrospective cohort study of 74 adult women with known AN compared with 48 control female subjects, asymmetric sensorineural hearing loss >15 dB at 3,000 Hz was found to be a useful predictor of acoustic neuroma (odds ratio [OR] 6.2; $p < 0.001$) [1] (see Fig. 5.2).

1. Saliba I. Asymmetric hearing loss: rule 3000 for screening vestibular schwannoma. Otol Neurotol. 2009;30:515.

Hearing loss is one of the classic characteristics of Waardenburg syndrome (WS).

Other typical features of this rare autosomal dominant hereditary disorder are heterochromia of the irises, a white forelock, and wide nasal bridge. The disease is named for Dutch ophthalmologist Petrus Johannes Waardenburg (1886–1979), who noted that people with irises of different colors often had hearing loss. About 60 % of patients with WS will have congenital sensorineural hearing loss, which may be profound [1–3].

Fig. 5.2 Acoustic neuroma. The tumor is centered and typically begins in the internal auditory canal extending into the cerebellopontine angle (*arrow*)

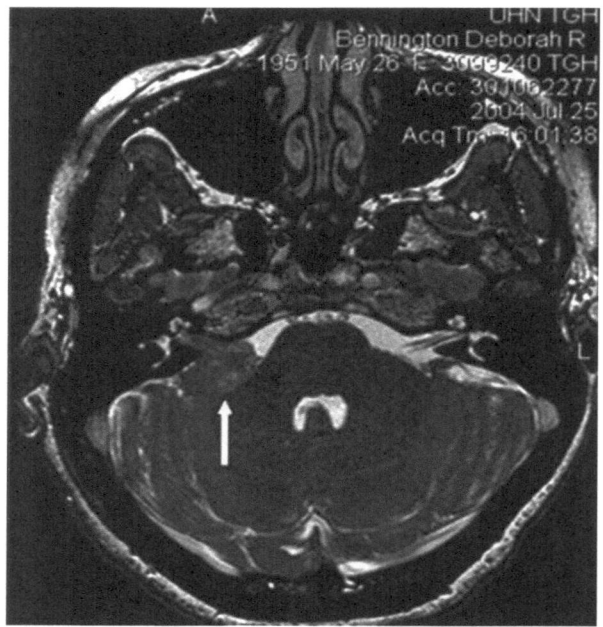

1. Tamayo ML, et al. Screening program for Waardenburg syndrome in Columbia: clinical definition and phenotypic variability. Am J Med Genetics. 2008;146:1026.
2. Teyebi N. Waardenburg syndrome type I in an Iranian female. Iranian J Pediatr. 2009;19:189.
3. Pingualt V, et al. Review and update of mutations causing Waardenburg syndrome. Hum Mutat. 2010;31:391.

A single screening question—*Do you have a hearing problem now?*—is useful in detecting unrecognized hearing loss in the elderly.

Gates et al. compared the global question to a ten-item instrument: the Hearing Handicap Inventory for the Elderly—Screening (HHIE-S). Compared to the HHIE-S, the global question had a greater sensitivity (71 % vs. 35 %) but a lower specificity (71 % vs. 94 %). With these findings, the global question has the edge as far as I am concerned, with greater sensitivity and the simplicity of use [1].

One might logically ask why the use of this handy question should be limited to the elderly.

Why not include this audiometric screening question in the routine care of adolescents, found in the Third National Health and Nutritional Examination Survey (NHANES III) to have a hearing loss prevalence of 19.5 %? [2].

1. Gates SA, et al. Screening for handicapping hearing loss in the elderly. J Fam Pract. 2003;52:56.
2. Shargorodsky J, et al. Change in prevalence of hearing loss in US adolescents. JAMA. 2010;304:772.

Dizziness and Vertigo

Dizziness—a symptom that can encompass lightheadedness, disequilibrium, presyncope, and vertigo—can have diverse origins, and the patient may have more than one cause.

Dizziness is a common complaint in primary care and is especially prevalent in the elderly, with balance problems reported by one-third of patients at age 70 years [1]. Suspect functional disease, anxiety or depression, in the patient with a complaint of lightheadedness. With disequilibrium, consider peripheral neuropathy or Parkinson disease. Presyncope may be related to medication effect, such as postural hypotension seen with some antihypertensives. Common causes of vertigo are benign paroxysmal positional vertigo, vestibular neuronitis, labyrinthitis, and Ménière disease. Of the four types noted above, vertigo occurs most commonly, present in about half of all patients with dizziness [2].

In a study of 100 patients with a mean age of 62 years with persistent dizziness, Kroenke et al. found vestibular disorders to be the most common cause (54 %), followed by psychiatric disorders (16 %) [3]. In a study of 417 elderly patients with dizziness, aged 65–95 years, Maarsingh et al. considered cardiovascular disease to be the most common cause (57 %), followed by peripheral vestibular disease (14 %). More than one cause, including drug effect, was found in 62 % of subjects [4].

1. Rangan S, et al. Dizziness in the elderly. Br J Hosp Med. 2011;72:M4.
2. Post RE, et al. Dizziness: a diagnostic approach. Am Fam Phys. 2010;82:361.
3. Kroenke K, et al. Causes of persistent dizziness: a prospective study of 100 patients in ambulatory care. Ann Intern Med. 1992;117:898.
4. Maarsingh OR, et al. Causes of persistent dizziness in elderly primary care patients. Ann Fam Med. 2010;8:196.

Benign paroxysmal positional vertigo (BPPV) is the most common cause of acute vertigo.

The most commonly occurring vestibular disorder accounts for one-third of "acute vertigo" referrals from one emergency department [1]. The diagnosis can be made clinically using the Dix–Hallpike maneuver, in which the clinician reclines the patient from sitting to a supine position. The head is turned 45° to one side and extended about 20° dorsally. A positive Dix–Hallpike test occurs when the maneuver prompts the onset of nystagmus [2].

A little-known clue may be the presence of the Tullio phenomenon—loud noises or sounds at a particular frequency cause vertigo and nystagmus—suggesting that the patient's vertigo has a peripheral cause [3].

1. Cutfield NJ, et al. Diagnosis of acute vertigo in the emergency department. Emerg Med. 2011;28:538.
2. Salvinelli F, et al. Benign paroxysmal positional vertigo: diagnosis and treatment. Clin Ter. 2004;155:395.
3. Labuguen RH, et al. Initial evaluation of vertigo. Am Fam Physician. 2006;73:244.

Tinnitus

Most patients with tinnitus have some hearing deficit.

Although I intuitively consider the figure to be high, Chan reports that tinnitus affects approximately 10 % of the population [1]. In a study of 520 consecutive patients with tinnitus, 297 (57 %) were found to have some degree of hearing loss, while 223 (43 %) had normal hearing. Subjects with impaired hearing reported more discomfort with the tinnitus and required higher masking levels than those with normal hearing [2].

1. Chan Y. Tinnitus: etiology, classification, characteristics, and treatment. Discov Med. 2009;42:133.
2. Savastano M. Tinnitus with and without hearing loss: are its characteristics different? Eur Arch Otorhinolaryngol. 2008;265:1295.

Unilateral tinnitus suggests the presence of significant disease.

Think of acoustic neuroma or Ménière disease. Henry et al. suggest that when unilateral tinnitus is encountered, the patient should have a hearing test. If there is unilateral hearing deficit, AN should be ruled out by magnetic resonance imaging (MRI), both with and without contrast [1].

1. Henry JA, et al. A triage guide for tinnitus. J Fam Pract. 2010;59:389.

Abnormalities of the External Ear

Diagonal earlobe creases suggest the presence of coronary artery disease (CAD).

Earlobe creases are sometimes called the Frank sign or Frank creases as a tribute to the physician who first described the connection between these findings and CAD [1] (see Fig. 5.3). Since then, his observation has been validated by a number of studies. Tranchesi studied 338 patients with CAD compared with 1,086 patients without CAD. Following adjustment for the usual confounders, the prevalence of creases was "58 % higher in patients with CAD than in control subjects ($p < 0.001$)" [2].

In a study of 520 autopsy cases, Edston found a strong correlation between external ear creases and CAD in both women and men ($p < 0.0001$), with a sensitivity of 75 % and positive predictive value of 68 %. He considers Frank creases to be "the strongest independent risk factor for CAD and sudden cardiac death apart from age and body mass index (both genders), as well as baldness and hair in the meatus externa (in males)" [3].

1. Frank ST. Aural sign of coronary artery disease. N Engl J Med. 1973;289:327.
2. Tranchesi B Jr, et al. Diagonal earlobe crease as a marker of the presence and extent of coronary atherosclerosis. Am J Cardiol. 1992;70:1417.
3. Edston E. The earlobe crease, coronary artery disease, and sudden cardiac death: an autopsy study of 520 individuals. Am J Forensic Med Pathol. 2006;27:129.

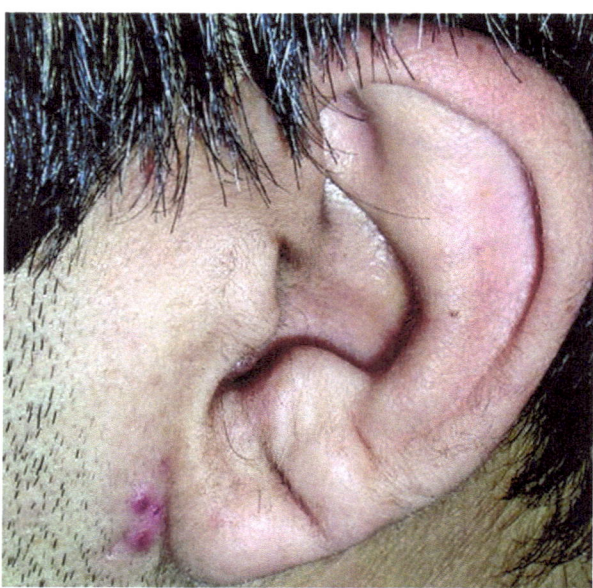

Fig. 5.3 Diagonal earlobe creases, aka Frank creases

Preauricular ear pits in an infant suggest the possible presence of hearing loss.

Preauricular sinuses, commonly called ear pits, occurring in about 1 % of newborns, should prompt audiologic evaluation. Ear pits may be sporadic or familial. Associated abnormalities may include deafness and the branchio-oto-renal (BOR) syndrome, involving the following: brachial cysts; ear pits, malformed ears, and hearing deficits; and renal abnormalities [1, 2]. In a study of 68,484 infants screened for hearing impairment, Roth et al. found permanent hearing impairment among 8/1,000 infants with preauricular skin tags or ear pits compared with 1.5/1,000 infants with no external ear abnormality [3].

1. Scheinfeld NS, et al. The preauricular sinus: a review of its clinical presentation, treatment, and associations. Pediatr Dermatol. 2004;21:191.
2. Bellini C, et al. Branchio-oto-renal syndrome: a report on nine family groups. Am J Kidney Dis. 2001;37:505.
3. Roth DA, et al. Preauricular skin tags and ear pits are associated with permanent hearing impairment in newborns. Pediatrics. 2008;122:e884.

The presence of the *red ear syndrome* (RES) in a child suggests the presence of pediatric migraine.

In the red ear syndrome, one or both ears become red and warm to the touch, associated with a burning sensation. Raieli et al. report of a study of 226 children ages 4–17 years with the complaint of headache, of whom 172 (76.4 %) had migraine. According to the authors, "RES was followed significantly more frequently by migraine, (23.3 %; $p < 0.0001$), and was characterized by high specificity and positive predictive value (96.3 and 95.3 % respectively)" [1].

1. Raieli V, et al. Prevalence of red ear syndrome in juvenile primary headaches. Cephalgia. 2010;31:597.

Atrophic Rhinosinusitis

Atrophic rhinosinusitis, often difficult to identify with certainty, may be diagnosed using proposed criteria.

Ly et al. studied 22 patients with atrophic rhinosinusitis compared with 22 patients with non-atrophic rhinosinusitis. According to these authors, atrophic rhinosinusitis, one of the more serious types of nonallergic rhinosinusitis, can be diagnosed with reasonable certainty upon finding that the patient has two or more of the following manifestations: nasal obstruction, recurrent epistaxis, episodic anosmia, nasal purulence, nasal crusting, chronic inflammatory disease such as sarcoidosis or Wegener granulomatosis, or a history or two or more sinus surgeries. Patients who have chronic rhinosinusitis and any two of these findings for 6 months or longer can be diagnosed as having atrophic rhinosinusitis with a sensitivity of 0.95 and a specificity of 0.77 [1, 2].

1. Ly TH, et al. Diagnostic criteria for atrophic rhinosinusitis. Am J Med. 2009;122:747.
2. Reed J, et al. Clinical features of sarcoid rhinosinusitis. Am J Med. 2009;123:856.

Nasal Polyps

Finding nasal polyps in a child should prompt testing for cystic fibrosis.

In one study of 23 older children with cystic fibrosis, nasal polyps were found in 39.1 % of subjects [1]. In another study of 605 patients, nasal polyposis was found in 157 subjects (25.9 %) and was the initial manifestation in 13 [2].

If the young patient does not have cystic fibrosis, other causes to be considered include aspirin sensitivity, asthma, Kartagener syndrome, or Young syndrome [3].

1. Weber SA, et al. Incidence and evolution of nasal polyps in children and adolescents with cystic fibrosis. Braz Otorhinolaryngol. 2008;74:16.
2. Stern RC, et al. Treatment and prognosis of nasal polyps in cystic fibrosis. Arch Pediatr Adol Med. 1982;136:1067.
3. Settipane GA. Nasal polyps: epidemiology, pathology, immunology, and treatment. Am J Rhinol. 1987;1:119.

Anosmia

Anosmia is characteristic of Kallmann syndrome and may occur with a number of other disorders as well.

The syndrome of hypogonadotropic hypogonadism and anosmia, named after German-American geneticist Franz Josef Kallmann, who first described the disease in 1944, is an inherited disorder with genetic heterogeneity [1]. Olfactory dysfunction can also occur as an early manifestation of Parkinson disease—during the so-called premotor phase [2].

Other possible causes of impairment of the sense of smell include allergic rhinitis, multiple sclerosis, pernicious anemia, diabetes mellitus, acute viral hepatitis, asthma, cirrhosis, sarcoidosis, Sjögren syndrome, Turner syndrome, head trauma, and zinc deficiency.

1. Rugarli EI, et al. Kallman syndrome: from genetics to neurobiology. JAMA. 1993;270:2713.
2. Tolosa E, et al. The premotor phase of Parkinson's disease. Parkinsonism Relat Disord. 2007;13:S2.

Epistaxis

Epistaxis is the most common presenting manifestation of hereditary hemorrhagic telangiectasia (HHT), aka Osler–Weber–Rendu disease.

In a study of 76 patients with HHT, 98 % had epistaxis as their presenting complaint [1].

Aspirin use may also cause epistaxis. Following a case control study of 326 patients hospitalized with epistaxis, Tay et al. found that patients using aspirin had a relative risk of hospital admission for epistaxis between 2.17 and 2.75, depending on the control group used for comparison [2].

In a more unexpected association, Page reports severe epistaxis following topiramate use [3]. Other possible causes include liver disease, myelosuppression, leukemia, trauma, and warfarin use.

1. Shah RK, et al. Hereditary hemorrhagic telangiectasia: a review of 76 cases. Laryngoscope. 2002;112:767.
2. Tay HL, et al. Aspirin, nonsteroidal anti-inflammatory drugs, and epistaxis: a regional record linkage case control study. Ann Otol Rhinol Laryngol. 1998;107:761.
3. Page RL. Intractable epistaxis associated with topiramate administration. Ann Pharmacother. 2006;40:1462.

Cheilitis

Include gastroesophageal reflux disease (GERD) in the differential diagnosis of cheilitis.

A report from France describes three patients in whom GERD may have been the cause of cheilitis [1]. Lipstick and flavored toothpaste have also been indicted as causes of cheilitis [2, 3].

Other possible offenders include alcoholism, vitamin deficiency, oral candidiasis, sprue, hypervitaminosis A, and iron deficiency anemia.

1. Mathelier-Fusade P. Cheilitis: a new manifestation of gastro-esophageal reflux? Ann Dermatol Venereol. 2009;136:887.
2. Zakon SJ, et al. Lipstick cheilitis. Arch Dermatol Syphilol. 1947;56:499.
3. Holmes G, et al. Cheilitis caused by contact urticaria to mint flavored toothpaste. Aust J Dermatol. 2001;42:43.

Abnormalities of the Oral Mucosa, Tongue, and Pharynx

The first sign of Wegener granulomatosis may be *mulberry-* or *strawberry-like* gingivitis.

Ruokonen et al. describe a patient with just such a gingivitis, which Sapira describes as a "pathognomonic feature of this condition" [1, 2] (see Fig. 5.4).

1. Ruokonen H, et al. "Strawberry-like" gingivitis being the first sign of Wegener's granulomatosis. Eur J Int Med. 2009;20:651.
2. Orient JM. Sapira's art and science of diagnosis. 3rd ed. Philadelphia: Lippincott, Williams & Wilkins; 2005. p. 267.

An erosive lesion of the oral mucosa may be the first sign of pemphigus vulgaris.

Shah reports that oral lesions, typically slow-healing erosions with poorly defined borders, are the initial manifestation of pemphigus in 50–70 % of cases. The lesion may occur on the buccal mucosa or palate [1, 2]. The presence of a one or more bullous skin lesions in such a patient makes pemphigus a strong diagnostic probability.

1. Shah HK. Case report: a sole persistent lesion of pemphigus vulgaris on the lower lip. Arch Dental Sci. 2010;1:66.
2. Sirois D, et al. Oral pemphigus vulgaris preceding cutaneous lesions: recognition and diagnosis. J Am Dent Assoc. 2000;131:1156.

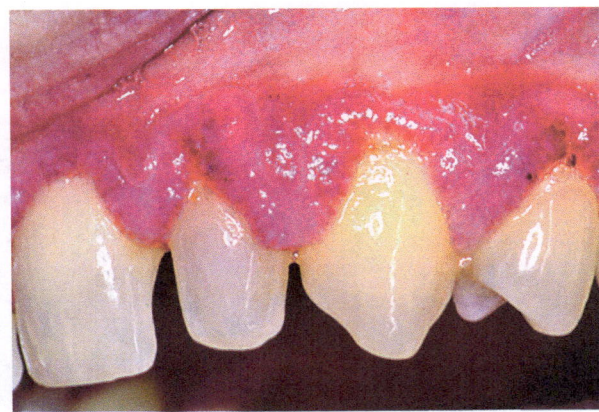

Fig. 5.4 *Mulberry* or *strawberry* gums, a rare but pathognomonic feature of Wegener granulomatosis, are due to vasculitis involving the interdental papillae, which results in gingival hyperplasia with clefting and petechiae. Such findings may occur at disease onset or with a flare of the disease

The first oral manifestations of Kaposi sarcoma are likely to be small red or purple patches on the oral mucosa.

The palate is the most common site of these sentinel lesions, which later become nodular and painfully ulcerated. Greenspan et al. point out that ketoconazole and zidovudine can also cause oral pigmentation, but this color change is more likely to be brown than red-purple [1].

1. Greenspan D, et al. HIV-related oral disease. Lancet. 1996;348:729.

Oral malignant melanoma is unlikely to be pigmented.

In a study of six patients with oral melanoma, only one-third (2) had pigmented lesions. The more consistent presentations were mass or discomfort [1]. The authors point out that oral melanoma is a rare disease, and hence, the numbers in this report are small. Nevertheless, it is sobering that a cancer we think of as *melanotic* is more likely to be unpigmented when it strikes the oral mucosa. Nevertheless, the authors caution that any pigmented lesion not reliably attributed to a specific source, such as an amalgam tattoo, should be biopsied [1].

1. Gorsky M, et al. Melanoma arising from the mucosal surface of the head and neck. Oral Surg Oral Med Oral Pathol Oral Radiol Endod. 1998;86:715.

Oral hairy leukoplakia, a painless pale lesion with vertical ridges and valleys typically found on the lateral border of the tongue, is often misdiagnosed as oral candidiasis (see Fig. 5.5).

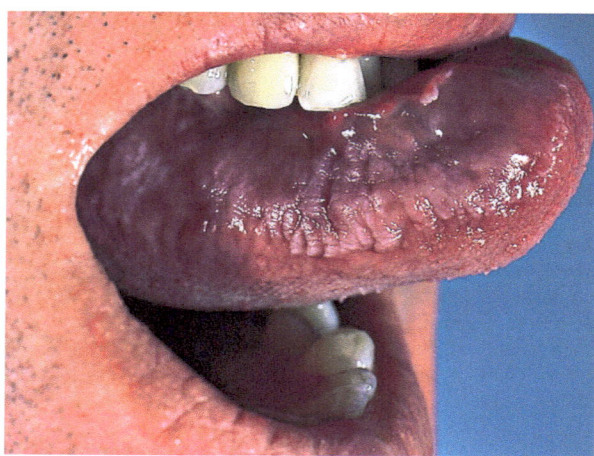

Fig. 5.5 Oral hairy leukoplakia of the tongue

Most cases occur in patients infected with the human immunodeficiency virus (HIV), and the onset of oral hairy leukoplakia is considered a poor prognostic sign that often heralds the beginning of acquired immunodeficiency syndrome [1, 2].

Oral hairy leukoplakia is also seen in patients with immunosuppression, such as renal transplant or chronic obstructive pulmonary disease patients on steroid therapy [3].

1. Resnick L, et al. Oral hairy leukoplakia. J Am Acad Dermatol. 1990;22:1278.
2. Alessi E, et al. Oral hairy leukoplakia. J Am Acad Dermatol. 1990;22:79.
3. Piperi E, et al. Oral hairy leukoplakia in HIV-negative patients: report of 10 cases. Int J Surg Pathol. 2010;18:177.

When a patient is found to have recurrent, severe aphthous stomatitis, think about the possibility of Behçet syndrome.

Also sometimes called malignant aphthosis or oculo-oral-genital syndrome, Behçet disease is fundamentally a vasculitis causing oral aphthous ulcers (the most commonly occurring manifestation), genital ulcers, and ocular inflammation which may take the form of conjunctivitis, keratitis, uveitis, optic neuritis, or retinal vessel occlusion [1, 2].

Of all countries, Turkey has the highest prevalence of Behçet disease, which is most common and most severe along the path of the old Silk Road traversed by Marco Polo in the thirteenth century and subsequently by merchants who followed in his path [2–4]. The eponymous name of the syndrome, which is of Turkish origin, is pronounced *bay-chet* [4].

1. Oh SH, et al. Comparison of the clinical features of recurrent aphthous stomatitis and Behçet's disease. Clin Exp Dermatol. 2009;34:e208.
2. Alli N, et al. Patient characteristics in Behçet disease: a retrospective analysis of 213 Turkish patients during 2001–2004. Am J Clin Dermatol. 2009;10:411.
3. Yurdakul S, et al. Behçet syndrome. Curr Opin Rheumatol. 2004;16:38.
4. Taylor RB. Essential medical facts every clinician should know. New York: Springer; 2011. p. 92.

Glossitis can be a manifestation of vitamin B12 deficiency.

One report describes atrophic glossitis, with a beefy, red smooth tongue, a presentation that was actually misdiagnosed as burning mouth disorder [1]. Another paper describes four patients with glossitis with linear lesions [2].

While on the subject of vitamin deficiency-induced tongue inflammation, glossitis was one of the manifestations seen in a 14-year-old girl with pellagra that developed as a result of anorexia nervosa [3].

1. Lehman JS, et al. Atrophic glossitis from vitamin B12 deficiency: a case misdiagnosed as burning mouth disorder. J Peridontol. 2006;77:2090.
2. Graells J, et al. Glossitis with linear lesions: an early sign of vitamin B12 deficiency. J Am Acad
   Dermatol. 2009;60:498.
3. Jagielska G, et al. Pellagra: a rare complication of anorexia nervosa. Eur Child Adolesc
   Psychiatry. 2007;16:417.

Oral gonococcal infection may present as tonsillitis.

Gonococcal pharyngitis is a well-recognized entity, but gonococcal tonsillitis occurs less commonly. In a series of 512 cases of oral gonococcal infection, 61 were described as tonsillitis. Of these, exudate in the tonsillar crypts was reported in 12 instances, while fever was present in 5 and cervical lymphadenopathy in 6 patients [1].

1. Balmelli C, et al. Gonococcal tonsillar infection: case report and literature review. Infection.
   2003;31:362.

Hoarseness

Hoarseness can be a manifestation of hypothyroidism.

Hoarseness has a long differential diagnosis, which includes some ominous possibilities. Just some of the conditions that can cause hoarseness are vocal abuse, infection, inhalation of steroids, spasmodic dysphonia, Sjögren disease, and irritants such as tobacco or alcohol. The clinician must also think of tumors such as squamous cell carcinoma, neuromuscular diseases such as myasthenia gravis and Parkinson disease, and a variety of systemic diseases. One of the latter category is hypothyroidism [1, 2].

And to just add a zebra diagnosis to the list, Khan et al. describe a 66-year-old woman who developed laryngeal tuberculosis with hoarseness as pulmonary tuberculosis was reactivated following steroid therapy for nephrotic syndrome [3].

1. Sonkin N. Voice changes in hypothyroidism. R I Med J. 1964;47:19.
2. Feierabend RH, et al. Hoarseness in adults. Am Fam Physician. 2009;80:363.
3. Khan NU, et al. Laryngeal tuberculosis: a diagnosis not to be missed. BMJ. 2009; pii:bcr11.2008.1228.

Selected Problems of the Ear, Nose, and Throat

When herpes zoster involves the skin near the tip of the nose, be concerned that the patient may subsequently develop herpes zoster ophthalmicus, one of the *must-not-miss diagnoses*.

The *tip of the nose* lesions which may presage herpes zoster ocular involvement was first described by English ophthalmologist Sir Jonathan Hutchinson (1828–1913), and the sign bears his name today: the Hutchinson sign [1]. The authors of one report studied 83 non-immunocompromised adults with acute herpes zoster ophthalmicus and a history of a skin rash within the prior week, concluding "Hutchinson's sign was a powerful predictor of ocular inflammation and corneal denervation in herpes zoster ophthalmicus (relative risks: 3.35 and 4.02, respectively)" [2].

In fairness, I must report a prospective cohort multicenter study by Adams et al. of 54 patients referred from primary care settings to ophthalmology. The authors conclude that there was a statistically significant association between eye redness and rash in the supratrochlear nerve distributions and the occurrence of significant ocular disease. But the authors report: "Hutchinson's sign (nasociliary nerve involvement) was not predictive of clinically relevant eye disease" [3].

Thus, some recent evidence seems to conflict with earlier studies and experiential lore. As for me as a primary care physician, I will continue to refer any patient with Hutchinson sign for ophthalmologic evaluation.

1. Hutchinson J. Clinical report on herpes zoster frontalis ophthalmicus (shingles affecting the forehead and nose). Ophth Hosp Rep J Royal London Ophth Hosp. 1864;3:865;1865;5:191.
2. Zaal MJ, et al. Prognostic value of Hutchinson's sign in acute herpes zoster ophthalmicus. Graefes Arch Clin Exp Ophthalmol. 2003;241:187.
3. Adam RS, et al. Triaging herpes zoster ophthalmicus patients in the emergency department: do all patients require referral? Acad Emerg Med. 2010;17:1183.

The patient with parotid gland enlargement may have lymphoma, especially if the patient has sicca syndrome or Sjögren syndrome.

Lymphoma is not uncommon in the major salivary glands, notably the parotid glands [1]. And there is an increased incidence of lymphoma in patients with sicca syndrome [2] and Sjögren syndrome [3].

1. Hyman GA, et al. Malignant lymphomas of the salivary glands. Review of the literature and report of 33 new cases, including four cases associated with the lymphoepithelial lesion. Am J Clin Pathol. 1976;65:421.
2. Kassan SS, et al. Increased risk of lymphoma in sicca syndrome. Ann Int Med. 1978;89:888.
3. Lazarus MN, et al. Incidence of cancer in a cohort of patients with primary Sjögren syndrome. Rheumatology. 2006;45:1012.

Patients with Sjögren syndrome often have early and rampant dental caries.

Decreased salivary production increases the incidence of dental caries. Things only get worse if the patient uses hard candy to relieve dry mouth symptoms [1] (see Fig. 5.6).

1. Matthews SA, et al. Oral manifestations of Sjögren syndrome. J Dent Res. 2008;87:308.

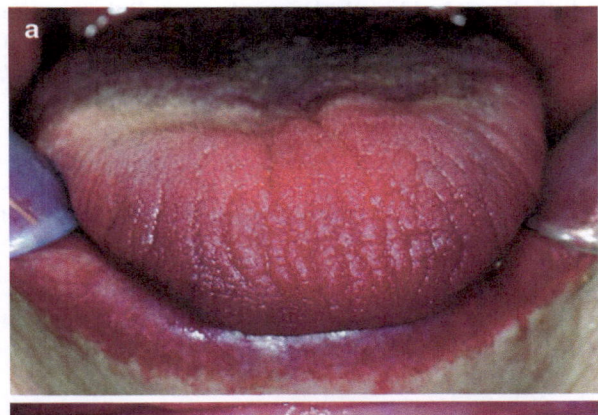

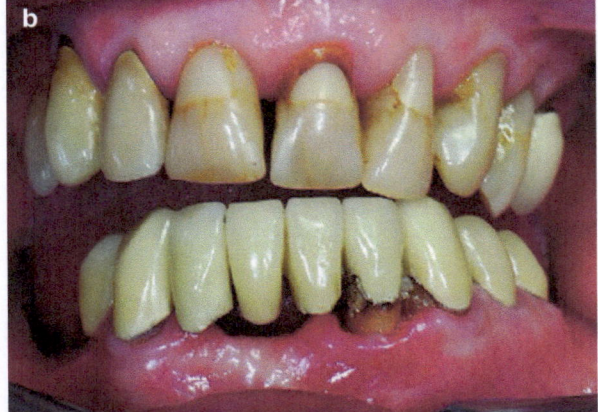

Fig. 5.6 Female patient with primary Sjögren syndrome. (a) Sensitive, depapillated tongue with fungal/yeast infection (candidiasis). Note also dry, atrophic lower lip. (b) Extensive dental caries experienced as indicated by fillings at atypical sites and abundant prosthetic restorations; buccal fillings in the upper jaw and a nine-unit bridge in the lower jaw. Recurrent cervical/root caries in the lower front indicate currently active caries disease. (c) Pronounced tooth wear/dental erosion on palatal and occlusal surfaces of the teeth

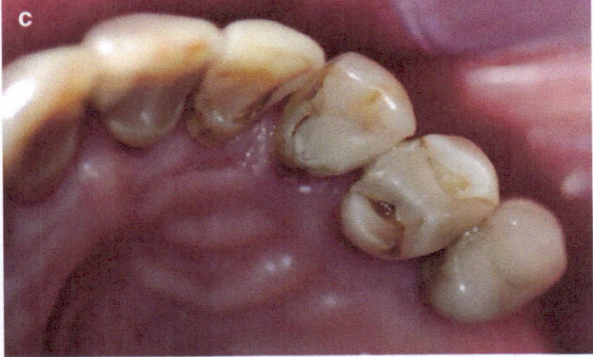

Halitosis may be a symptom of GERD.

Up to half of all US adults report having "bad breath" at some time in their lives [1]. Two recent studies have linked halitosis to GERD, especially in patients wearing dentures [2, 3]. Moshkowitz et al. found that the link between halitosis and GERD did not extend to functional dyspepsia, peptic ulcer disease, and *H. pylori* infection [3].

There are, of course, other causes of halitosis, including certain foods, tobacco use, dry mouth, and poor oral hygiene. There is an interesting report from the multidisciplinary bad breath clinic in Leuven, Belgium. (Yes, there is actually a halitosis clinic.) These clinicians found that 16 % of 2,000 patients who visited their clinic merited the diagnosis of *pseudo-halitosis/halitophobia* [4].

1. Lee SS, et al. Halitosis update: a review of causes, diagnoses, and treatments. J Calif Dent Assoc. 2007;35:258.
2. Struch F, et al. Self-reported halitosis and gastro-esophageal reflux disease in the general population. J Gen Intern Med. 2008;23:260.
3. Moshkowitz M, et al. Halitosis and gastro-esophageal reflux disease: a possible association. Oral Dis. 2007;13:581.
4. Quirynen M, et al. Characteristics of 2000 patients who visited a halitosis clinic. J Clin Peridontol. 2009;36:970.

Chapter 6
The Cardiovascular System

The tragedies of life are largely arterial.
Sir William Osler (1849–1919) [1]

Contents

R.B. Taylor, *Diagnostic Principles and Applications,*
DOI 10.1007/978-1-4614-1111-6_6, © Springer Science+Business Media, LLC 2013

As I began work on this chapter, I reflected on Osler's aphorism presented above and concurred that, yes, many of our leading causes of morbidity and mortality involve some disorder of the arteries—heart attacks, strokes, vascular dementia, arterial occlusions of the extremities, and even the arterial "tension" in hypertension. In this chapter I will cover diseases of the heart, arteries, and veins, while some of specific manifestations of arterial (and venous) diseases—such as occlusion of the central retinal artery, mesenteric ischemia, and testicular torsion—are covered elsewhere in the book.

Knowing the diagnostic pathways in the land where heart disease may lurk is especially important because cardiovascular disease remains the leading cause of death both in the US and worldwide. Furthermore, of interest to primary care clinicians is the following: In a 2010 study of closed malpractice claims against family physicians, the most common allegation was diagnostic error, with myocardial infarction leading the list of diagnoses allegedly missed [2].

1. Osler W. Cardiovascular diseases. In: Osler W, McCrae T, editors. Modern medicine: its theory and practice. Philadelphia: Lea & Febiger; 1908. p. 431.
2. Flannery FT, et al. Characteristics of medical professional liability claims in patients treated by family medicine physicians. J Am Board Fam Med. 2010;23:753.

High Blood Pressure

The sphygmomanometer in your office (or mine) may not be as accurate as you think.

For middle-aged and older persons, hypertension is the most common diagnosis reported in the US primary care office setting, with more than 274 million visits to physicians of all types as reported by the National Ambulatory Medical Care Survey for 2003–2005 [1, 2]. For a visit type so prevalent, with hypertension a known risk factor for heart attack and stroke and with our devices to measure blood pressure (BP) both low cost and low tech, we might assume that our sphygmomanometers are quite accurate. This, however, is not necessarily the case.

Writing in 1975, Thulin et al. found that in every tenth aneroid sphygmomanometer studied, there was a 10 Hg or greater error when compared with a mercury manometer [3]. In a more recent (2010) report, authors tested various types of blood-pressuring devices. They found that when using the European calibration standard of ±3 mmHg, the failure rates were mercury, 6 % (1/18); aneroid, 31 % (19/62); and automated devices, 26 % (12/47) [4].

1. Ma J, et al. Screening, treatment, and control of hypertension in US private physician offices, 2003–2004. Hypertension. 2008;51:1275.
2. Fang J, et al. Heath care service provided during physician office visits for hypertension: differences by specialty. J Clin Hypertens. 2010;12:8.
3. Thulin T, et al. Measurement of blood pressure: a routine test in need of standardization. Postgrad Med J. 1975;51:390.
4. de Greeff A, et al. Calibration accuracy of hospital-based non-invasive blood pressure measuring devices. J Hum Hypertens. 2010;24:58.

Either side of the acoustic stethoscope—diaphragm or bell—can be used in determining blood pressure.

Kantola et al. compared bell and diaphragm of the acoustic stethoscope in measurement of BP in 250 adults, finding no statistically significant differences in determining systolic pressure or diastolic pressure [1].

1. Kantola I, et al. Bell or diaphragm in the measurement of blood pressure? J Hypertens. 2005;23:499.

White coat hypertension is truly influenced by physician measurement.

It is important to distinguish between white coat hypertension and sustained hypertension, because the latter confers significantly greater risk of death [1]. For this reason, the following is noteworthy.

Ogedegbe et al. studied 238 hypertensive patients with measurements in the waiting area, in the examination room (with or without the physician present), and with the physician taking the blood pressure. Anxiety scores were recorded before and after each BP measurement. They found that patients with white coat hypertension had significantly higher anxiety scores ($p < 0.01$) than normotensive, sustained hypertension, or masked hypertension patients, with the highest anxiety scores noted when the physician performed the blood pressure determination [2].

1. Dawes MG, et al. Comparing the effects of white coat hypertension and sustained hypertension on mortality in a UK primary care setting. Ann Fam Med. 2008;6:390.
2. Ogedegbe G, et al. The misdiagnosis of hypertension: the role of patient anxiety. Arch Intern Med. 2008;168:2459.

The most common cause of secondary hypertension in middle-aged adults is aldosteronism.

When a hypertensive patient has hypokalemia, the aldosterone/renin ratio should be determined. Other causes of persistent hypertension to be considered are renal artery stenosis and pheochromocytoma. An abdominal bruit suggests renal artery stenosis, and episodic flushing, headache, sweating, and palpitations are characteristic of pheochromocytoma [1, 2] (see Fig. 6.1).

1. Viera AJ, et al. Diagnosis of secondary hypertension: an age-based approach. Am Fam Physician. 2010;82:1471.
2. Hager C, et al. Pheochromocytoma: an easily overlooked cause of secondary hypertension. WV Med J. 2009;105:10.

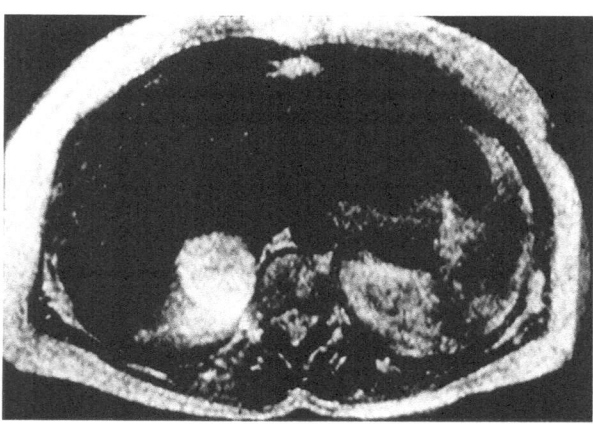

Fig. 6.1 Computed tomography scan in pheochromocytoma

The young adult woman with difficult-to-control hypertension may have renovascular hypertension owing to fibromuscular dysplasia (FD) of the renal artery.

FD, which most commonly affects the renal and carotid arteries, is familial in about one case in ten. Extrarenal manifestations include asymptomatic bruit, transient ischemic attacks, and stroke [1]. In decreasing order of accuracy, the noninvasive tests for FD are computed tomography angiography, magnetic resonance angiography, and ultrasonography [2].

1. Plouin PF, et al. Fibromuscular dysplasia. Orphanet J Rare Dis. 2007;2. doi:10.1186/1750-1172-2-28.
2. Olin JW. Recognizing and managing fibromuscular dysplasia. Cleveland Clin J Med. 2007; 74:273.

Consider the diagnosis of paroxysmal hypertension (pseudopheochromocytoma) in the patient with repeated episodes of blood pressure elevation in the absence of emotional stress.

Pheochromocytoma is one of those maladies for which *many are called and few are chosen*. Up to 98 % of patients suspected of having pheochromocytoma do not have the tumor [1]. In these individuals in whom sporadic hypertension is accompanied by flushing, headache, and palpitations, think of the diagnosis of paroxysmal hypertension. This disease, more common in women, can have paroxysms lasting a few minutes to a few days and reoccurring at intervals varying from daily to every few weeks. The blood pressure elevation, which may be alarmingly high, and accompanying symptoms and signs appear suddenly and without apparent reason [2]. Mann suggests a psychologic basis for some cases of labile hypertension, related to repressed emotions or a repressive (nonemotional) coping style [1].

1. Mann SJ. Severe paroxysmal hypertension (pseudopheochromocytoma). Arch Intern Med. 1999;159:670.
2. Mann SJ. The clinical spectrum of labile hypertension: a management dilemma. J Clin Hypertens. 2009;11:491.

Chest Pain

The patient with chest pain is most likely to have a musculoskeletal cause.

Chest pain is a very common complaint, accounting for more than 5 % of emergency department visits, second only to abdominal pain [1].

In a study of 672 patients presenting with chest pain, the leading causes were chest wall syndrome (43 %), coronary artery disease (12 %), and anxiety (7 %). Only four subjects had acute myocardial infarction [2]. These snippets of epidemiologic data are slightly reassuring but must be considered in context of acute myocardial infarction being a *must-not-miss diagnosis*. The gravity of the potentially missed heart attack makes the evaluation of a chest pain complaint a vital clinical skill.

1. Pitts SR, et al. National Hospital Ambulatory Medical Survey: 2006 emergency department summary. Natl Health Stat Rep. 2008;7:1.
2. Verdon F, et al. Chest pain in daily practice: occurrence, causes and management. Swiss Med Wkly. 2008;14:340.

Hand gestures may be some help in distinguishing cardiac from noncardiac chest pain but must be interpreted cautiously.

These time-honored clinical indicators, one of which ever bears an eponymous title, have been passed from one generation of clinicians to the next. Here is the where we stand today: A patient with chest pain may illustrate the pain in several ways: holding the clenched fist to the chest (the Levine sign), holding the flat of the hand to the chest (the *palm sign*), and holding both hands flat in the middle of the chest and then drawing them outward. Or the patient might point to a specific spot on the chest (the *pointing sign*).

In 1995 Edmondstone reported his study of 203 consecutive chest pain patients, 138 of whom had cardiac pain, 21 of whom had noncardiac pain, and 44 of whom had pain of uncertain origin. Of the patients with cardiac pain, 110 (80 %) used one of the three hand-to-chest gestures described above, while only 33 (51 %) of the patient with noncardiac pain or pain of uncertain origin used one of these signs ($p < 0.01$) [1].

Later, in 2000, Albarran et al. studied 267 chest pain patients, of whom 118 had myocardial infarction (MI) and 149 did not. They studied manual gestures, choice of verbal descriptors, and extent of pain radiation and concluded that "it is currently impossible to draw any conclusions as to whether the variables studied can be judged as reliable indicators of MI" [2].

More recently (2007), Marcus et al. studied 202 chest pain patients, finding the following prevalence of gestures: the Levine sign (11 %), the palm sign (35 %), the arm sign (describing pain by touching the left arm) (16 %), and the pointing sign (4 %). They found the Levine and arm signs to have specificities between 78 % and 88 % but with positive predictive values that did not exceed 55 %. They found, however, that the pointing sign had a 98 % specificity for nonischemic chest pain [3].

1. Edmondstone WM. Cardiac chest pain: does the body language help in diagnosis? BMJ. 1995;311:1660.
2. Albarran JW, et al. Are manual gestures, verbal descriptors, and pain radiation as reported by patients reliable indicators of myocardial infarction? Preliminary findings and implications. Intensive Crit Care Nurs. 2000;16:98.
3. Marcus GM, et al. The utility of gestures in patients with chest discomfort. Am J Med. 2007;120:83.

Chest pain relieved by sublingual nitroglycerine is not necessarily caused by cardiac disease.

The above was the conclusion reached following a prospective study of 664 chest pain patients in whom a cardiac cause was identified in 122 individuals (18 %). All 664 patients were given an empiric dose of sublingual nitroglycerine, following which there was "no significant difference in any subgroup of numeric descriptive scale response to sublingual nitroglycerin administration in patients with and without a diagnosis of cardiac chest pain" [1].

1. Diercks DB, et al. Changes in numeric descriptive scale for pain after sublingual nitroglycerin do not predict cardiac etiology of chest pain. Ann Emerg Med. 2005;45:581.

A cluster of independent predictors can help identify the origin of chest wall pain.

In a series of 1,212 adults with chest pain, attending physicians diagnosed chest wall pain in almost half (46.6 %). The reported location of the pain tended to be left-sided (69.2 %) and/or retrosternal (52.0 %). The authors propose four determinants—localized muscle tension, stinging pain, pain reproducible by palpation, and absence of cough—and suggest that a patient who has chest pain with three of the these characteristics has a likelihood ratio of 3.0 that the cause is chest wall pain [1].

1. Bösner S, et al. Chest wall syndrome in primary care patients with chest pain: presentation, associated features and diagnosis. Fam Pract. 2010;27:363.

Be suspicious of coronary artery disease in the person with chest pain—think young adult—who might be a cocaine user.

Carillo et al. describe 478 patients age ≤50 years admitted to a coronary care unit over 8 years. Of these, 56 (11.7 %) were cocaine users, with the prevalence increasing over the 7-year period of the study. Among patients age <30 years, 25 % were cocaine users. The investigators found that cocaine users had larger infarcts (measured by troponin levels), lower left ventricular ejection fraction, and increased hospital mortality [1].

Other cardiac effects of cocaine may be seen: arrhythmias, heart failure, and sudden cardiac death [2].

1. Carillo X, et al. Acute coronary syndrome and cocaine use: 8-year prevalence and inhospital outcomes. Eur Heart J. 2011;32:1244.
2. Lippi G, et al. Cocaine in acute myocardial infarction. Adv Clin Chem. 2010;51:53.

In a patient with chest pain, a negative troponin level means that the cause is likely to be something other than coronary artery disease.

In the paper, described above, on the utility of gestures in patients with chest discomfort, Marcus et al. found that a positive predictive value of 88 % for nonischemic chest discomfort when the patient had a negative troponin [1].

While on the subject of troponin, Mills et al. suggest that we lower the diagnostic threshold of plasma troponin. In a study of various diagnostic levels of plasma troponin, "lowering the diagnostic threshold to 0.05 ng/mL was associated with a lower risk of death and recurrent MI (from 39 to 21 %) in patients with troponin concentrations of 0.05–0.19 ng/mL (OR 0.42; CI 95 %, 0.24–0.84; $p=0.01$)" [2].

In fact, the sensitive troponin assay can indicate an increased risk of heart failure and cardiovascular death in patients with stable coronary artery disease and even the presence of structural heart disease and subsequent risk for all-cause mortality in a population-based cohort [3, 4]. All of which suggests that perhaps we should follow our post-MI patients with episodic troponin testing.

1. Marcus GM, et al. The utility of gestures in patients with chest discomfort. Am J Med. 2007;120:83.
2. Mills NL, et al. Implementation of a sensitive troponin I assay and risk of recurrent myocardial infarction and death in patients with suspected acute coronary syndrome. JAMA. 2011;305:1210.
3. Omland T, et al. A sensitive cardiac troponin T assay in stable coronary artery disease. N Engl J Med. 2009;361:2538.
4. de Lemos JA, et al. Association of troponin T detected with a highly sensitive assay and cardiac structure and mortality risk in the general population. JAMA. 2010;304:2503.

The patient with chest pain accompanied by dyspnea and syncope should be evaluated for the presence of aortic stenosis.

This worrisome valvular disease affects 3 % of persons >65 years of age. The presence of the classic manifestations described above means the patient has become *symptomatic* and that without aortic valve replacement has a life expectancy of 2–3 years [1]. The recommended initial test is Doppler echocardiography.

1. Grimard BH, et al. Aortic stenosis: diagnosis and treatment. Am Fam Physician. 2008;78:717.

Anterior chest pain relieved by leaning forward may be due to pericarditis.

Pericarditis classically causes a pleuritic type of chest pain, sometimes referred to the left shoulder, which may be relieved by leaning forward. Most cases of this inflammation of the pericardium are caused by viral infection. In most patients with pericarditis, a friction rub will be found at some time during the course of the disease [1, 2].

1. Goyle KK, et al. Diagnosing pericarditis. Am Fam Physician. 2002;66:1695.
2. Lange RA, et al. Acute pericarditis. N Engl J Med. 2004;351:2195.

Disorders of Heart Rate and Rhythm

Increased heart rate (HR) is an unfavorable prognostic finding, one to be considered in many diagnostic assessments.

This holds true for both patients with heart disease and persons in general. Fox et al. report on patients with stable coronary artery disease and left ventricular dysfunction. There were 2,693 patients with heart rates of 70 beats per minute (bpm) or greater and 2,745 patients with heart rates below 70 bpm. They found an increase risk of adverse cardiovascular outcomes, especially heart failure and coronary events, in the cohort with heart rates ≥70 bpm [1].

What's more, Zhang et al. tell that in numerous studies of individuals and their heart rates, "increased HR is universally associated with a greater risk of death" [2].

1. Fox K, et al. Heart rate as a prognostic risk factor in patients with coronary artery disease and left-ventricular systolic dysfunction (BEATIFUL): a subgroup analysis of a randomized controlled trial. Lancet. 2008;372:817.
2. Zhang GQ, et al. Heart rate, lifespan, and mortality risk. Ageing Res Rev. 2009;8:52.

In a patient complaining of palpitations, tapping out the cadence of the heart rhythm may aid diagnosis.

Tapping the rhythm cadence might be done by either the patient or the clinician. If the patient has a sense of the rhythm and rate, ask the person to *tap it out* with the fingers. What is offered may be a classic pattern of atrial fibrillation, a regular irregularity of the beat, or even a tachyarrhythmia that might be *too fast to tap out*. Alternatively, the clinician might tap out a few of the common rhythms causing palpitations, to see if the patient recognizes the pattern.

In addition, of course, the diagnostic approach includes a history, physical examination, and 12-lead electrocardiogram (ECG).

If further investigation is indicated, the next step would be ambulatory ECG monitoring and electrophysiologic studies. Giada reports that continuous Holter monitoring, recommended when the patient reports daily palpitations, has a low sensitivity and that a higher sensitivity is found with event recorders, used when a compliant patient describes infrequent events lasting long enough to trigger event recording and with external loop recorders, indicated in instances of short-lasting but infrequent symptoms associated with hemodynamic dysfunction [1, 2]. One paper suggests the use of an implantable loop recorder in patients with infrequent palpitations and without severe heart disease, holding the approach to be both safe and cost-effective [3]. We might, however, reflect upon the cost difference between finger tapping and the use of implantable loop recorders.

1. Giada F, et al. Diagnostic management of patients with palpitations of unknown origin. Ital Heart J. 2004;5:581.
2. Giada F, et al. Diagnostic management of patients with palpitations. G Ital Cardiol. 2010;11:S9.
3. Giada F, et al. Recurrent unexplained palpitations (RUP) study comparison of implantable loop recorder versus conventional diagnostic strategy. J Am Coll Cardiol. 2007;49:1951.

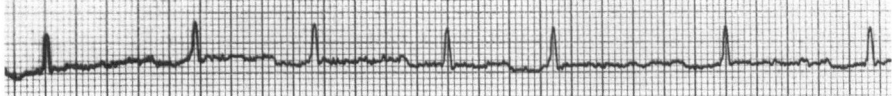

Fig. 6.2 Electrocardiogram of a patient with atrial fibrillation

Atrial fibrillation (AF) may be the first sign of hyperthyroidism.

Atrial fibrillation, the most common of the cardiac arrhythmias, may be the bell-wether manifestation of hyperthyroidism. Indicator symptoms of AF include palpitations, lightheadedness, fatigue, dyspnea, and chest pain [1] (see Fig. 6.2). Selmer et al. studied 139,521 patients with a mean age of 73.5 years who had new-onset AF. They found a significantly increased risk of hyperthyroidism in new-onset AF patients compared to controls (HR 2.98; 95 % CI 2.84–3.12) [2]. AF is found in up to 15 % of hyperthyroid patients (any stage of disease), compared to a 4 % of patients without thyroid disease [3].

1. Gutierrez C, et al. Atrial fibrillation: diagnosis and treatment. Am Fam Physician. 2011;83:61.
2. Selmer C, et al. New-onset atrial fibrillation is an independent long-term risk factor for hyperthyroidism. Circulation. 2010;122:A12505.
3. Bielecka-Dabrowa A, et al. The mechanisms of atrial fibrillation in hyperthyroidism. Thyroid Res. 2009;2:4.

Count atrial fibrillation among the possible presenting signs of pulmonary embolus (PE).

Several reports have described this link, and one, by Szwast et al., describes atrial fibrillation as the presenting manifestation of PE in a 17-year-old previously healthy boy [1–3].

1. O'Toole L, et al. Pulmonary embolism presenting with atrial fibrillation. Lancet. 1993;342: 1050.
2. Gutierrez C, et al. Atrial fibrillation: diagnosis and treatment. Am Fam Physician. 2011;83:61.
3. Szwast A, et al. Atrial fibrillation and pulmonary embolism. Ped Emerg Care. 2007;23:826.

The patient with a cardiac arrhythmia with a ventricular rate of approximately 150 beats per minute is likely to have atrial flutter (see Fig. 6.3).

Atrial flutter has an estimated incidence of 88/100,000 person-years and is associated with the following risk factors: age, male gender, heart failure, and chronic obstructive lung disease [1]. In flutter, there is classically held to be a rapid, regular atrial rhythm at about 300 beats per minute. Actually the number is a little less, 240–338 beats per minute, mean 293 beats per minute, but using 300 makes the

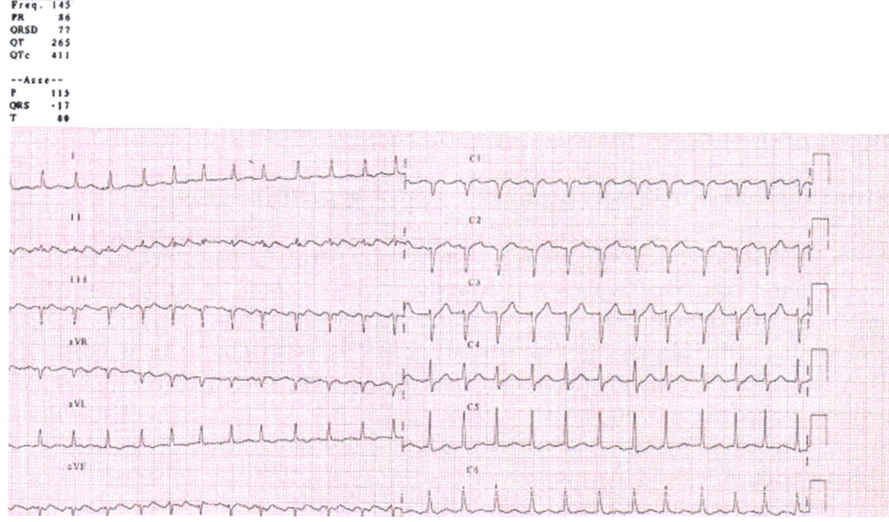

Freq. 145
PR 86
QRSD 77
QT 265
QTc 411

--Axis--
P 115
QRS -17
T 80

Fig. 6.3 Electrocardiogram showing atrial flutter

math a little easier. Then consider that flutter typically involves 2:1 conduction across the atrioventricular (AV) node. Do the math: $300/2 = 150$ beats per minute. Even ratios (2:1 and 4:1) occur much more often than odd-number ratios such as 3:1 and 5:1 [2, 3]. One report describes eight patients with 1:1 conduction, with ventricular rates of 218 ± 18 bpm [4].

1. Granada J, et al. Incidence and predictors of atrial flutter in the general population. J Am Coll Card. 2000;36:2242.
2. Wells JL, et al. Characterization of atrial flutter: studies in man after open heart surgery using fixed atrial electrodes. Circulation. 1979;60:665.
3. Dhar S, et al. Current concepts and management strategies in atrial flutter. South Med J. 2009;102:917.
4. Kawabata M, et al. Clinical and electrophysiological characteristics of patients having atrial flutter with 1:1 atrioventricular conduction. Europace. 2008;10:284.

Heart Murmurs

The newborn infant with congenital heart disease (CHD) may not have a murmur.

In a study of 812 neonates, 15 were found to have CHD accompanied by a murmur, and seven had CHD without a detectable murmur. All diagnoses of CHD were confirmed on echocardiography [1].

1. Hoque M, et al. Importance of cardiac murmur in diagnosing congenital heart disease in neonatal period. Bangladesh J Child Health. 2008;32:102.

A newly heard murmur is the most common initial physical finding in hypertrophic cardiomyopathy (HCM) of children.

Why should clinicians seeing children and adolescents be concerned about HCM? It is because the disorder is both "the most common inherited cardiovascular disorder and the leading cause of sudden cardiac death in young people in the United States" [1]. These facts underpin why we do routine school physicals, especially of young athletes. Dadlani reports that in some countries, screening with history and physical examination is supplemented by routine electrocardiography [1].

1. Dadlani GH. Diagnosis and screening of hypertrophic cardiomyopathy in children. Prog Pediatr Card. 2011;31:21.

A newly heard murmur at the base of the heart in an adult suggests the presence of aortic stenosis (AS).

Several reasons explain why aortic stenosis is the most prevalent heart valve lesion in the USA. First of all, the post-rheumatic heart disease valvular abnormalities we older clinicians learned about in medical school are now largely historical curiosities. Secondly, AS is a disease of aging and we all know what is happening to the population. Thirdly, up to 2 % of the Americans have a congenital bicuspid aortic valve, prone to stenosis [1].

The typical murmur of AS is a harsh ejection murmur best heard at the base of the heart, specifically at the upper right sternal border and radiating to the neck [1]. Following a study of 250 subjects with AS, Wood reports that the aortic systolic murmur is invariably found in AS and that in the absence of valvular incompetence and heart failure, the duration of the murmur is indicative of the degree of stenosis [2].

Things are often different in the elderly, and in older patients with aortic stenosis, the right-sided basal murmur may be difficult to auscultate, and you may hear a musical systolic murmur at the apex [3].

Fig. 6.4 Transthoracic
echocardiography showing
the left atrial myxoma
attached to the anterior mitral
valve leaflet

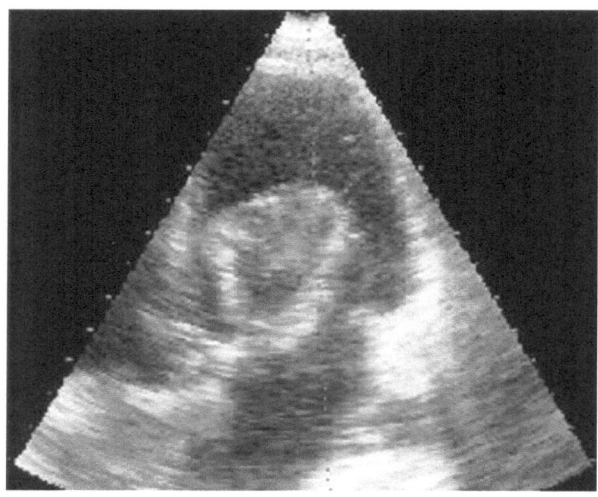

1. Carabello BA. Aortic stenosis. N Engl J Med. 2002;346:677.
2. Wood P. Aortic stenosis. Am J Cardio. 1958;1:553.
3. Roberts WC, et al. Severe valvular aortic stenosis in patients over 65 years of age: a clinico-pathologic study. Am J Cardiol. 1971;5:497.

A heart murmur that changes with body position might be caused by a heart tumor.

Granted, primary heart tumors are rare, found in only 0.0017–0.19 % of patients at autopsy. Most are benign tumors, most of these are myxomas, and most occur in the atria (see Fig. 6.4). Reynen reports that more than half of patients with cardiac myxomas will have detectable murmurs, but because the character of the murmur varies with the location of the tumor and even the patient's body position, the murmur of myxoma defies precise characterization and may be either systolic or diastolic [1]. For example, Urata et al. describe a 67-year-old woman with a heart tumor who was found to have a grade II/VI, low-pitched diastolic rumble along the left sternal border, which intensified before the first heart sound [2].

1. Reynen K. Cardiac myxomas. N Engl J Med. 1995;333:1610.
2. Urata M, et al. A murmur of a tumor. Circulation. 2009;120:e77.

Heart Failure

In the patient with acute dyspnea, prompt determination of brain natriuretic peptide (BNP) can help identify—or rule out—the diagnosis of heart failure (HF).

The chief cause of acute dyspnea in the emergency room setting is HF [1]. A review of 22 previously published studies examined the diagnostic merits of various manifestations of heart failure. They concluded that the most useful test was finding a serum BNP less than 100 pg/mL (negative LR 0.11; 95 % CI, 0.07–0.16) [2]. Maisel et al. studied 1,586 persons presenting to the emergency department with dyspnea, concluding, "The negative predictive value of B-type natriuretic peptide at levels of less than 50 pg/mL was 96 %" [3].

1. Ray P, et al. Differential diagnosis of acute dyspnea: the value of B natriuretic peptides in the emergency department. QJM. 2008;101:831.
2. Wang CS, et al. Does this dyspneic patient in the emergency department have congestive heart failure? JAMA. 2005;294:1944.
3. Maisel AS, et al. Rapid measurement of B-type natriuretic peptide in the emergency diagnosis of heart failure. N Engl J Med. 2002;18:161.

Elevated uric acid levels can help differentiate between acute decompensated heart failure and noncardiac causes of dyspnea.

The diagnostic utility of serum uric acid in the assessment of dyspnea was the subject of a study of 743 unselected patients presenting to the emergency department with a chief complaint of dyspnea. Reichlin et al. found that uric acid levels were higher in patients with acute decompensated heart failure (51 % of the cohort) as compared with patients with noncardiac causes ($p < 0.001$) [1].

1. Reichlin T, et al. Diagnostic and prognostic value of uric acid in patients with acute dyspnea. Am J Med. 2009;122:1054.

Thromboembolic Disease

Despite the utility of the Wells score and D-dimer test, clinical assessment remains useful in the diagnosis of deep vein thrombosis (DVT).

In ruling in or out DVT in the patient with calf pain, we rely heavily on our favored diagnostic tools: In patients with a pretest probability of DVT based on the Wells score or an elevated D-dimer result, duplex ultrasonography can help confirm the diagnosis. On the other hand, patients with a low clinical probability of DVT, a negative D-dimer result obviates the need for further testing [1].

Nevertheless, the wise clinician attends to clinical clues. Goodacre et al. conducted a systematic review of studies related to clinical assessment of DVT. Here is what they found: "Only malignancy (likelihood ratio [LR], 2.71), previous DVT (LR, 2.25), recent immobilization (LR, 1.98), difference in calf diameter (LR, 1.80), and recent surgery (LR, 1.76) were useful for ruling in DVT, while only absence of calf swelling (LR, 0.67) or difference in calf diameter (LR, 0.57) was useful for ruling out DVT." The foregoing notwithstanding, the authors go on to point out that the Wells score is superior to clinical characteristics in assessment of possible DVT [1].

1. Jacobs LG, et al. Office management of deep vein thrombosis in the elderly. Am J Med. 2009;10:904.
2. Goodacre S, et al. Meta-analysis: the value of clinical assessment in the diagnosis of deep vein thrombosis. Ann Intern Med. 2005;143:129.

Some physical examination maneuvers can help clarify the picture in suspected DVT of the lower extremity.

The most common symptom reported by patients with DVT is aching in the affected calf, although this complaint is hardly sensitive or specific. Calf muscle induration, limb swelling, and a positive Homan sign are other helpful findings [1]. Here are some diagnostic approaches, less commonly used today, that might prove useful:

Cuff sign: Apply a blood pressure cuff to the thigh and inflate to a pressure of 4 mmHg. Ortiz-Ramirez et al. describe pain following this maneuver in 100 % of 32 patients with DVT, compared with a reported sensitivity of 81.2 % for the Homan sign [2].

Cord sign: The saphenous vein should be palpated for cords, which if found, are highly specific (98 %) for DVT, even if they have a low sensitivity (10 %) [3].

Lisker sign: This describes tenderness and pain upon percussion of tibia medial to the crest, reported to be present in approximately 65 % of patients with DVT [1, 4].

1. Knox EW. Deep vein thrombophlebitis of the lower limbs. 1964;33:28.
2. Ortiz-Ramirez T, et al. New early diagnostic sign of phlebitis. Am Heart J. 1955;50:366.
3. Kahn SR. The clinical diagnosis of deep venous thrombosis: integrating incidence, risk factors, symptoms and signs. Arch Intern Med. 1998;158:2315.
4. Orient JM, editor. Sapira's art and science of diagnosis. 3rd ed. Philadelphia: Lippincott, Williams & Wilkins; 2005. p. 437.

Fig. 6.5 Chest radiograph of a
patient with pulmonary embolus.
There is an area of opacification in
the lower right zone of the lung

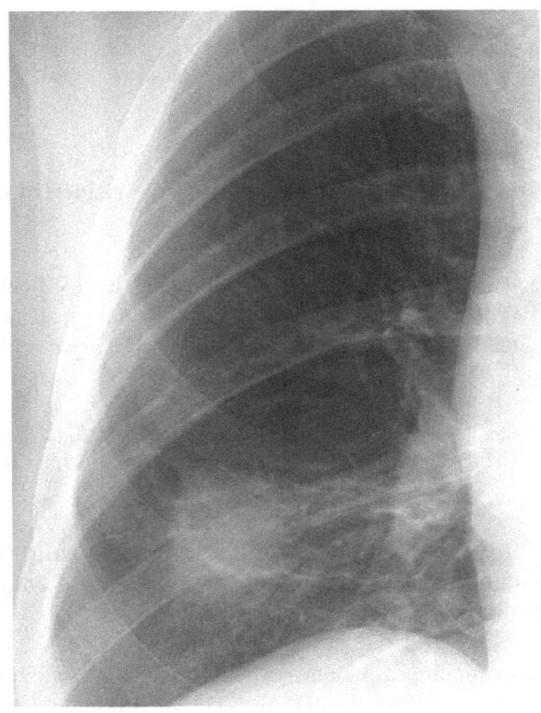

**Dyspnea, sometimes present only on exertion, may be the only symptom of
pulmonary embolism** (see Fig. 6.5).

In the setting of acute pulmonary embolism, shortness of breath may develop rapidly, although this is not always the case. In some patients, there will also be pleuritic pain, cough, and/or orthopnea. The most common physical sign of PE is
tachypnea, present in about half of all patients [1]. In one study, dyspnea and tachypnea ($\geq$ 20/min) occurred in 105 (90 %) of 117 PE patients [2].

These findings, especially the symptoms, are ominous. Laporte et al. report a
study in which they found that patients with symptomatic non-massive PE ($n = 6{,}264$)
had a 5.42-fold higher risk of death compared with patients with deep vein thrombosis without symptomatic PE ($n = 9{,}008$). The risk of fatal outcome was "multi-
plied by 17.5 in patients presenting with a symptomatic massive PE ($n = 248$)" [3].

In additions, Marik reminds us that unsuspected PE may be manifested as worsening heart failure or chronic obstructive pulmonary disease (COPD) [4].

1. Stein PD, et al. Clinical characteristics of patients with acute pulmonary embolism: data from
   PIOPED II. Am J Med. 2007;120:871.
2. Stein PD, et al. Clinical, laboratory, roentgenographic, and electrocardiographic findings in patients
   with acute pulmonary embolism and no pre-existing cardiac or pulmonary disease. Chest. 1991;100:598.

3. Laporte S, et al. Clinical predictors for fatal pulmonary embolism in 15,520 patients with venous thromboembolism. Circulation. 2008;117:1711.
4. Marik PE. Deep vein thrombosis. In: Handbook of evidence-based critical care. New York: Springer; 2010. p. 246.

Sometimes in pulmonary embolism arising from deep veins of the leg, the deep vein thrombosis is undetectable.

Not finding the expected evidence of deep vein thrombosis does not rule out the diagnosis of pulmonary embolism. It may just mean that the entire thrombus has detached and made its way to the pulmonary circulation [1].

1. Sandler DA, et al. Autopsy proven pulmonary embolism in hospital patients: are we detecting enough deep vein thrombosis? J R Soc Med. 1989;82:203.

The utility of simplified clinical decision rules (CDRs) and D-dimer testing in excluding PE is similar to the use of more comprehensive decision rules and D-dimer testing.

In evaluating a patient with suspected PE, which decision rules are best? Douma et al. tested four of them in 807 consecutive patients with suspected PE: the Wells rule, revised Geneva score, simplified Wells rule, and simplified Geneva score. The authors report, "All four CDRs show similar performance for exclusion of acute PE in combination with a normal D-dimer result" [1].

1. Douma RA, et al. Performance of 4 clinical decision rules in the diagnostic management of acute pulmonary embolism. Ann Intern Med. 2011;7:709.

Selected Problems of the Cardiovascular System

The pulse pressure (PP), easily noted each time blood pressure is determined, can be a useful source of diagnostic clues.

The pulse pressure, technically the systolic pressure measured in mmHg minus the diastolic pressure, is typically in the range of 40; think of a blood pressure of 120/80. A narrow pulse pressure suggests the presence of aortic stenosis or perhaps congestive heart failure, shock, or even cardiac tamponade. In the case of aortic stenosis, the decreased pulse pressure may be the first evidence noted; in the other three disorders noted, other, often quite obvious, clinical signs help point to the diagnosis [1, 2].

A wide pulse pressure, on the other hand, is found when there is a high stroke volume, classically in patients with aortic insufficiency. Sometimes called a *Watson water hammer pulse* or, when detected in the carotid artery, Corrigan pulse. A wide pulse pressure may have diverse causes. Other cardiovascular origins include systolic hypertension, not uncommon in the elderly, and patent ductus arteriosus. Noncardiac causes of a wide pulse pressure include fever, anemia, and hyperthyroidism. Increased pulse pressure is a general index of arterial stiffening and is a harbinger of heart failure in the elderly, with a 14 % increased risk of heart failure for each 10 mmHg elevation in pulse pressure [3].

1. Varadarajan P, et al. Clinical profile and natural history of 453 nonsurgically managed patients with severe aortic stenosis. Ann Thorac Surg 2006;82:2115.
2. Roberts WC, et al. Severe valvular aortic stenosis in patients over 65 years of age: a clinico-pathologic study. Am J Cardiol. 1971;5:497.
3. Chase U, et al. Increased pulse pressure and risk of heart failure in the elderly. JAMA. 1999;281:634.

There exist both pulsus paradoxus and reversed pulsus paradoxus, and both are sometimes useful indicators of underlying disease.

Pulsus paradoxus, often still mentioned in physical examination lectures, describes an exaggeration of the normal inspiratory decrease in systolic blood pressure and pulse wave amplitude and may occur in constrictive pericarditis, cardiac tamponade, obstructive sleep apnea, COPD, and asthma. Why the term *paradoxus*? We use the Latin term for paradox because, in this setting, one can detect beats on cardiac auscultation during inspiration that cannot be palpated at the radial pulse [1, 2].

What about reversed pulsus paradoxus? This term describes an inspiratory increase in the systolic and diastolic blood pressures, considered to be related to an increase in left ventricular stroke volume upon inspiration. Massumi et al. describe three causes of reversed pulsus paradoxus: "idiopathic hypertrophic subaortic stenosis, isorhythmic ventricular rhythms, and during intermittent inspiratory positive-pressure breathing in the presence of left ventricular failure" [2].

1. Khasnis A, et al. Clinical signs in medicine: pulsus paradoxus. J Postgrad Med. 2002;48:46.
2. Abu-Hilal M, et al. Pulsus paradoxus: historical and clinical perspectives. Int J Cardiol. 2010;138:229.
3. Massumi RA, et al. Reversed pulsus paradoxus. N Engl J Med. 1973;289:1272.

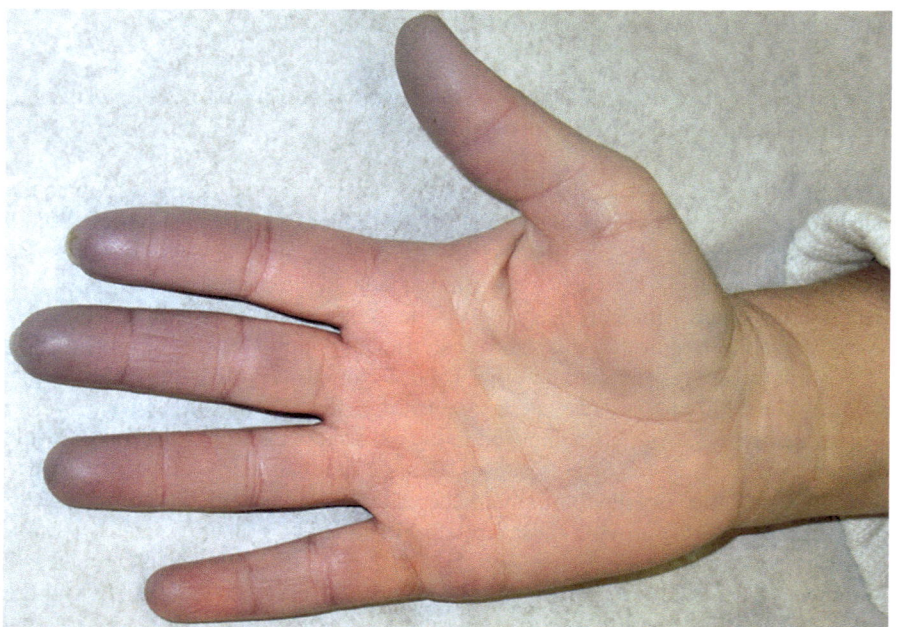

Fig. 6.6 Raynaud phenomenon (cyanotic phase) in a patient with limited scleroderma

Unilateral Raynaud phenomenon (RP) suggests the presence of local or regional vascular disease [1].

Priollet points out that unilateral RP is uncommon and may have an underlying cause [1]. RP has a 3–5 % prevalence in the general population, and in 80 % of instances, no specific cause is found and these cases are hence termed primary RP. The chief causes of secondary RP are connective tissue disorders, notably systemic sclerosis [2] (see Fig. 6.6).

Priollet et al. studied 96 consecutive RP patients, with 73 participating in long-term follow-up, finding 24 patients with suspected secondary disease of whom 14 were eventually found to have a definitive diagnosis, generally connective tissue diseases. The authors emphasize: "The study proved that Raynaud's phenomenon without an underlying cause must be followed up for more than 2 years, contrary to what was recommended previously, before it can be rightly diagnosed as primary Raynaud's phenomenon" [3].

1. Priollet P. Raynaud's phenomena: diagnostic and treatment study. Rev Pract. 1998;48:1659.
2. Vilella T, et al. Raynaud's phenomenon. Med Clin. 2009;132:712.
3. Priollet P, et al. How to classify Raynaud's phenomenon. Long-term follow-up of 73 cases. Am J Med. 1987;83:494.

Not all acute, severe chest pain is caused by coronary artery disease; an occasional chest pain patient will have acute aortic dissection.

The 43-year-old male patient's symptoms were severe chest pain, dyspnea, sweating, and dry mouth. According to the legal complaint, the patient's physician failed to consider a dissecting aortic aneurysm in the differential diagnosis; the patient died 48 h after admission. The failure-to-diagnose case was settled for $250,000 [1].

Although we are all familiar with the classic acute aortic dissection presentation with the sudden onset of *tearing* thoracic or abdominal pain and mediastinal or aortic widening seen on chest roentgenography, clinical presentations may be diverse and initial studies may be misleading [2]. Here are two tips that may prove helpful in identifying acute aortic dissection:

New murmurs: The patient with acute aortic dissection may develop a new diastolic murmur in the aortic area or an abdominal vascular murmur [3].

D-dimer test: The D-dimer test may be elevated in acute aortic dissection [4, 5].

1. Sussman JL. Missed dissecting aortic aneurysm proves fatal. J Fam Pract. 2011;60:434.
2. Hagan PG, et al. The International Registry of Acute Aortic Dissection (IRAD): new insights into an old disease. JAMA. 2000;283:897.
3. Zhang LL, et al. Clinical analysis of 30 cases on aortic dissecting. J SW Univ Nationalities. 2010;36:691.
4. Martin T, et al. D-dimer elevated in acute aortic dissection. BMJ Case Reports. 2010; doi:10.1136/bcr.04.2010.2943.
5. Suzuki T, et al. Diagnosis of acute aortic dissection by D-dimer. Circulation. 2009;119:2645.

Even a small abdominal aortic aneurysm (AAA) can rupture.

Sir William Osler (1849–1919) observed, "No disease is more conducive to clinical humility than aneurysm of the aorta" [1]. A small, often previously undetected, aortic bulge can suddenly become a painful surgical emergency [2]. Ruptured AAA, although considered by some to occur infrequently and thus be accorded a low rank on the differential diagnosis list in patients with abdominal pain, is described by Choke as "the 13th commonest cause of death in the Western World" [3] (see Fig. 6.7).

Fig. 6.7 Contrast-enhanced magnetic resonance angiogram in a patient with an abdominal aortic aneurysm. A modest-sized aneurysm is seen originating below the renal arteries (*long arrows*) and extending to the level of the aortic bifurcation. The renal arteries and iliac arteries (*arrowheads*) are well visualized without evidence of disease. The visualization of the renal veins (*short arrows*) and renal perfusion on this study was due to later imaging after contrast injection. *Ao* aorta

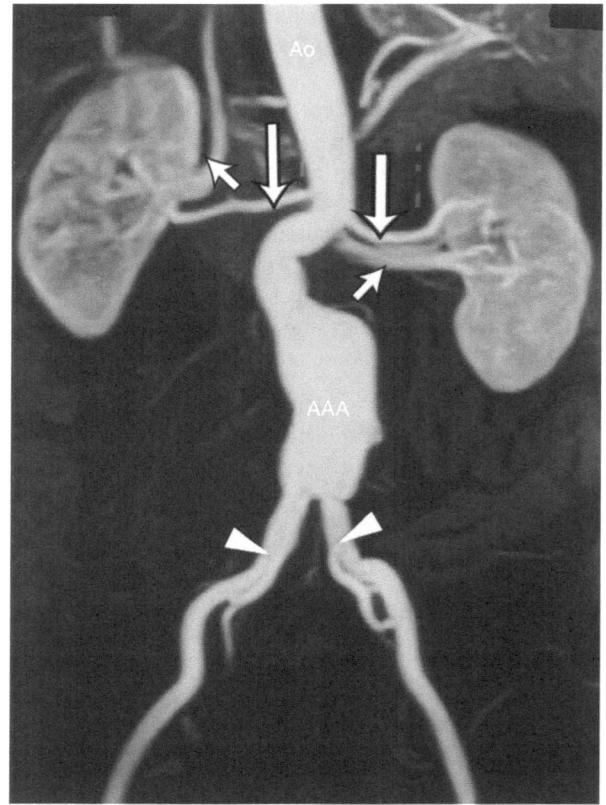

1. Osler W. Quoted in Bean RB, Bean WB, editor. Aphorisms by Sir William Osler. New York: Henry Schuman; 1950. p. 1950.
2. Inzili F, et al. Biomechanical factors in abdominal aortic aneurysm rupture. Eur J Vasc Surg. 1993;7:667.
3. Choke E, et al. A review of biological factors implicated in abdominal aortic aneurysm rupture. Eur J Vasc Endovasc Surg. 2005;30:227.

Chapter 7
The Respiratory System

Breathing is the greatest pleasure in life.
Italian author Giovanni Papini (1881–1956) [1]

Contents

R.B. Taylor, *Diagnostic Principles and Applications*,
DOI 10.1007/978-1-4614-1111-6_7, © Springer Science+Business Media, LLC 2013

Papini had a colorful literary career, writing collections of poetry and an essay titled *If Dante Were Alive*. I found the aphorism above in a book of medical quotations (reading these collections is one of my vices) and attempted to find its exact source and context. Although my quest for why Papini penned these words was unsuccessful, I decided to use the quotation anyway, apologetically citing the secondary source. But, after all, breathing is what the respiratory system is all about, and any patients with acute asthma or pulmonary edema would likely agree that, for them, normal breathing is their greatest wish. And as a favorite adage of medical students reminds us, air goes in and out, blood goes round and round, and urine runs downhill.

1. Papini G. Quoted in MacDonald P. The Oxford dictionary of medical quotations. New York: Oxford Univ Press; 2004. p. 75.

Cough

When evaluating a patient with chronic cough, think of the following causes first: postnasal drip syndrome, asthma, and gastroesophageal reflux disease (GERD).

Following a search of reported studies published over a 30-year time span, D'Urzo et al. found the three entities noted above, or even a combination of these, to be the most common sources of chronic cough [1]. Patients with chronic cough as the chief manifestation of cough-variant asthma may, in fact, have absent wheeze and dyspnea [2]. Other causes of chronic cough include bronchiectasis, chronic fungal infection, lung abscess, and tuberculosis (discussed below). Chest roentgenography is needed to identify the chronic cough patient with bronchogenic carcinoma. In the patient with asthma, bronchiectasis, or chronic bronchitis, pulmonary function testing typically shows an obstructive pattern, while a restrictive ventilatory defect is seen in sarcoidosis, pneumoconiosis, and idiopathic pulmonary fibrosis [3].

1. D'Urzo A, et al. Chronic cough: three most common causes. Can Fam Physician. 2002; 48:1311.
2. Abouzgheib W, et al. Cough and asthma. Curr Opin Pulm Med. 2007;13:44.
3. Braman SS, et al. Chronic cough: diagnosis and treatment. Prim Care. 1985;12:217.

Tuberculosis (TB), a cause of cough seen in countries around the globe, often is associated with a delay in diagnosis.

A review of 52 published studies found an average *patient delay* of 28.7 days and a subsequent *health system delay* of 25 days [1]. Another systematic review—this one of 58 studies—associated diagnostic delay with a variety of factors including human immunodeficiency virus (HIV) infection, rural residence, poverty, female sex, alcohol and substance abuse, low educational level, self-treatment, and stigma. Falsely negative sputum smears occurred in some cases. The core problem in delayed diagnosis of TB, according to the authors, "seemed to be a vicious cycle of repeated visits at the same healthcare level, resulting in nonspecific antibiotic treatment and failure to access specialized TB services" [2]. See Fig. 7.1.

1. Smeeramareddy CT, et al. Time delays in diagnosis of pulmonary tuberculosis: a systematic review of literature. BMC Infect Dis. 2009;11:9.
2. Storia DG, et al. Diagnostic delay in tuberculosis. BMC Pub Health. 2008;14:8.

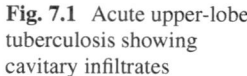
Fig. 7.1 Acute upper-lobe
tuberculosis showing
cavitary infiltrates

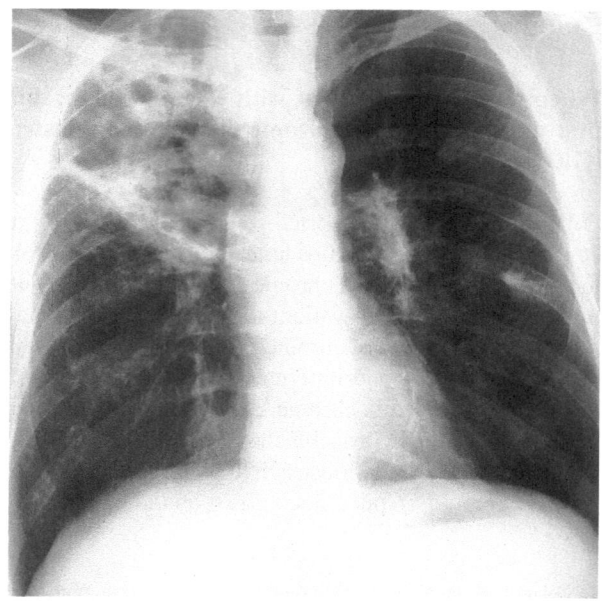

**Our ability to identify the presence of pneumonia by traditional chest
examination is open to question**.

Despite my advocacy for knowledge and use of physical signs, some concern has
been raised in regard to chest examination and pneumonia: "Traditional chest physical examination alone is not sufficiently accurate on its own to confirm or exclude
the diagnosis of pneumonia." The quotation above is the conclusion of Wipf et al.,
who studied 52 male patients with symptoms suggestive of pneumonia. All were
examined by three physicians who did not know the patients' histories, laboratory
results, or x-ray findings. The three examiners had a "highly variable" degree of
interobserver agreement regarding various physical findings, and their diagnoses
of pneumonia had a sensitivity of 47–69 % and a specificity of 58–75 % [1].

In a somewhat similar study, physicians both interviewed patients and performed a physical examination and then compared their diagnoses to x-ray
findings. The physicians' diagnoses of pneumonia had a sensitivity of 74 %
(49–90 %) and a specificity of 84 % (78–88 %), with a negative predictive value
of 97 % (94–99 %) and a positive predictive value of only 27 % (16–42 %).
Perhaps the difference from the Wipf et al. study was having access to the clinical
history. Whatever the difference, Lieberman et al. conclude "that the ability of

physicians to negate x-ray confirmed pneumonia by clinical assessment in febrile adult respiratory tract infections is good, but that their ability to successfully predict this condition is poor" [2].

1. Wipf JE, et al. Diagnosing pneumonia by physical examination: relevant or relic? Arch Intern Med. 1999;159:1082.
2. Lieberman D, et al. Diagnosis of ambulatory community-acquired pneumonia: comparison of clinical assessment versus chest x-ray. Scand J Prim Health Care. 2003;21:57.

Elderly patients with community-acquired pneumonia may not exhibit the classic symptoms and signs of cough, fever, and chest pain.

Osler termed pneumonia "captain of the men of death", and this insight is especially pertinent in the elderly patient, whose pneumonia may present as general lethargy and a decline in functional and/or mental status [1]. In a study of 1,812 patients ages 18–75 and older employing a linear regression analysis and controlling for patient demographics and other variables, Metlay et al. found older age to be associated with lower symptom scores ($p < 0.001$) [2].

1. Lim WS, et al. Pneumonia Guidelines Committee of the BTS Standards of Café Committee. BTS guidelines for the management of community acquired pneumonia in adults: update 2009. Thorax. 2009;64(suppl 3):1.
2. Metlay JP, et al. Influence of age on symptoms at presentation in patients with community acquired pneumonia. Arch Intern Med. 1997;157:1453.

Wheezing and Stridor

Detecting wheezing on maximal forced exhalation is not a reliable sign of asthma.

To restate the aphorism I used to begin the preface to this book: All that wheezes is obstruction, but not all that wheezes is asthma. Wheezing, reported to occur in nearly half of all US children by age 6 and also noted in many adults, has a wide spectrum of causes other than asthma. These include allergy, infection, foreign body aspiration, vocal cord dysfunction, bronchiectasis, Wegener granulomatosis, cystic fibrosis, and tumors [1].

As for the use of maximal forced exhalation to detect wheezing and thus make a diagnosis of asthma, I must report that although forced exhalation will, indeed, often reveal wheezes not detected with normal breathing, concluding that these wheezes represent asthma seems to be a plastic pearl—a cherished technique that has not passed the evidence-based test. King et al. studied 44 patients suspected of having asthma referred for methacholine challenge to confirm or rule out asthma. Of the 14 patients with wheezing on maximal forced exhalation, eight had a positive methacholine challenge test (sensitivity = 57 %); of 30 subjects with a negative methacholine challenge test, 11 had no evidence of wheezing on maximal forced exhalation (specificity = 37 %) [2].

1. Weiss LN. The diagnosis of wheezing in children. Am Fam Physician. 2008;77:1109.
2. King DK, et al. Wheezing on maximal forced exhalation in the diagnosis of atypical asthma: lack of sensitivity and specificity. Ann Intern Med. 1989;110:451.

In the patient with asthma, the character and timing of wheezing can provide important clues regarding disease severity.

Here, based on a study of 93 patients examined on 320 occasions with determination of peak expiratory flow rate (PEFR), are three facts to keep in mind [1]:

Wheezing presence: Wheezing, whether reported by history or found on physical examination, was associated with a significantly decreased PEFR.
Wheezing phases: Biphasic wheezing (heard during both inspiration and expiration) was found to be associated with a lower PEFR than expiratory wheezing alone.
Wheezing characteristics: The most severe obstruction was found in patients with loud and high-pitched wheezes.

A potentially ominous sign may be the disappearance of wheezing in an asthma patient who still seems to be acutely ill, a *must-never-miss* scenario that may signal respiratory failure with insufficient air movement to produce audible sound.

1. Shim CS, et al. Relationship of wheezing to the severity of obstruction in asthma. Arch Intern Med. 1983;143:890.

Vocal cord dysfunction (VCD), which may be caused by psychological stress, can be misdiagnosed as asthma.

Both VCD and asthma can present with wheezing and dyspnea. One difference is that the wheezes of VCD have central origins, while asthmatic wheezes are generated more peripherally. Murphy et al. suggest use of automated lung sound analysis to distinguish between these conditions [1].

McFadden et al. describe seven elite athletes with VCD causing wheezing and dyspnea during competition—what sports fans call *choking*. Athletes with this syndrome risk the misdiagnosis of exercise-induced asthma [2].

1. Murphy RL, et al. Method of differential diagnosis of centrally and peripherally generated wheezes. Chest. 2009;136:731A.
2. McFadden ER, et al. Vocal cord dysfunction masquerading as exercise-induced asthma: a physiologic cause for "choking" during athletic activities. Am J Respir Crit Care Med. 1996; 153:942.

Few afebrile children with wheezing have pneumonia.

Matthews et al. studied 526 children, of whom 247 (47 %) had a history of wheezing. In wheezing but afebrile children, defined as having a temperature of <38 °C, pneumonia was diagnosed radiographically in only 2.2 % (CI 95 %: 1.0–4.7) [1].

1. Matthews B. Clinical predictors of pneumonia among children with wheezing. Pediatrics. 2009; 124(1):e29.

The next patient you see with acute epiglottitis is likely to be an adult.

Although much of the literature on acute epiglottitis describes pediatric subjects, an epidemiologic study in Denmark leads to the conclusion that, owing to the widespread use of *H. influenzae* type B vaccine in children, acute epiglottitis is now rare in the pediatric age group, while the incidence in adults has remained unchanged [1].

For those who enjoy medical history, it is speculated that George Washington died in 1796 of epiglottitis, although many also argue that he really died of the robust bleeding and purging administered by his physicians [2].

1. Guldfred LA, et al. Acute epiglottitis: epidemiology, clinical presentation, management and outcome. J Laryngol Otol. 2008;122:818.
2. Taylor RB. White coat tales: medicine's heroes, heritage, and misadventures. New York: Springer; 2008. p. 215.

Soft-tissue lateral neck roentgenograms can be helpful in the diagnosis of acute epiglottitis or could be misleading.

The classic finding in lateral neck films is the *thumb sign*, representing swelling of the epiglottis until it resembles the thumb of an adult [1]. In a retrospective study of 57 adults with acute epiglottitis, soft-tissue neck x-rays were abnormal in 88.1 % of patients, but there was a 12 % false-negative rate [2].

1. Solomon P, et al. Adult epiglottitis: the Toronto Hospital experience. J Otolaryngol. 1998; 27:332.
2. Schampl S, et al. Radiological findings in acute adult epiglottitis. Eur Radiol. 1999;9:1629.

Dyspnea

Dyspnea—the subjective experience of breathlessness, shortness of breath, or breathing discomfort—is a worrisome symptom that may lead to one of a number of serious diagnoses.

Pulmonary causes of dyspnea include asthma, chronic obstructive pulmonary disease (COPD), pulmonary embolism, foreign body in the airway, or interstitial lung disease. Cardiac disease may also cause dyspnea, and Ray et al. state that congestive heart failure is the main cause of acute dyspnea in the emergency department patient (although I might challenge this assertion based on the number of acutely asthmatic patients I have encountered in the emergency setting) [1, 2]. The presence of dyspnea has been suggested as a good predictor of early diagnosis of COPD [3].

1. Dyer DS, et al. ACR appropriateness criteria on chronic dyspnea: suspected pulmonary origin. J Thor Imaging. 2010;25:w21.
2. Ray P, et al. Differential diagnosis of acute dyspnea: the value of B natriuretic peptides in the emergency department. QJM. 2008;101:831.
3. Hernandez-Zenteno R, et al. Dyspnea is a good predictor for early diagnosis of COPD: a comparison of a symptoms-based versus non-symptoms based strategies to detect smokers with COPD. Am J Respir Crit Care Med. 2011;183:A4604.

The tall, thin person with sudden onset of dyspnea accompanied by chest pain may have a spontaneous pneumothorax (SP).

Luh reports that SP occurs more commonly in men than in women [1]. See Fig. 7.2. There are, however, a number of papers describing catamenial (related to the menses) SP as well as SP during pregnancy. In the papers describing catamenial SP, diaphragmatic defects and endometriosis are described in some patients [2]. An SP may occur primarily (no known antecedent disease) or may be caused by a variety of chronic lung diseases, notably bullous emphysema. I found one report of SP in a 31-year-old man with bronchopulmonary sequestration [3].

1. Luh SP. Diagnosis and treatment of primary spontaneous pneumothorax. J Zhejiang Univ Sci B. 2010;11:735.
2. Alifano M, et al. Catamenial pneumothorax: a prospective study. Chest. 2003;124:1004.
3. Togal T, et al. An unusual cause of spontaneous pneumothorax. BMJ Case Reports. 2011. doi:10.1136/bcr.08.2010.3209.

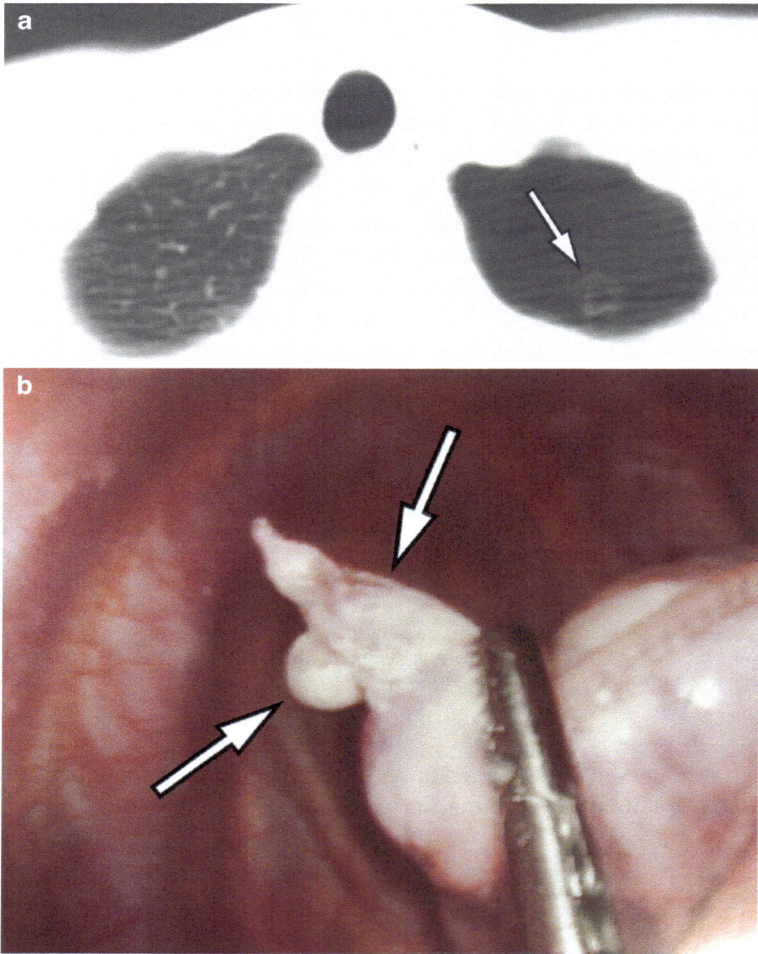

Fig. 7.2 Right apical bleb with associated pneumothorax in a 14-year-old boy. (**a**) CT image through the upper thorax shows a bleb on the left (*arrow*) and surrounding pneumothorax. (**b**) Thorascopic image shows a bleb (*arrows*)

Four diagnoses account for two-thirds of cases of chronic dyspnea: asthma, chronic obstructive pulmonary disease, interstitial lung disease, and cardiomyopathy.

The conclusion stated above resulted from a study of 85 patients referred to a pulmonary subspecialty clinic with a chief complaint of dyspnea, a cohort in whom there was 100 % success in identifying the cause of dyspnea. In 66 % of instances, the diagnosis was made on clinical impression alone [1]. In another study, investigators assessed 123 patients with a chief complaint of dyspnea present for >8 weeks, concluding that in 47 % of patients, the cause of dyspnea was *nonrespiratory* [2].

1. Pratter MR, et al. Cause and evaluation of chronic dyspnea in a pulmonary disease clinic. Arch Intern Med. 1989;149:2277.
2. Pratter MR, et al. An algorithmic approach to chronic dyspnea. Respir Med. 2011;105:1014.

A patient with chronic dyspnea and *Velcro rales* heard late in inspiration may have an interstitial lung disease (ILD).

The interstitial lung diseases are a collection of disorders considered together because they all somehow originate in the pulmonary interstitium. Examples of interstitial lung diseases include alveolar proteinosis, sarcoidosis, Goodpasture syndrome, Wegener granulomatosis, amyloidosis, asbestosis, silicosis, idiopathic pulmonary fibrosis, and Gaucher disease. The *tearing crackles* described as Velcro rales are found in many types of ILD, although they are less likely to be noted in the granulomatous diseases [1]. Patients with asbestosis, sarcoidosis, polymyositis, and idiopathic pulmonary fibrosis may have clubbing of the digits, generally indicating disease at an advanced stage [2].

1. Hilman BC. Interstitial and hypersensitivity pneumonitis and their variants. Pediatr Rev. 1980;1:229.
2. Grathwohl KW, et al. Digital clubbing associated with polymyositis and interstitial lung disease. Chest. 1995;108:1751.

Breathlessness is a leading symptom of the hyperventilation syndrome (HVS).

Anxiety and somatic symptoms induced in part or wholly by voluntary overbreathing are other features of the hyperventilation syndrome [1]. Although I cannot document the following assertion in the literature, I have found that patients with the HVS often describe feeling "unable to take a full breath".

Weinberger et al. remind us that HVS and asthma may coexist, and patients with this comorbidity may have difficulty distinguishing between symptoms due to HVS and airway obstruction (asthma) [2]. Also, many patients with HVS have agoraphobia, and many agoraphobic patients have symptoms of HVS [3].

HVS is common in music performance artists, notably among wind musicians and singers [4]. And in a study I find a little troubling, Karavidas et al. found in-flight dysfunctional breathing or frank HVS in 45 % of 55 airline pilots surveyed [5].

1. Lewis RA, et al. Definition of the hyperventilation syndrome. Bull Eur Physiopathol Respir. 1986;22:201.
2. Weinberger M, et al. Pseudo-asthma: when cough, wheezing, and dyspnea are not asthma. Pediatrics. 2007;120:855.
3. Garssen B, et al. Agoraphobia and the hyperventilation syndrome. Behav Res Ther. 1983;21:643.
4. Studer R, et al. Hyperventilation complaints in music performance anxiety among classical music students. J Psychosom Res. 2011;70:557.
5. Karavidas MK, et al. In-flight hyperventilation among airline pilots. Aviation Space Environ Med. 2009;80:495.

Hemoptysis

Hemoptysis is an alarm symptom that may be an early sign of lung cancer.

A review of the records of 762,325 patients over 6 years identified four alarm symptoms: The new onset of hemoptysis, dysphagia, hematuria, or rectal bleeding was associated with an increased risk of a diagnosis of cancer, especially in men and in patients over the age of 65 [1].

I will return to this study as we consider other body systems in later chapters. For this chapter, it is noteworthy that in the study reported, the investigators found 4,812 new episodes of hemoptysis leading to 220 diagnoses of respiratory tract cancer in men (PPV 7.5 %, 6.6–8.5 %) and 81 in women (PPV 4.3 %, 3.4–5.3 %) [1].

In a study in Jerusalem by Hirshberg et al. of 208 patients with hemoptysis, the most common cause was bronchiectasis (20 %), followed by lung cancer (19 %), bronchitis (18 %), and pneumonia (16 %). Active tuberculosis accounted for only 1.4 % of cases of hemoptysis [2]. A recent study by Uzon et al. of 178 hemoptysis patients found lung cancer to be the most common diagnosis (28.6 %), followed by pulmonary embolism (12.9 %) [3].

1. Jones R, et al. Alarm symptoms in early diagnosis of cancer in primary care: cohort study using General Practice Research Database. BMJ. 2007;334:1040.
2, Hirshberg B, et al. Hemoptysis: etiology, evaluation, and outcome in a tertiary referral hospital. Chest. 1997;112:440.
3. Uzon O, et al. A prospective evaluation of hemoptysis cases in a tertiary referral hospital. Clin Respir J. 2010;4:131.

In a patient with hemoptysis and a normal chest radiograph, think of the diagnosis of pulmonary embolism (PE).

In the Uzon et al. study described above of 178 patients, the investigators found that the most frequent diagnosis in patients with hemoptysis in the setting of a normal chest x-ray was pulmonary embolism, found in seven of the patients studied [1].

1. Uzon O, et al. A prospective evaluation of hemoptysis cases in a tertiary referral hospital. Clin Respir J. 2010;4:131.

Hemoptysis in children has its own differential diagnosis, with tracheobronchitis topping the list.

Other causes of childhood hemoptysis include cystic fibrosis, bronchiectasis, foreign body aspiration, arteriovenous malformation, hereditary telangiectasia, vocal cord laceration, aspiration of blood, and pneumonia [1].

1. Fabian MC, et al. Hemoptysis in children: the hospital for sick children experience. J Otolaryngol. 1996;25:44.

Pleuritis and Pleural Effusion

Think of pulmonary embolism in a patient presenting with pleuritic chest pain.

Pulmonary embolism is found in 5–20 % of emergency department patients presenting with pleuritic chest pain and is the most common life-threatening cause of this relatively common symptom. Other causes to consider include pneumonia, pericarditis, pneumothorax, and acute myocardial infarction [1].

1. Kass SM, et al. Pleurisy. Am Fam Physician. 2007;75:1357.

The chief cause of pleural effusion in the USA is heart failure.

Other common causes of pleural effusion include pneumonia, cancer, pulmonary embolism, and viral disease. See Fig. 7.3. Don't overlook the diagnosis of cirrhosis of the liver in the patient who uses alcohol heavily [1]. Five percent of patients with active *M. tuberculosis* infection will have a tuberculous pleural effusion [2]. Porcel advises that almost all patients with newly discovered pleural effusion should have a diagnostic thoracentesis [3], although Duysinx cautions that in the case of malignant pleurisy, thoracentesis "has a diagnostic sensibility not exceeding 62 %" [4].

Some patients presenting with pleural effusion will have uncommon causes, such as sarcoidosis [5] or coccidioidomycosis [6]. And just to add a zebra diagnosis, pleural effusions were found in 46 % of 41 consecutive patients with yellow nail syndrome, a rare disorder characterized by yellow nails, lymphedema, and/or pulmonary manifestations [7].

1. Light RW. Clinical practice: pleural effusion. N Engl J Med. 2002;346:1971.
2. Goopy A, et al. Diagnosis and treatment of tuberculous pleural effusion. Chest. 2007;131:880.
3. Porcel JM. Pearls and myths in pleural fluid analysis. Respirology. 2011;16:44.
4. Duysinx B, et al. How do I explore a pleural disease? Rev Med Liege. 2008;63:615.
5. Akcay S, et al. The diagnosis of sarcoidosis pleurisy by medical thoracoscopy: report of three cases. Tuberk Toraks. 2008;56:429.
6. Afshar K, et al. Exudative pleurisy of coccidioidomycosis: a case report and review of the literature. J Med Case Reports. 2008;3:291.
7. Maldonado F, et al. Yellow nail syndrome: analysis of 41 consecutive patients. Chest. 2008; 134:375.

Fig. 7.3 Chest x-ray of a
patient with heart failure. (**a**)
Cardiomegaly and bilateral
pleural effusion at initial
presentation. (**b**) Bilateral
pleural effusion resolved after
treatment

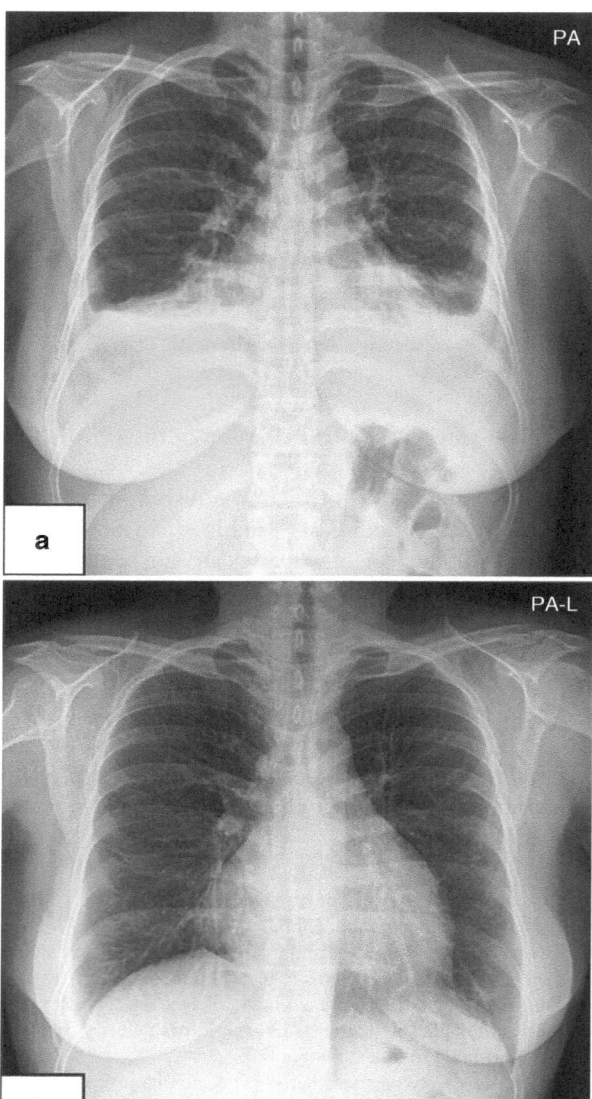

Lung Cancer

Most lung cancer patients have symptoms at the time of diagnosis; however, early manifestations can be diverse, and there are no symptoms specific to lung cancer.

Lung cancer, the leading cause of cancer-related death in the USA, has an average 5-year survival rate of 15 % [1]. Here is a list of just some of the possible manifestations of lung cancer: cough, hemoptysis, wheezing, pneumonia (distal to an obstructing mass), dyspnea, hoarseness, chest pain, pleural effusion, dysphagia, night sweats, fatigue, weight loss, fever, bone pain, pathologic fracture, neurologic deficit, hepatomegaly, Cushing syndrome, or syndrome of inappropriate antidiuretic hormone syndrome [2].

One indicator may be sudden, effortless smoking cessation. Reporting at the 13th World Conference on Lung Cancer (San Francisco, 2009), Campling described 55 patients who quit smoking before being diagnosed with lung cancer; 49 (89 %) of these subjects were asymptomatic at the time of quitting [3].

1. Collins LG, et al. Lung cancer: diagnosis and management. Am Fam Physician. 2007;75:56.
2. Hammerschmidt S, et al. Lung cancer: current diagnosis and treatment. Dtsch Arztebl Int. 2009; 106:809.
3. Campling B. Easy smoking cessation may signal lung cancer. Pulmonary Med. 2009;9:47.

There is often a preventable delay in the diagnosis of lung cancer.

In a retrospective cohort study of 587 patients with lung cancer, investigators found missed diagnostic opportunities in 222 (37.8 %). They report, "The median time to diagnosis in cases with and without missed opportunities was 132 and 19 days, respectively, ($p < 0.001$)." The most common cause of a missed diagnostic opportunity? An abnormal chest radiograph [1]. See Fig. 7.4. I believe that early lung cancer is a *must-never-miss diagnosis*.

1. Singh H, et al. Characteristics and predictors of missed opportunities in lung cancer diagnosis: an electronic health record-based study. Presented at 32nd annual meeting of Society of General Internal Medicine, Miami, 13–16 May 2009.

Lung cancer screening and the evaluation of the patient with suspected lung cancer involve diverse and evolving modalities.

Recognizing that lung cancer diagnostic methods are being developed and refined as I write this page, here are some data from recently published papers:

Fig. 7.4 Chest x-ray of a patient with a right upper-lobe non-small-cell lung cancer. The patient has moderate COPD as evidenced by the hyperinflation of the lungs and the narrow cardiac silhouette

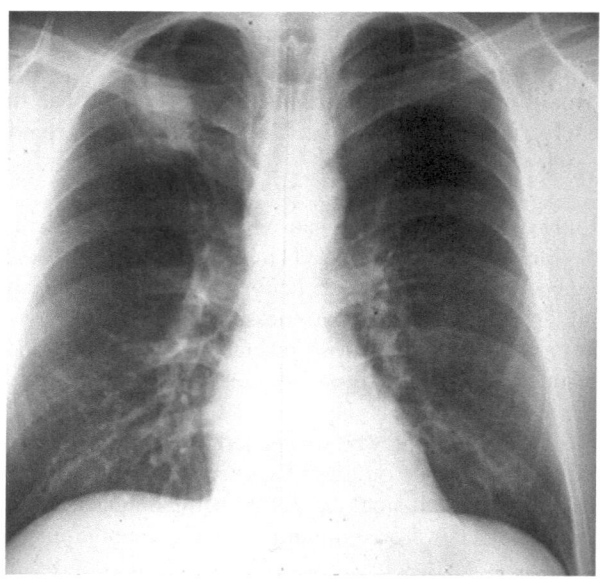

Low-dose computed tomographic (CT) screening reduces lung cancer mortality. In a study of 53,454 patients at high risk for lung cancer, when compared with radiography, there was a 20 % relative reduction in the rate of lung cancer deaths in the low-dose CT group [1].

In the diagnosis of lung cancer, sputum cytology has a pooled sensitivity of 0.66 and a specificity of 0.99 [2].

The overall sensitivity of flexible bronchoscopy (FB) for lung cancer diagnosis is 0.88. However, the diagnostic yield is much better for proximal endobronchial lesions than for peripheral tumors. The use of endobronchial ultrasound increases the diagnostic yield of FB [2].

Transthoracic needle aspiration has a pooled sensitivity of 0.90 in lung cancer diagnosis, with better yields in proximal than in peripheral lesions [2].

Use of a panel of serum biomarkers may prove useful in identifying lung cancer. In a study of sera of 100 patients, 50 with lung cancer and 50 matched controls, four markers—carcinoembryonic antigen, retinol binding protein, alpha-1 antitrypsin, and squamous cell carcinoma antigen—collectively classified the majority of lung cancer and control patients (sensitivity, 89.3 %; specificity, 84.7 %) [3].

1. National Lung Screening Trial Research Team. Reduced lung-cancer mortality with low-dose computed tomographic screening. New Engl J Med. 2011;365:395.
2. Rivera MP, et al. Initial diagnosis of lung cancer: ACCP evidence-based clinical practice guidelines. 2nd ed. Chest. 2007;132;s1315.
3. Patz EF, et al. Panel of serum biomarkers for the diagnosis of lung cancer. J Clin Oncol. 2007; 25:5578.

Selected Problems of the Respiratory System

Loud snoring and daytime sleepiness suggest the presence of obstructive sleep apnea (OSA).

The suspected diagnosis is further supported by reports by the bed partner of observed apneas [1]. Be especially suspicious in the patient with older age, obesity, large neck circumference, hypertension, menopause, a family history of OSA, and/or who uses alcohol or cigarettes. Present in an estimated 3–7 % of the population, OSA increases the risk of hypertension, cardiovascular diseases including stroke, and impaired glucose metabolism [1, 2]. Although OSA is traditionally considered to be more common in men, Ye et al. suggest that the disease may be underdiagnosed in women because of differing disease manifestations in female patients [3].

According to McNicholas, laboratory-based polysomnography is the *gold standard* in the diagnosis of OSA. See Fig. 7.5. However, the author goes on to report "growing evidence that limited sleep studies focused on respiratory and cardiac variables are adequate in most cases, and are particularly suited to home assessment" [4].

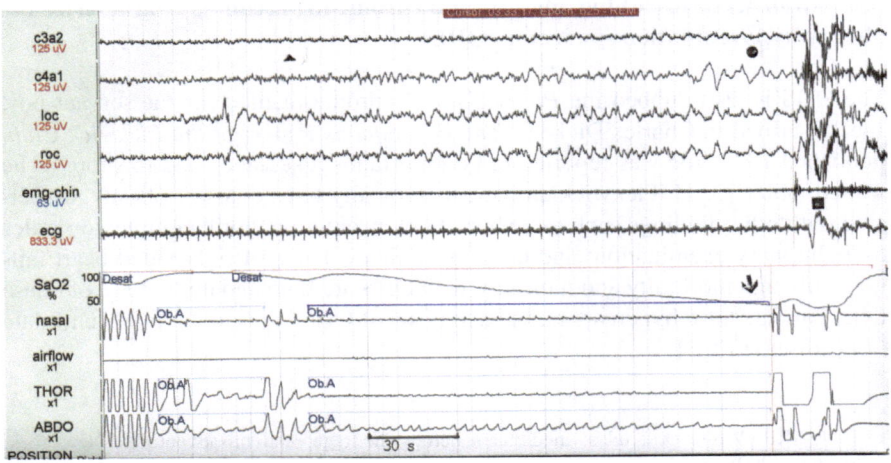

Fig. 7.5 Sleep study showing an episode of prolonged obstructive apnea with severe desaturation (see SaO$_2$ and *arrow*), which resulted in diffuse slowing of the EEG (see c4a1) from a classic rapid eye movement sleep pattern (see *triangle*) to a diffuse delta slow-wave pattern (see *circle*) compatible with cerebral hypoxia. The episode was terminated by the sleep technician's attempt to arouse the patient (diffuse movement artifact; see *square*) to prevent the episode from evolving into a cardiopulmonary arrest. c3a2 and c4a1 electroencephalogram, loc and roc right and left electrooculogram, emg-chin mentalis electromyogram, Sa2 (%) oxygen saturation, nasal airflow, *THOR* thoracic respiratory effort, *ABDO* abdominal respiratory effort, *Ob.A* obstructive apnea

1. Punjabi NM. The epidemiology of adult obstructive sleep apnea. Proc Am Thor Soc. 2008; 5:136.
2. Kapur VK. Obstructive sleep apnea: diagnosis, epidemiology, and economics. Resp Care. 2010; 55:1155.
3. Ye L, et al. Gender differences in the clinical manifestations of obstructive sleep apnea. Sleep Med. 2009;10:1075.
4. McNicholas WT. Diagnosis of obstructive sleep apnea. Proc Am Thor Soc. 2008;5:154.

In the male patient with benign prostatic enlargement (BPE), nocturia may suggest the coexistence of OSA.

In a study of 59 men with BPE, investigators found the following: "The odds ratio for symptomatic OSA gradually increased from 1.00 in patients with no nocturia to 2.44, 5.75, and 12.3 in patients reporting 1, 2–3, and >3 episodes of nocturia per night, respectively" [1].

1. Tandeter H, et al. Nocturic episodes in patients with benign prostatic enlargement may suggest the presence of obstructive sleep apnea. J Am Board Fam Med. 2011;24:146.

Sleep disordered breathing, obesity, and chronic hypercapnia characterize the obesity hypoventilation syndrome (OHS).

The OHS is also dubbed the *Pickwickian* syndrome, named for the servant boy, Joe, described in Charles Dickens' *The Posthumous Papers of the Pickwick Club*, published 1837. Joe was reported to go on errands fast asleep and to snore as he waited tables [1, 2]. Pickwickian patients typically have colossal obesity, associated with other findings such as a short, thick neck; a plethoric complexion; rales on pulmonary examination; and hemodynamic evidence of right-sided heart failure. Although morbidity and mortality with OHS are high and up to 20 % of obese OSA patients have hypercapnia, the diagnosis of OHS is often not made until late in the disease [2, 3].

1. Taylor RB. White coat tales: medicine's heroes, heritage, and misadventures. New York: Springer; 2008. p. 92.
2. Mokhlesi B, et al. Recent advances in obstructive hypoventilation syndrome. Chest. 2007;132:1322.
3. Littleton SW, et al. The Pickwickian syndrome--obstructive hypoventilation syndrome. Clin Chest Med. 2009;30:467.

The patient who seems to *forget to breathe* when asleep may have hypoventilation owing to impaired autonomic control of ventilation, aka the Ondine curse.

This rare disease is named for a mythical water nymph who married a mortal, Sir Lawrence. Her bridegroom promised that his "every waking breath shall be my pledge of love and faithfulness to you." When he proved unfaithful, remembering his own words, the betrayed nymph cursed the wayward husband with an affliction such that he could breathe readily while awake but would fail to breathe and die if he fell asleep [1, 2]. A Japanese physician colleague who returned to his homeland to help with disaster relief following the 2011 tsunami told me of encountering one such patient who, having lost the electricity needed to support her breathing apparatus, communicated her problem to the doctor with the one breathless word, *Ondine*. Fortunately for the patient, the doctor recognized the clue.

Ondine syndrome may coexist with Hirschsprung syndrome, a comorbidity eponymously termed Haddad syndrome [1].

1. Taylor RB. White coat tales: medicine's heroes, heritage, and misadventures. New York: Springer; 2008. p. 96.
2. Samdani PG, et al. Congenital central hypoventilation syndrome. Ind J Pediatr. 2007;74:953.
3. Verloes A, et al. Ondine-Hirschsprung syndrome (Haddad syndrome): further delineation in two cases and review of the literature. Eur J Pediatr. 1993;152:75.

The most common cause of acute respiratory failure (ARF), cardiogenic pulmonary edema, may be underdiagnosed in the emergency setting.

Respiratory failure is the inability to sustain normal oxygen and carbon dioxide tensions when breathing room air. When this situation occurs acutely, it is termed ARF. In a prospective, observational study of 514 patients age 65 or greater with ARF, the chief causes were cardiogenic pulmonary edema (43 %), community-acquired pneumonia (35 %), acute exacerbation of chronic respiratory disease (32 %), pulmonary embolism (18 %), and acute asthma (3 %). Almost half of these patients had more than two diagnoses. The authors report, "The accuracy of diagnosis of the emergency physician ranged from 0.76 for cardiogenic pulmonary edema to 0.96 for asthma." The outcome of the errant diagnoses was inappropriate therapy in 32 % of patients, leading to a 25 % mortality rate in the inappropriate treatment group versus 11 % in the appropriate treatment group ($p < 0.001$) [1]. See Fig. 7.6.

Fig. 7.6 Frontal portable chest radiograph showing bilateral central hazy opacities, pulmonary vascular congestion, indistinctness of the pulmonary hila, and enlarged heart, consistent with cardiogenic pulmonary edema

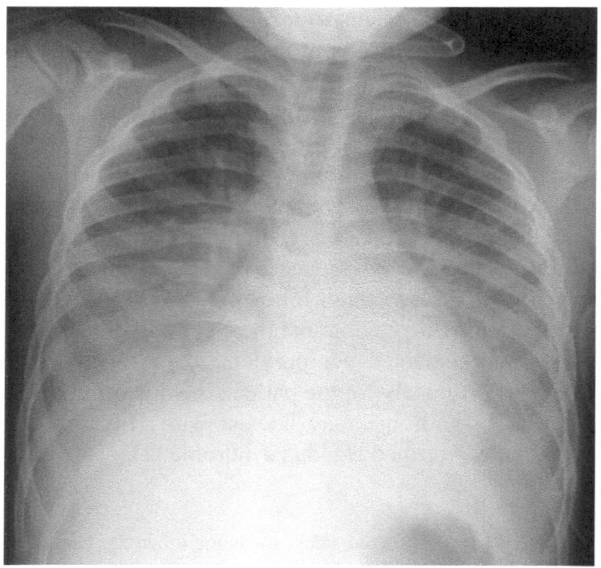

1. Ray P, et al. Acute respiratory failure in the elderly: etiology, emergency diagnosis and prognosis. Crit Care. 2006;10:151.

Chapter 8
The Digestive System

*The longer I live, the more I am convinced that the apothecary
is of more importance than Seneca; and that half the
unhappiness in the world proceeds from little stoppages, from a
duct choked up, from food pressing in the wrong place, from a
vext duodenum, or an agitated pylorus.*

English clergyman and
author Sydney Smith (1771–1845) [1]

Contents

R.B. Taylor, *Diagnostic Principles and Applications*,
DOI 10.1007/978-1-4614-1111-6_8, © Springer Science+Business Media, LLC 2013

Smith barely suggested the full spectrum of digestive disorders to which humankind is subject. Despite his piety, erudition, and insight into the workings of the gastrointestinal (GI) tract, the Reverend may be best remembered for his rhyming recipe for salad dressing. Here are the first few lines:

> Two boiled potatoes strained through a kitchen sieve,
> Softness and smoothness to the salad give.
> Of mordant mustard take a single spoon,
> Distrust the condiment that bites too soon!. . .

1. Smith S. Quoted in: A memoir of the reverend Sydney Smith by his daughter, Lady Holland, with a selection from his letters. New York: Harper; 1855. Chap. 6.

Abdominal Pain

Our increased use of imaging in the assessment of acute abdominal pain has afforded a small increase in diagnostic specificity, but has had little impact on missed surgical illness, while hospital admission rates have actually increased.

Abdominal pain is the leading chief complaint in emergency department (ED) visits in the USA [1], and the numbers of abdominal-pain visits seem to be increasing [2]. As our quest for diagnoses has become more sophisticated, largely involving imaging, visit times and cost per visit have escalated. The use of ultrasonography in right upper quadrant (RUQ) pain and computed tomography (CT) in right and left lower quadrant pain has become almost routine [3]. But to what end?

Hastings et al. compared what happened to 1,000 consecutive adult patients presenting to the ED with abdominal pain in 1972, 1993, and 2007. By 2007, imaging was used in 42 % of encounters. Here, in tabular form, is what they found in the latest two series [4]:

Year	Specific diagnosis (%)	Hospitalized (%)	Missed surgical disease (cases/thousand)
1993	75	18.3	1 case
2007	79	24.7	2

1. Pitts ER, et al. National Hospital Ambulatory Medical Care Survey: 2006 emergency department summary. Natl Health Stat Rep. 2008;7:1.
2. Bhuiya FA, et al. Emergency department visits for chest pain and abdominal pain: United States, 2008. NCHS Data Brief. 2010;43:1.
3. Cartwright SL, et al. Evaluation of acute abdominal pain in adults. Am Fam Physician. 2008;77:971.
4. Hastings RS, et al. Abdominal pain in the ED: a 35-year retrospective. Am J Emerg Med. 2010;29:711.

The older patient with marked periumbilical pain that seems unsupported by the physical examination may have acute mesenteric ischemia (AMI).

A potentially catastrophic and *must-never-miss diagnosis*, AMI should be suspected in patients presenting with acute abdominal pain who also have congestive heart failure, atrial fibrillation, or peripheral arteriosclerosis. There may be a hypercoagulable condition leading to mesenteric vein thrombosis [1–3].

While on the subject of abdominal pain, Lyon et al. remind us that in appendicitis in the older patient, we make the correct initial diagnosis only half the time [1].

1. Lyon C, et al. Diagnosis of acute abdominal pain in older patients. Am Fam Physician. 2006;74:1537.
2. Ragsdale L, et al. Acute abdominal pain in the older adult. Emerg Med. 2011;29:429.
3. Cappell MS. Intestinal (mesenteric) vasculopathy. N Am. 1998;27:783.

The patient's posture can provide clues to the cause of abdominal pain.

The patient with peritonitis resists movement, as pain results when bowel rubs against the inflamed peritoneum. This is in contrast to the patient with bowel obstruction, who may be moving restlessly. Think of acute pancreatitis when a patient lies on the exam table in a fetal position. The patient lying supine with the hip rotated and knee flexed, who reports pain when the hip is extended, has the psoas sign (aka the Obraztsova sign), traditionally suggesting peritonitis although other causes include local bleeding or abscess [1–3].

In addition, watch the patient's eyes during your palpation of the abdomen. With minor, nonspecific pain, patients tend to close their eyes—almost restfully—during the examination. In contrast, patients with more severe, and more painful, abdominal disease are likely to keep their eyes open, anticipating palpation that might aggravate the pain [4].

1. Silen W, editor. Cope's early diagnosis of the acute abdomen. 22nd ed. New York: Oxford; 2010.
2. Orient JM, editor. Sapira's art and science of diagnosis. 3rd ed. Philadelphia: Lippincott, Williams & Wilkins; 2005.
3. McGee S. Evidence-based physical diagnosis. Philadelphia: W. B. Saunders; 2001.
4. Gray DW, et al. The closed eyes sign: an aid to diagnosing nonspecific abdominal pain. BMJ. 1988;297:837.

Three credible reports indicate that judicious use of analgesics in patients with undifferentiated acute abdominal pain (AAP) does not interfere with diagnostic efforts.

The latest of these reports (2011) describes a review of eight studies identified through the Cochrane Controlled Trials Register regarding the use of opioid analgesics in patients with abdominal pain. The authors conclude as follows: "The use of opioid analgesics in the therapeutic diagnosis of patients with AAP does not increase the risk of diagnosis error or the risk or error in making decisions regarding treatment" [1]. Two earlier systematic reviews support this conclusion [2, 3].

1. Manterola C, et al. Analgesia in patients with acute abdominal pain. Cochrane Database Syst Rev. 2011;19:CD005660.
2. Thomas SH, et al. Effect on diagnostic efficiency of analgesia for undifferentiated abdominal pain. Br J Surg. 2003;90:5.
3. McHale PM, et al. Narcotic analgesia in the acute abdomen—a review of prospective trials. Eur J Emerg Med. 2001;8:131.

Fig. 8.1 (**a**) McBurney point marked for mini-incision. (**b**) Incision appearance on postoperative day four

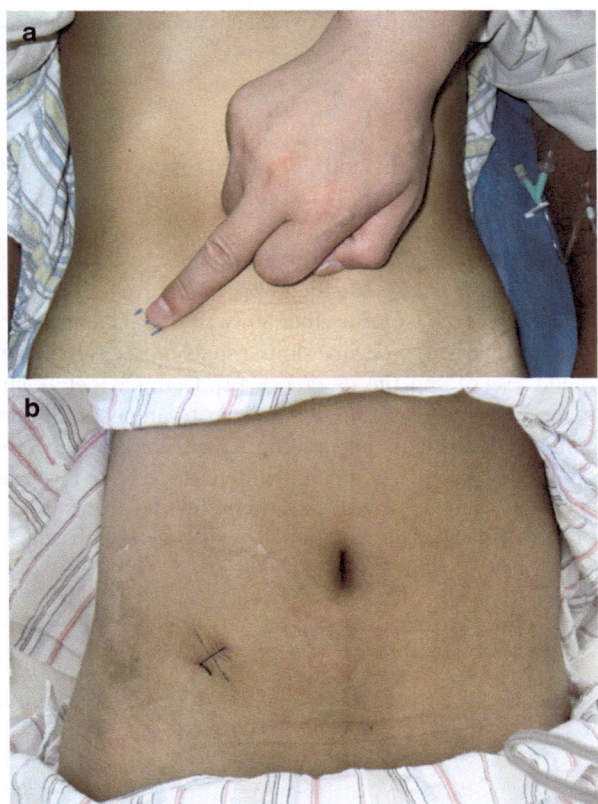

If you had to base a diagnosis of appendicitis on a single symptom or sign, make it the finding of tenderness at the McBurney point.

McBurney point is classically described as being located one-third of the distance on a line extending from the right anterior superior iliac spine to the umbilicus. See Fig. 8.1. The patient can often localize this site with a single finger, especially after coughing [1]. A study of 54 patients with appendicitis found lower abdominal tenderness present in all. Also, among these patients, there was guarding in 81.5 % and rebound tenderness in 77.7 %. Rovsing sign, in which deep palpation in a counterclockwise manner beginning in the left iliac fossa causes pain in the right lower quadrant of the abdomen, was noted in 50 % of patients [2].

Other telltale signs of appendicitis include the obturator sign (hypogastric pain caused by flexion and internal rotation of the hip), Dunphy sign (exacerbation of right lower pain on coughing), and Blumberg sign (which is another name for rebound tenderness).

1. McGee S. Evidence based physical diagnosis. 2nd ed. Philadelphia: Saunders; 2007.
2. Adesunkanmi AR. Acute appendicitis: a prospective study of 54 cases. West Afr J Med. 1993;12:197.

Be sure to ask the patient with suspected appendicitis about possible loss of appetite.

Although some may question the merits of the clinical pearl that patients with appendicitis tend to lose their appetites, I found three papers to support the thesis.

Gonclaves et al. report that 86 % of 267 patients operated on for appendicitis had anorexia [1]. In a somewhat similar study of 54 cases of acute appendicitis, Adesukanmi found loss of appetite in 77.7 % [2]. Cetinkaya et al. studied levels of appetite hormone (ghrelin) in serum and saliva of patients with appendicitis, cholecystitis, and controls. In patients undergoing appendectomy, they found decreased preoperative ghrelin levels when compared with postoperative levels and with control levels. They speculate that the lower levels of ghrelin may be a causative factor in the loss of appetite observed in acute inflammatory disorders such as acute appendicitis [3].

1. Gonclaves M, et al. Acute appendicitis in children. Acta Med Port (Portugal). 1993;6:377.
2. Adesunkanmi AR. Acute appendicitis: a prospective study of 54 cases. West Afr J Med. 1993;12:197.
3. Cetinkaya Z, et al. Changes in appetite hormone (ghrelin) levels in saliva and serum in acute appendicitis cases before and after operation. Appetite. 2009;52:104.

The rectal examination is probably unnecessary when evaluating a patient with suspected appendicitis.

When I was in training, woe to any house officer assessing a patient with right lower quadrant pain who failed to do a digital rectal examination. But is this intrusive examination really useful in these patients? Kremer et al. studied records of 477 patients with documented acute appendicitis who received rectal examinations. During rectal examination, 13.7 % of these subjects experienced right-sided pain and 7.4 % had pain in the pouch of Douglas. Nevertheless, the investigators report that "none of the rectal examination parameters was statistically significant for the diagnosis of acute appendicitis." They conclude that in evaluation of suspected appendicitis, rectal examination is *superfluous* [1]. A review of published studies by Muris et al. led to the conclusion that the rectal examination "does not seem useful in diagnosing appendicitis" [2].

1. Kremer K, et al. The diagnostic value of rectal examination of patients with acute appendicitis. Langenbecks Arch Chir Suppl Kongressbd. 1998;115:1120.
2. Muris JW, et al. The diagnostic value of rectal examination. Fam Pract. 1993;10:34.

Abdominal pain is the most common symptom of acute intermittent porphyria.

Other possible manifestations of the disease that may have caused the *madness* of *King George III* include tachycardia, hypertension, nausea, vomiting, and abdominal distension. Psychiatric manifestations are common, and dark urine may be an important clue to the diagnosis [1, 2].

1. Bylesjö I, et al. Clinical aspects of acute intermittent porphyria in northern Sweden: a population based study. Scand J Clin Lab Invest. 2009;69:612.
2. Macalpine I, et al. The "insanity" of King George 3rd: a classic case of porphyria. BMJ. 1966;8:65.

Nausea and Vomiting

The most common cause of acute nausea and vomiting is noninfectious gastrointestinal disease.

In a study of 169 patients with nausea and vomiting, most diagnoses were made on clinical grounds, with only seven subjects requiring specific diagnostic procedures. Three-quarters of these patients were prescribed medication as therapy [1].

The wise clinician keeps in mind that the most common endocrinologic cause of nausea and vomiting in women is pregnancy [2].

1. Frese T, et al. Nausea and vomiting as the reasons for encounter. J Clin Med Res. 2011;3:23.
2. Scorza K, et al. Evaluation of nausea and vomiting. Am Fam Physician. 2007;76:76.

The patient with chronic, recurrent episodes of acute nausea may have the cyclic vomiting syndrome (CVS).

Patients with CVS may feel quite well between episodes, although attacks may be severe [1]. Patients may sometimes be treated with antimigraine therapy, which, although I have not seen this speculation in print, might help to clinch the diagnosis.

Chronic cannabis use can cause a cannabinoid hyperemesis syndrome, with features resembling CVS. Sontineni reports one patient in whom the symptom of intense nausea was improved using hot baths. Of course, ceasing cannabis use also eliminates the problem [2].

1. Talley NJ. Functional nausea and vomiting. Aust Fam Physcian. 2007;36:694.
2. Sontineni SP, et al. Cannabinoid hyperemesis syndrome: clinical diagnosis of an underrecognized manifestation of chronic cannabis abuse. World J Gastroenterol. 2009;15:1264.

Dysphagia and Dyspepsia

The first step in the assessment of the patient with dysphagia is determining if the problem is oropharyngeal or esophageal.

The most common cause of oropharyngeal dysphagia is a stroke. Other causes include structural abnormalities of the oropharynx and a variety of neurologic and muscular disorders [1]. One of these is myasthenia gravis.

In patients with myasthenia gravis, dysphagia (which may include both solids and liquids) is a common symptom caused by buccopharyngeal muscle weakness [2]. To help clinch the diagnosis, check for binocular diplopia and asymmetric ptosis described in Chap. 2.

1. Mujica VR, et al. When it's hard to swallow: what to look for in patients with dysphagia. Postgrad Med. 1999;107:131, 141.
2. Viets HR. Diagnosis of myasthenia gravis in patients with dysphagia. JAMA. 1947;134:987.

Rapidly progressing dysphagia, especially if involving first solids and later both solids and liquids, is an alarm symptom suggesting carcinoma of esophagus or gastric cardia.

In contrast, Castell et al. suggest that dysphagia that begins by involving both solids and liquids suggests the presence of a motility disorder [1]. Even then one is not on safe ground: In a prospective long-term study of 448 patients with achalasia—a motor disorder of the lower esophageal sphincter with impaired relaxation on swallowing—15 (3.3 %) developed esophageal cancer over a mean follow-up of 9.6 years [2]. See Fig. 8.2.

1. Castell DO, et al. Evaluation of dysphagia: a careful history is crucial. Dysphagia. 1987;2:65.
2. Leeuwenburgh I, et al. Long-term esophageal cancer risk in patients with primary achalasia: a prospective study. Am J Gastroenterol. 2010;105:2144.

Not all dyspepsia is functional.

Dyspepsia—epigastric distress or bloating, often described as *indigestion*—is the most common GI symptom, with a worldwide prevalence of 7–45 % [1]. Gastroesophageal reflux disease (GERD) is a common cause, sometimes also causing cough. Even more serious causes occur: Upper GI distress occurs in approximately 80 % of patients with documented peptic ulcer disease [2], and in one study, 91 % of 45 subjects with early gastric cancer described dyspepsia [3].

Fig. 8.2 Esophagogram showing a stricture caused by esophageal cancer in the middle thoracic portion of the esophagus

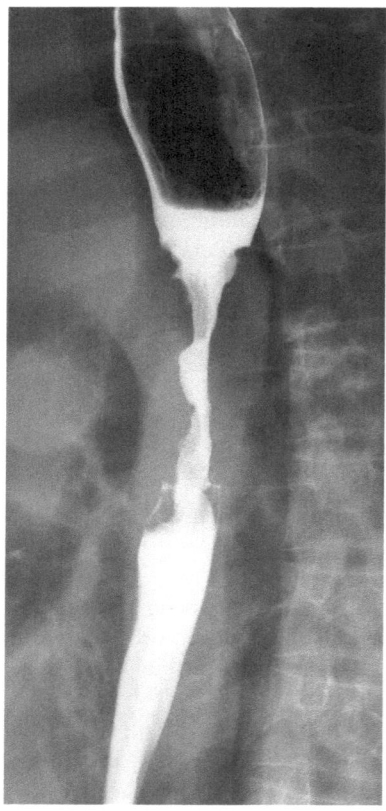

1. Buzas GM. Functional dyspepsia: the past, the present, and the Rome III classification. Orv Hetil. 2007;148:1573.
2. Barkun A, et al. Systematic review of the symptom burden, quality of life, impairment and costs associated with peptic ulcer disease. Am J Med. 2010;123:358.
3. Sue-Ling HM, et al. Early gastric cancer: 46 cases treated in one surgical department. Gut. 1992;33:1318.

Gastrointestinal Bleeding

Upper gastrointestinal (UGI) bleeding is likely to be painless.

Typically manifested as hematemesis, melena, or both, UGI bleeding accounts for 300,000 US hospital admissions annually. In most instances, the bleeding is painless [1]. Even when the cause is ulceration induced by nonsteroidal anti-inflammatory drugs, the bleeding is painless in approximately half the cases [2]. At the end of the diagnostic trail, the causes of UGI bleeding, according to one report, are likely to be duodenal ulcer (34 %), ruptured portal varices (16 %), neoplasm (10 %), gastric ulcer (8 %), and gastric erosion (6 %) [3]. Parenthetically, I find the 10 % incidence of neoplasms in patients with UGI bleeding to be very concerning.

1. Cappell MS, et al. Initial management of acute upper gastrointestinal bleeding: from initial evaluation up to gastrointestinal endoscopy. Med Clin N Am. 2008;92:491.
2. Cappell MD, et al. Acute nonvariceal upper gastrointestinal bleeding: endoscopic diagnosis and therapy. Med Clin N Am. 2008;92:511.
3. Ahmed MU, et al. Etiology of upper gastrointestinal hemorrhage in a teaching hospital. J Teachers Assoc. 2008;21:53.

Some unlikely disorders can cause UGI bleeding.

In 85–90 % of patients, the source of UGI bleeding can be detected [1]. Sometimes what is found is not on the list of *usual suspects*. One report describes UGI bleeding caused by a gastric arteriovenous malformation [2]. Other possible bleeding sources include the Mallory–Weiss tear (See Fig. 8.3.), gastric antral vascular ectasia, and the Dieulafoy lesion—an aberrant arteriole typically found in the gastric fundus [3, 4].

1. Bresci G. Occult and obscure gastrointestinal bleeding: causes and diagnostic approach in 2009. Word J Gastrointest Endosc. 2009;15:3.
2. Ng SC, et al. Gastric arteriovenous malformation: a rare cause of upper GI bleed. Gastrointest Endosc. 2009;69:155.
3. Sablijak P, et al. Less frequent causes of upper gastrointestinal bleeding. Acta Chir Iugosl. 2007;54:119.
4. Al-Mishlab T, et al. Dieulafoy lesion: an obscure cause of GI bleeding. J R Coll Surg Edinb. 1999;44:222.

Fig. 8.3 Longitudinal tear (*arrows*) in the esophagogastric junction following repeated vomiting in a case of chronic alcoholism with fatal bleeding (Mallory–Weiss syndrome)

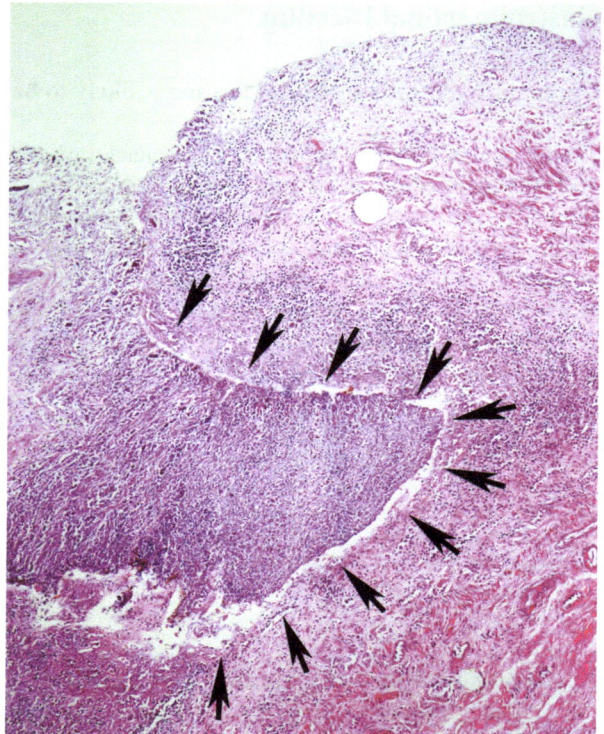

Diarrhea and Malabsorption

Think of intestinal parasites if you have adequately, but unsuccessfully, treated a returning voyager for traveler's diarrhea (TD).

Bacteria such as enterotoxigenic *E. coli*, enteroaggregative *E. Coli*, Salmonella, Campylobacter, or Shigella cause most, but not all, traveler's diarrhea. Parasites, although less common causes of TD, will be found in some individuals reporting persistent loose stools [1, 2]. Think about giardiasis, isosporiasis, cyclosporiasis, or, perhaps, blastocystosis [3, 4].

1. Brunette GW, editor. CDC Health information for international travel 2010: the yellow book. New York: Oxford; 2011.
2. Yates J. Traveler's diarrhea. Am Fam Physician. 2005;71:2095.
3. Keystone JS. Blastocystis hominis and traveler's diarrhea. Clin Infect Dis. 1995;21:102.
4. Fathy FM. A study of Blastocystis hominis in food-handlers: diagnosis and potential pathogenicity. J Egypt Soc Parasitol. 2011;41:433.

Consider the possibility of celiac disease (CD) when you encounter a patient with fatigue, iron deficiency anemia, and what seems to be irritable bowel syndrome (IBS).

Once termed celiac sprue, derived from the Dutch word *Sprue*, CD is an autoimmune enteropathy triggered by ingestion of gluten—found in wheat, barley, and rye—by genetically predisposed persons. The gold standard for diagnosis is biopsy of the small bowel mucosa [1]. Sanders et al. studied 1,200 subjects, finding 12 new cases of CD. In this population, the prevalence of CD was 1 %. However, within the sample, they report as follows: "The prevalence of celiac disease was 3.3 % (4/123) in participants with irritable bowel syndrome, 4.7 % (3/64) in participants with iron deficiency anemia, and 3.3 % (3/92) in participants with fatigue" [2].

1. Green PHR, et al. Celiac disease. N Engl J Med. 2007;357:1731.
2. Sanders DS, et al. A primary care cross-sectional study of undiagnosed adult celiac disease. Eur J Gastroenterol Hepatol. 2003;15:407.

Celiac disease may occur in patients with a variety of other disorders.

Patients with CD may develop small intestine adenocarcinoma or enteropathy-associated T-cell lymphoma as complications [1]. Aphthous ulcers occur commonly [1]. Older patients often develop iron deficiency anemia or osteoporosis [2]. CD can also be associated with any of a number of autoimmune disorders: Graves disease of the thyroid, Addison disease, autoimmune liver disease, and type 1 diabetes mellitus. (3) At highest risk are children with Down syndrome, who have a 20-fold greater increased risk of developing CD compared to the general population [4].

1. Green PHR, et al. Celiac disease. N Engl J Med. 2007;357:1731.
2. Freeman H, et al. Celiac disease. Best Pract Res Clin Gastroenterol. 2002;16:37.
3. Catassi C, et al. Celiac disease: more common than once thought. US Pharm. 2008;33:24.
4. Hill ID, et al. Guideline for the diagnosis and treatment of celiac disease in children: recommendations of the North American Society for Pediatric Gastroenterology, Hepatology and Nutrition. J Pediatr Gastroenterol Nutr. 2005;40:1.

Diseases of the Pancreas

Consider the diagnosis of acute pancreatitis in the patient with mid-epigastric pain, nausea, and vomiting. See Fig. 8.4.

Be especially suspicious of the diagnosis of acute pancreatitis if the patient has biliary disease or is a heavy user of alcohol. Also, there may be an increased risk of acute pancreatitis in patients with type 2 diabetes mellitus [1]. Mild acute pancreatitis, recognized early and managed with intravenous hydration, has a low mortality rate. Failure to respond to therapy over time should prompt a search for a complication such as an abscess or pseudocyst [2, 3].

1. Noel RA, et al. Increased risk of acute pancreatitis and biliary disease observed in patients with type 2 diabetes: a retrospective cohort study. Diab Care. 2009;32:834.
2. Gupta PK, et al. Acute pancreatitis: diagnosis and management. Am Fam Physician. 1995;52:435.
3. Carroll JK, et al. Acute pancreatitis: diagnosis, prognosis, and treatment. Am Fam Physician. 2007;75:1513.

Painless jaundice, the classic presentation of pancreatic cancer, may actually be a favorable prognostic sign.

Pancreatic cancer offers a dismal 5-year survival rate of 4 %, worse than that of lung cancer. In a study of 393 patients with pancreatic cancer, those ($n=21$) who had potentially curable resection tended to have the smallest lesions, located in the head of the pancreas. Of these patients with the most favorable outlook, 52 % first presented with painless jaundice. Patients with lesions less amenable to resection

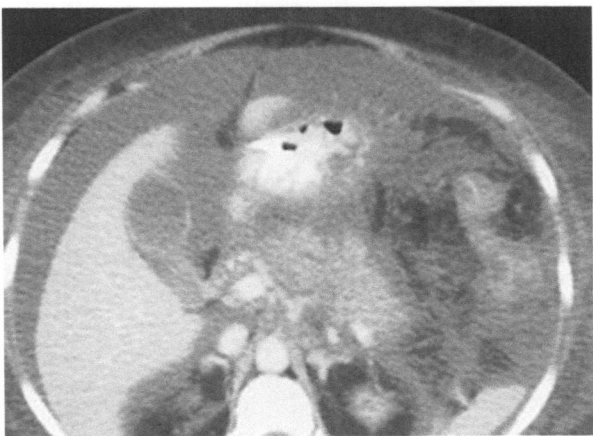

Fig. 8.4 CT scan showing enlarged, heterogeneously enhancing pancreas, due to acute pancreatitis

tended to have pain (80–85 %), often a dull abdominal ache radiating to the back, which may be associated with jaundice [1].

1. Kaiser MH, et al. Pancreatic cancer: assessment of prognosis by clinical presentation. Cancer. 1985;56:397.

Two diverse groups of patients have an increased risk of pancreatic cancer: diabetics and persons with a non-O blood group.

Chari et al. studied 2,122 diabetic patients age 50 years and older, of whom approximately 1 % developed pancreatic cancer within the first 3 years following the diagnosis of diabetes [1]. And, based on data from two large studies involving 927,995 person-years of follow-up, Wolpin et al. report, "Overall, 17 % of the pancreatic cancer cases were attributable to inheriting a non-O blood group (blood group A, B, or AB)" [2].

1. Chari ST, et al. Probability of pancreatic cancer following diabetes: a population-based study. Gastroenterology. 2005;129:504.
2. Wolpin BM, et al. ABO blood group and the risk of pancreatic cancer. J Natl Can Inst. 2009;101:424.

Diseases of the Liver

Our ability to detect hepatomegaly is less than stellar.

In a study of 57 generalist physicians who agreed to have an encounter with an unannounced standardized patient with hepatomegaly presenting with a complaint of abdominal pain, only four (7 %) detected the liver enlargement. For the record, older, more experienced physicians were more likely to detect the hepatomegaly [1]. The result was even worse in a study of the detection of liver enlargement in obese children. In this study involving 11 obese children examined by 18 primary care physicians and pediatric gastroenterologists, hepatomegaly was detected in only 1.4 % of encounters [2].

Add to this the fact that, according to Naylor, half of all palpable livers are not enlarged at all, necessitating measurement of the vertical span to accurately assess liver size [3].

1. Borrel-Carrió F, et al. Family physicians' ability to detect a physical sign (hepatomegaly) from an unannounced standardized patient (incognito SP). Eur J Gen Pract. 2011;17:95.
2. Fishbein M, et al. Undetected hepatomegaly in obese children by primary care physicians: a pitfall in the diagnosis of pediatric nonalcoholic fatty liver disease. Clin Pediatr. 2005;44:135.
3. Naylor CD. Physical examination of the liver. JAMA. 1994;271:1859.

When a large liver is found, be sure to auscultate for a bruit.

Cook holds that a large hard nodular liver associated with a bruit is virtually confirmatory for liver cancer [1]. In one series, a bruit over the liver was audible in 25 % of patients with hepatocellular cancer [2]. Arterial bruits over the liver can also occur in alcoholic hepatitis [3].

1. Cook GC. Hepatocellular carcinoma: one of the world's most common malignancies. Q J Med. 1985;57:705.
2. Desai HN. Clinical aspects of hepatocellular carcinoma in man. S Afr Med J. 1976;50:1611.
3. Clain D, et al. Abdominal arterial murmurs in liver disease. Lancet. 1966;2:516.

When faced with a jaundiced patient, think first of cancer, gallstones, or alcoholic liver disease.

These were the most common causes of jaundice in a prospective study of 720 jaundiced patients age 16 or greater. The incidence was pancreatic or biliary carcinoma (20 %), gallstone disease (13 %), and alcoholic liver disease (10 %) [1].

The astute mathematician will note that the three categories above account for only 43 % of jaundiced subjects in the study. Other causes of jaundice cover a wide panorama. Here are comments on just a few of them:

Sepsis/shock: One study found sepsis/shock to be the cause of jaundice in 27 of 121 icteric subjects [2].

Drugs: A number of drugs have been implicated as causes of jaundice: These include probenecid (Benemid), rifampin (Rifadin), and chlorpromazine (Thorazine). A study in rural England found drugs to be the culprit in 8.1 % of patients with jaundice in the absence of biliary obstruction; the leading offenders were amoxicillin–clavulanate (Augmentin) and flucloxacillin/floxacillin (Floxapen) [3].

Gilbert syndrome: Do not overlook the diagnosis of Gilbert syndrome, with elevated levels of unconjugated bilirubin in the absence of bile in the urine [4].

Malaria: Jaundice may accompany the other manifestations of malaria [5].

1. Reisman Y, et al. Clinical presentation of (subclinical) jaundice: the Euricterus project in The Netherlands. Hepatogastroenterology. 1996;43:1190.
2. Whitehead MW, et al. The cause of obvious jaundice in South West Wales: perceptions versus reality. Gut. 2001;48:409.
3. Hussaini S, et at. Antibiotic therapy: a major cause of drug-induced jaundice in southwest England. Eur J Gastroenterol Hepatol. 2007;19:15.
4. Gilbert A, et al. La cholamae simple familiale. Sem Med. 1901;21:241.
5. Anand AC, et al. Jaundice in malaria. J Gastroenterol Hepatol. 2005;20:1322.

Our ability to visually assess neonatal jaundice is not very good.

Moyer et al. describe 122 healthy term infants whose bilirubin was estimated by experienced nurse practitioners, pediatric residents, and attending physicians. They found poor agreement (0–23 % agreement beyond chance) regarding the presence of jaundice at each specific body site. They also found poor agreement (Pearson correlation coefficient, 0.37) between estimated bilirubin concentrations and slightly better (Pearson correlation coefficient, 0.43) between estimated and actual bilirubin values [1].

1. Moyer VA, et al. Accuracy of clinical judgment in neonatal jaundice. Arch Ped Adol Med. 2000;154:391.

Colorectal Disorders

Abdominal bloating and distension, commonly reported by patients with functional GI disorders, can be an early warning clue to the diagnosis of ovarian cancer.

In one study, of 542 irritable bowel syndrome patients, 76 % reported abdominal bloating [1]. And about half of IBS patients with bloating also note distension—an increase in abdominal girth [2]. However, somewhere among these patients are women with abdominal bloating and distension related to ovarian cancer. In a study by Matsuo et al. of 276 cases, 93.5 % of women with ovarian cancer were symptomatic at the time of diagnosis. Leading complaints were abdominal pain (40.6 %), abdominal distension (33.7 %), and bloating (21.7 %) [3].

1. Chang L, et al. Sensation of bloating and visible abdominal distension in patients with irritable bowel syndrome. Am J Gastroenterol. 2001;96:3341.
2. Agrawal A, et al. Abdominal bloating and distension in functional gastrointestinal disorders: epidemiology and exploration of possible mechanisms. Aliment Pharmacol Ther. 2008;27:2.
3. Matsuo K, et al. Patient-reported symptoms and survival in ovarian cancer. Int J Gynecol Cancer. 2011;21:1555.

Think of toxic megacolon (TM) in the setting of a patient with acute or chronic diarrhea and massive abdominal distension.

TM is a potentially lethal, *must-not-miss disorder* "characterized by total or segmental non-obstructive colonic dilatation of at least 6 cm associated with systemic toxicity" [1]. Classically associated with inflammatory bowel disease, TM may also occur in patients with infectious colitis, ischemic colitis, diverticulitis, volvulus, obstructive colon cancer, and pseudomembranous enterocolitis [1, 2]. Risk factors include recent colonoscopy and the use of anticholinergic medications [2]. See Fig. 8.5.

1. Sheth SG, et al. Toxic megacolon. Lancet. 1998;351:509.
2. Levine CD. Toxic megacolon: diagnosis and treatment challenges. AACN Clin Issues. 1999;10:492.

We clinicians miss far too many opportunities to detect colorectal cancer (CRC), another *must-not-miss diagnosis*.

In a study of 513 patients with CRC, investigators found at least one missed opportunity in 161 patients (31.3 %). The most common missed clues were suspected or confirmed iron deficiency anemia, positive fecal occult blood testing (FOBT), and

Fig. 8.5 Toxic megacolon:
Colonic dilatation (without
air insufflation) with
intraluminal air and fluid. (**a**)
The luminal contour is
distorted and anhaustral.
Diffuse slight wall thickening
with increased CM
enhancement of the whole
colon and ill-defined nodular/
pseudopolypoid surface (**b**)

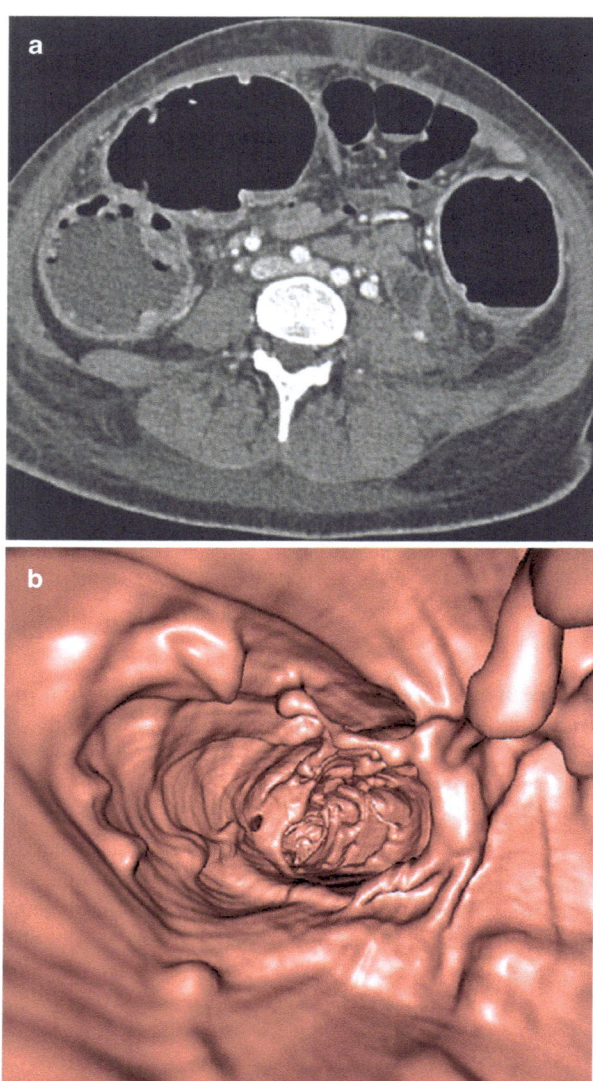

hematochezia (passage of blood-containing stool). For patients with anemia, the
median time to endoscopic referral was 393 days. Patients at greatest risk of missed
opportunities to diagnose CRC were those age >75 [1]. In a subsequent report, this
same team quantified the referral median delays for other clues: positive fecal occult
blood test, 92 days ($p < 0.0001$); hematochezia, 75 days ($p = 0.02$); and for history of
polyps, 221 days ($p = 0.0006$) [2].

1. Singh H, et al. Missed opportunities to initiate endoscopic evaluation for colorectal cancer diagnosis. Am J Gastroenterol. 2009;104:2543.
2. Singh H, et al. Reducing referral delays in colorectal cancer diagnosis: is it about what you ask? Qual Saf Health Care. 2010;19:1.

Rectal bleeding is an alarm symptom for possible colorectal cancer (CRC).

In a study of 762,325 patients age 15 years and older (cited several times in this book as we come to the symptoms described in the chapter), there were 15,289 episodes of rectal bleeding reported, leading to 184 diagnoses of CRC in men (PPV, 2.4 %, 2.1–2.8 %) and 154 in women (PPV 2.0 %, 1.7–2.3 %) [1].

1. Jones R, et al. Alarm symptoms in early diagnosis of cancer in primary care: cohort study using General Practice Research Database. BMJ. 2007;334(7602):1040.

Low-dose aspirin use may actually increase the sensitivity of immunochemical fecal occult blood testing.

In a study of 24 persons using low-dose aspirin and 181 nonusers, the increasingly available immunochemical fecal occult blood test was found to have a higher sensitivity for detecting advanced colorectal cancer when the patient was using low-dose aspirin. How? The answer lies in the test chemistry. Traditional guaiac-based FOBT is subject to falsely positive results when the patient has taken aspirin. Not so with immunochemical FBOT, which reacts to globin, which is degraded by proteases in the colon, and which seems to enjoy enhanced sensitivity when the patient has consumed aspirin [1].

1. Brenner H, et al. Low-dose aspirin use and performance of immunochemical fecal occult blood tests. JAMA. 2010;304:2513.

Abrupt and *gripping* anorectal pain awakening the patient at night and then subsiding in a few minutes describes proctalgia fugax (PF), an underappreciated clinical entity.

According to one astute author, "Proctalgia fugax was long thought to be a disease of young professional males, because only doctors had the temerity to describe their symptoms in letters to the editor of Lancet" [1]. According to various reports, the prevalence of PF in the general population is somewhere between four and 18 % [2]. A wide spectrum of remedies have been proposed, ranging from warm baths to albuterol inhalation to Botox injections.

1. Thompson WG. The road to Rome. Gastroenterol. 2006;130:1552.
2. Jeyarajah S, et al. Proctalgia fugax, an evidence-based management pathway. Int J Colorect Dis. 2010;25:1037.

Selected Problems of the Digestive System

Early in the disease, the person with gastric cancer may lose his or her appetite for meat.

Described by some as the second most common cause of cancer death worldwide, gastric cancer is especially common in developing countries [1]. A helpful clue to early diagnosis may be an impaired appetite, especially for meat [1, 2].

1. Sintara K, et al. Gastric cancer: the experimental models. J Physiol Sci. 2008;21:33.
2. Herschel G. The diagnosis of cancer of the stomach in its early stage. Presidential address to the West Kent Medico-Churgical Society in 1903. London: H. J. Glaishhen; 1903. p. 2.

Campylobacter enteritis is the leading precursor of Guillain–Barré syndrome (GBS).

Tam et al. conducted a 10-year nested case-control study and concluded that Campylobacter enteritis was associated with a 60-fold excess risk of GBD and that one case of GBS in five was attributable to this infection. Their findings also supported the previous reports of an association of GBS with recent Epstein–Barr infection and influenza-like illness. As an aside, these authors report that influenza vaccine may offer some protection against GBS [1].

1. Tam CC, et al. Guillain-Barré syndrome and preceding infection with Campylobacter, influenza, and Epstein-Barr virus in the General Practice Database. PLoS ONE. 2007;2(4):e344.

The patient who is very obese can be misdiagnosed as having ascites.

Incorrectly labeling the obese person as having ascites could lead to inappropriate diagnostic procedures—think diagnostic paracentesis—and unnecessary diuretic therapy. How can we tell the difference? Here is where classical physical findings can be especially useful. Look for bulging of the flanks. Palpate fluid in the peritoneal cavity using the fluid wave technique. Percuss the abdomen, seeking periumbilical hyperresonance as gas-filled bowel rises to the top. Continue percussing, looking for shifting dullness as the patient is turned from supine to a lateral position. Use the *puddle sign*, having the patient stand for a few minutes, and then use auscultatory percussion (listening below while percussing at various sites) to detect a dependent fluid level [1]. See Fig. 8.6.

Once the presence of ascites has been confirmed, a search begins for the cause. Following paracentesis, the next diagnostic step is determination of the serum-ascites

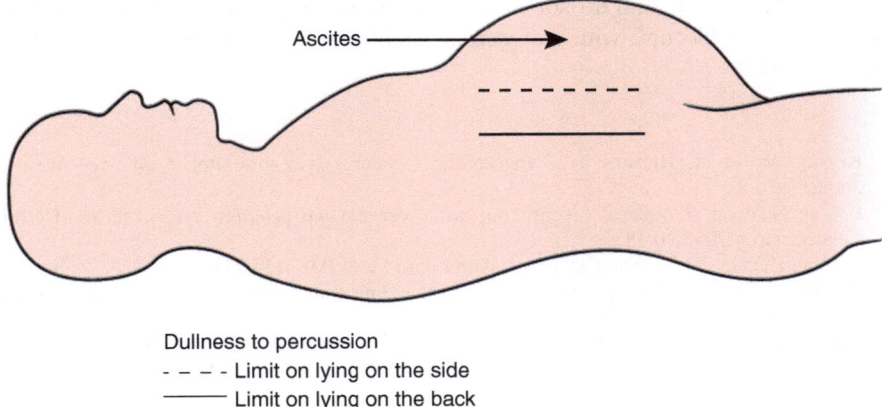

Dullness to percussion
- – – - Limit on lying on the side
———— Limit on lying on the back

Fig. 8.6 Bulging of flanks in ascites. At least 2 L of fluid must be present in the abdominal cavity before it can be detected clinically. The earliest signs of ascites present in the abdominal cavity are bulging of the flanks and dullness to percussion in the flank. The latter can be confirmed by the shifting of the percussion dullness when the patient changes position

albumin gradient [2, 3]. The odds are high that the eventual diagnosis will be cirrhosis of the liver, responsible for approximately 80 % of cases of ascites. Less common causes are cancer, heart failure, and tuberculosis. Rare causes of ascites that have been reported include hemorrhagic ascites as the presentation of endometriosis [4] and chylous ascites as a manifestation of the battered child syndrome [5].

1. Orient JM, editor. Sapira's art and science of bedside diagnosis. Philadelphia: Lippincott, Williams & Wilkins; 2005. p. 454.
2. Hou W, et al. Ascites: diagnosis and management. Med Clin N Am. 2009;93:801.
3. Runyon BA, et al. The serum-ascites albumin gradient is superior to the exudate-transudate concept in the differential diagnosis of ascites. Ann Intern Med. 1992;117:215.
4. Palayekar M, et al. Recurrent hemorrhagic ascites: a rare presentation of endometriosis. Obstet Gynecol. 2007;110:521.
5. Boysen BE. Chylous ascites: manifestation of the battered child syndrome. Am J Dis Child. 1975;129:1338.

Hiccups can be a symptom of myocardial ischemia.

Krysiak et al. present just such a patient, a 62-year-old man with recurrent hiccups upon exertion as part of his presentation with myocardial ischemia [1]. In fact, myocardial ischemia is just one of the almost 100 causes of hiccups. Another is hiccups as an atypical manifestation of gastrointestinal reflux disease [2]. Hiccups occur commonly in patients with achalasia [3] and have been reported in a patient with gastric volvulus [4]. And do not forget medications as possible, although uncommon, causes of hiccups, with oral steroids and benzodiazepines leading the list in one review [5].

1. Krysiak W, et al. Hiccups as a myocardial ischemia symptom. Pol Arch Med Wewn. 2008;118:148.
2. Pooran N, et al. Protracted hiccups due to severe erosive gastritis: a case series. J Clin Gastroenterol. 2006;40:183.
3. Seeman H, et al. Hiccups and achalasia. Ann Intern Med. 1991;115:711.
4. McElreath DP, et al. Hiccups: a subtle sign in the clinical diagnosis of gastric volvulus and a review of the literature. Dig Dis Sci. 2008;53:3033.
5. Giudice M. Drugs may induce hiccups in rare cases. Can Pharmacol J. 2007;140:124.

Might the "Haagen-Dazs test" catch on as a useful method to distinguish between symptoms of peptic ulcer disease and cholecystitis?

Proposed in a letter by a physician in Buffalo, New York, the "Haagen-Dazs test" (which was self-administered by the physician, based on the advice of her MD father) is performed as follows. The patient with undiagnosed abdominal pain eats a pint of Haagen-Dazs ice cream. This ingestion should either sooth an inflamed ulcer or aggravate acute cholecystitis. For what it is worth, it did point to the correct diagnosis in the case of the doctor describing the test. The test has the merits of being low cost, low tech, and reasonably safe, if we disregard the caloric content involved [1].

1. Rolston KL. We narrowed the differential with the "Haagen-Daz test." (Letter) J Fam Pract. 2011;60:453.

The Collins sign may be helpful in the diagnosis of acute cholecystitis.

While on the subject of cholecystitis, a useful clue can be the Collins sign, described by Professor Paddy Collins of the Royal College of Surgeons in Ireland. According to the professor, patients with gallstone pain often illustrate their discomfort by placing their hand behind the back, pointing to the tip of the scapula with the thumb extended superiorly. See Fig. 8.7. In a case-control study, the sign was positive in 51.5 % of 202 patients and in 7.5 % of control subjects [2].

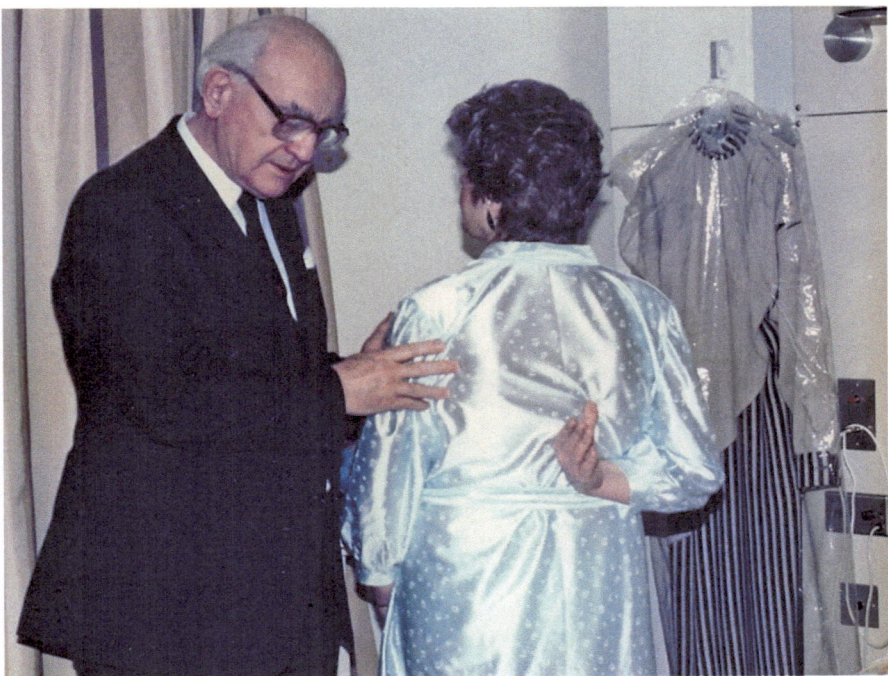

Fig. 8.7 Collins sign demonstrated to Professor Collins by patient with a hand behind the back and the thumb pointing upward

1. Gilani SN. Collins' sign: validation of a clinical sign in cholelithiasis. Irish J Med Sci. 2009; 178:397.

Chapter 9
The Kidney and Male Genitourinary System

*Bones can break, muscles can atrophy, glands can loaf, even
the brain can go to sleep, without immediately endangering
our survival; but should the kidneys fail. . . neither bone,
muscle, gland, nor brain could carry on.*

American physiologist and part-time philosopher
Homer William Smith (1895–1962) [1]

Contents

R.B. Taylor, *Diagnostic Principles and Applications*,
DOI 10.1007/978-1-4614-1111-6_9, © Springer Science+Business Media, LLC 2013

Described in his obituary as the "acknowledged dean of renal physiology," Smith certainly had a heroic view of the urinary system [2]. In the book cited [1], Smith describes the key role of renal function in allowing early evolutionary survival in water and subsequently on land as we pursued the long journey toward our current status as ambulatory, sapient human beings. But of course, there is more to the story than the kidney, and survival of the species truly depends on the integrity of the entire genitourinary system.

1. Smith HW. From fish to philosopher. New York: Doubleday; 1961.
2. Fishman AP. Homer W. Smith (In memoriam). Circulation. 1962;26:984.

Dysuria

The physical examination and urine analysis are not needed in the evaluation of most women presenting with acute dysuria suggesting a urinary tract infection (UTI).

A study by Bent et al. of published articles, textbooks, and expert opinion yielded the following conclusion: "In women who present with one or more symptoms of UTI, the probability of infection is approximately 50 %. Specific combinations of symptoms (e.g., dysuria and frequency without vaginal discharge or irritation) raise the probability of UTI to 90 %, effectively ruling in the diagnosis based on history alone." The authors go on to report that when a patient presents with one or more of symptoms suggesting cystitis, the usual assessment—clinical history, physical examination, and dipstick urinalysis—cannot reliably lower the posttest probability of disease to a level where UTI can be ruled out [1].

Gonzales et al. concur regarding urine analysis, holding that in women with multiple and typical symptoms of UTI, urinalysis has insufficient negative predictive value to exclude culture-confirmed urinary tract infection. They suggest that urinalysis is probably overutilized in the evaluation of dysuria [2].

With the above considered, it seems to me that many women with clear-cut symptoms of acute uncomplicated UTI can be managed over the telephone.

1. Bent S, et al. Does this woman have an acute uncomplicated urinary tract infection? JAMA. 2002;287:2701.
2. Gonzales R, et al. Dysuria. In: McPhee SJ, et al., editors. Current medical diagnosis and treatment. New York: McGraw-Hill; 2010.

The young, single, sexually active male with dysuria is more likely to have urethritis than cystitis.

The diagnostic implications of a chief complaint of acute dysuria in men versus women have to do with the gender differences in plumbing. Other symptoms of male urethritis include urethral discharge (although the patient may be unaware of this manifestation), penile tingling or itching, and urinary frequency [1, 2]. Finding ten or more white blood cells (WBCs) per high power field in the urinary sediment confirms the diagnosis of urethritis, as does confirming the presence of a urethral discharge or noting a positive result on a leukocyte esterase test in a first-void urine specimen [2].

1. Sonnex C. Sexual health and genital medicine in clinical practice. New York: Springer; 2007. p. 74.
2. Brill JR. Diagnosis and treatment of urethritis in men. Am Fam Physician. 2010;81:873.

About half of all women with interstitial cystitis/painful bladder syndrome will have dysuria at the onset.

This syndrome, a common cause of chronic pelvic pain (see Chap. 10), began with burning or pain on urination in 75 (54 %) of 138 female patients surveyed in one study [1].

1. Warren JW, et al. Dysuria at onset of interstitial cystitis/painful bladder syndrome in women. Urology. 2006;68:477.

Hematuria

Hematuria is one of the four alarm symptoms highlighted in a large study published in 2007.

Also mentioned in previous chapters, this study of 762,325 persons over 6 years identified hematuria as one of the four alarm symptoms—along with hemoptysis, dysphagia, and rectal bleeding—associated with an increased likelihood of cancer, especially in men and patients over age 65 [1]. In a study of 264 patients with gross hematuria, 10 % had tumors [2].

1. Jones R, et al. Alarm symptoms in early diagnosis of cancer in primary care: cohort study using General Practice Research Database. BMJ. 2007;334:1040.
2. El-Galley R, et al. Practical use of investigations in patients with hematuria. J Endourol. 2008;22:51.

Gross and microscopic hematuria share the same differential diagnosis of most likely causes: tumor, infection, or stone.

While the definition of gross hematuria is visual and intuitive, microscopic hematuria requires a definition. Patel et al. consider microscopic hematuria present if the patient has more than three red blood cells (RBCs) per high power field (HPF) [1]. Another group uses a cutoff of five or more RBC/HPF [2].

As physicians, our response to finding hematuria has been less than inspiring. Current guidelines recommend urologic evaluation for hematuria of any degree. In one study of 788 primary care physicians in two cities, 77 and 69 % of gross hematuria patients were referred for urologic evaluation, while in both cities only 36 % of primary care physicians referred patients with microscopic hematuria for evaluation [3]. Delays in diagnosis of bladder cancer affect mortality, with patients in whom the diagnosis of bladder cancer was delayed 9 months were more likely to succumb to their disease than those diagnosed within 3 months (HR 1.34; 95 % CI 1.20–1.50) [4].

1. Patel JV, et al. Hematuria: etiology and evaluation for the primary care physician. Can J Urol. 2008;15 Suppl 1:54.
2. El-Galley R, et al. Practical use of investigations in patients with hematuria. J Endourol. 2008;22:51.
3. Nieder AM, et al. Are patients with hematuria appropriately referred to urology? A multi-institutional questionnaire based survey. Urol Oncol. 2010;28:500.
4. Hollenbeck BK, et al. Delays in diagnosis and bladder cancer mortality. Cancer. 2010;116:5235.

Bladder cancer-induced hematuria is intermittent.

For this reason, a single urinalysis may overlook a tumor of the bladder, and effective screening necessitates repetitive testing [1].

1. Messing EM, et al. Hematuria screening for bladder cancer. J Occup Med. 1990;32:838.

A rare cause of hematuria is the nutcracker syndrome.

Caused by entrapment of the left renal vein between the aorta and the superior mesenteric artery leading to left renal hypertension and subsequent development of perirenal bleeding varicosities, the nutcracker syndrome can also cause proteinuria and flank pain [1, 2]. See Fig. 9.1.

1. Hanna HE, et al. Nutcracker syndrome: an underdiagnosed cause for hematuria? S D J Med. 1997;50:429.
2. Genc G, et al. A rare cause of recurrent hematuria in children: nutcracker syndrome. J Trop Pediatr. 2010;56:275.

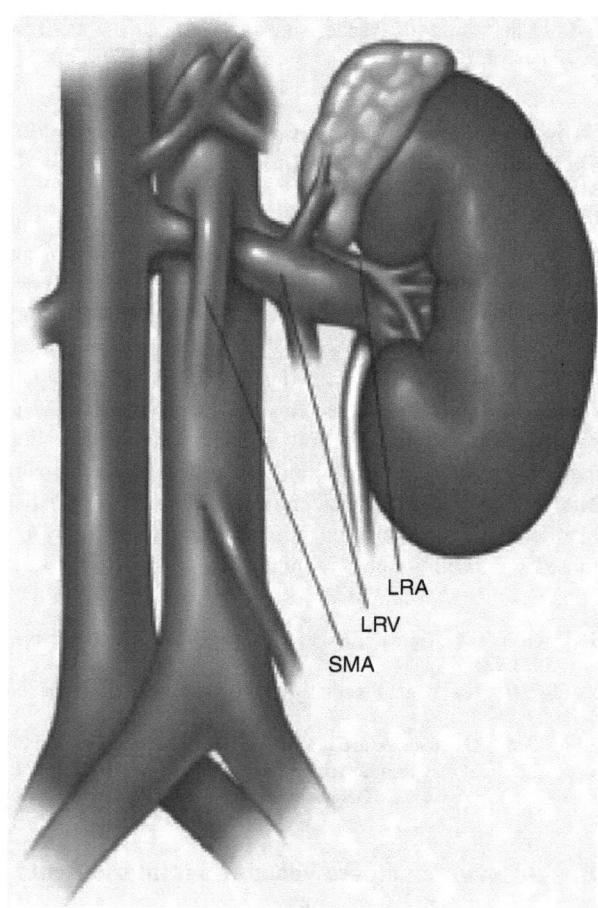

Fig. 9.1 Anatomy of the nutcracker syndrome. Superior mesenteric artery (*SMA*) drapes over the left renal vein (*LRV*). *LRA* left renal artery

Urinary Frequency, Nocturia, and Incontinence

Nocturia is the leading cause of disturbed sleep in older individuals.

In a study of 1,424 patients ages 55–84, 53 % reported problem of nocturia, more than four times the frequency of pain (12 %), the next most common cause of disturbed sleep [1]. Nocturia is, however, not only a problem for older individuals. Up to 20 %, perhaps more, of younger individuals wake consistently to void at least twice per night [2].

Nocturia can be due to a variety of causes including lower urinary tract obstruction, diabetes mellitus, anxiety, cardiovascular disease, and sleep apnea [3]. Especially noteworthy is the association between the frequency of nocturia and the severity of sleep apnea in older individuals [4]. In addition, in a study of 1,820 men ages 52 ± 9 years, nocturia twice or more often per night was found to be an age-independent risk factor for hip fractures in men ($p = 0.03$, chi^2 test) [5].

1. Bliwise DL, et al. Nocturia and disturbed sleep in the elderly. Sleep Med. 2009;10:540.
2. Bosch JL, et al. The prevalence and causes of nocturia. J Urol. 2010;184:440.
3. Weiss JP, et al. New aspects of the classification of nocturia. Curr Urol Rep. 2008;9:362.
4. Endeshaw YW, et al. Sleep-disordered breathing and nocturia in older adults. J Am Geriatr Soc. 204;52:957.
5. Temml C, et al. Nocturia is an age-independent risk factor for hip fractures in men. Neurourol Urodyn. 2009;28:949.

Even in younger men, asking about incontinence will yield a positive response in almost 1 in 20 individuals.

In a study of 5,297 men ages 20 years or older, the overall prevalence of moderate to severe urinary incontinence was 4.5 % (95 % CI 3.8, 5.4). Of course, the prevalence increased with age, up to 16 % in men age 75 years and older. The authors identify a variety of potential associated factors, including, in addition to age, chronic disease, race/ethnicity, education, depression, and prior diagnosis of enlarged prostate or cancer of the prostate [1].

In a study of 50 women, a 1-week urinary diary was found to be "a reliable method for assessing the frequency of voluntary micturitions and involuntary episodes of urine loss." Subjects kept the diaries for two consecutive weeks, which were compared. The authors report that key variables—diurnal and nocturnal micturition frequency and number of incontinent episodes—were reproducible and did not differ by urodynamic cause [2].

1. Markland AD, et al. Prevalence of urinary incontinence in men: results from the National Health and Nutrition Examination Survey. J Urol. 2010;184:1022.
2. Wyman JF, et al. The urinary diary in evaluation of incontinent women: a test-retest analysis. Obstet Gynecol. 1998;71:812.

Renal Failure

Acute renal failure (ARF), often iatrogenically caused, occurs more often than has been generally believed.

William Heberden (1710–1801) wrote: "The most dangerous ischuria is that in which the kidneys secrete no urine from the blood" [1]. Acute renal failure, aka acute kidney injury, is a somewhat poorly defined clinical diagnosis associated with an abrupt rise in the serum creatinine level. In a study of 748 cases of ARF, the cause was acute tubular necrosis in 45 %, prerenal disease in 21 %, acute-onset chronic renal failure in 12.7 %, and obstructive uropathy in 10 % [2]. ARF caused by obstructive uropathy requires bilateral blockage if the patient has two normal kidneys, and the most common cause in this setting is prostatic hypertrophy or cancer.

There may be a variety of comorbidities, including, in a study of 618 patients with ARF, coronary artery disease, 37 %; chronic kidney disease, 30 %; diabetes mellitus, 29 %; and chronic liver disease, 21 % [3].

1. Heberden W. Commentaries on the history and cure of diseases. 4th ed. London: Payne; 1802. Chap. 55.
2. Liaño F, et al. Epidemiology of acute renal failure: a prospective, multicenter, community-based study. Kidney Int. 1996;50:811.
3. Mehta RL, et al. Spectrum of acute renal failure in the intensive care unit: the PICARD experience. Kidney Int. 2004;66:1613.

If you had to choose just one noninvasive test to help identify the cause of ARF, it should be microscopic examination of the urine sediment.

ARF patients whose urine sediment contains granular and epithelial cell casts probably have acute tubular necrosis. Just one red cell cast indicates the presence of glomerulonephritis or vasculitis, which also may cause proteinuria, lipiduria, and dysmorphic RBCs. See Fig. 9.2. Abundant pyuria indicates infection, while a normal urinalysis in the setting of acutely elevated creatinine levels suggests other possibilities such as prerenal disease, obstructive uropathy, heart failure, or cirrhosis of the liver [1–3].

1. Lameire N, et al. Acute renal failure. Lancet. 2005;365:417.
2. Schrier RW, et al. Acute renal failure: definitions, diagnosis, pathogenesis, and therapy. J Clin Invest. 2004;114:5.
3. Chesney RW. Acute renal failure: diagnosis. Peds Rev. 1995;16:101.

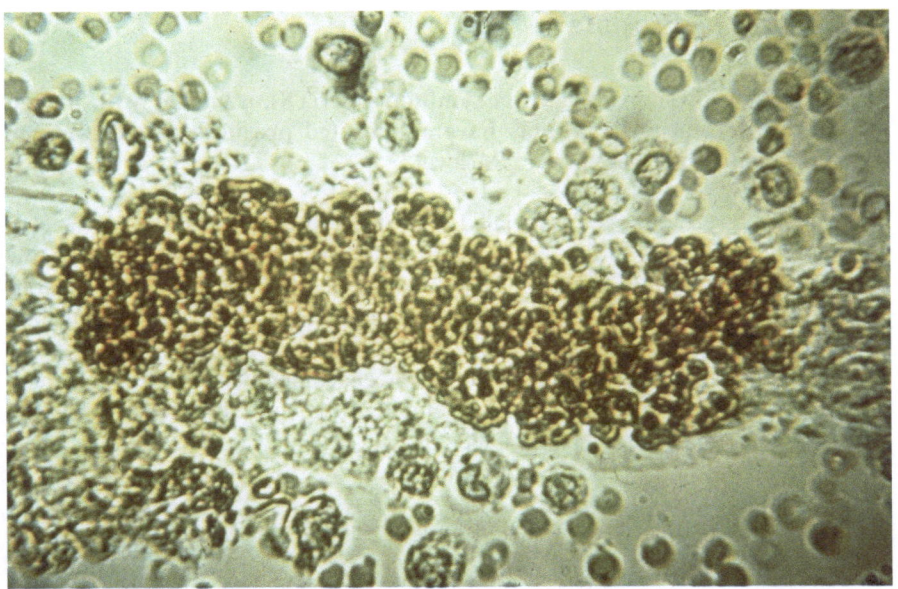

Fig. 9.2 Red blood cell cast in acute poststreptococcal glomerulonephritis

The lowly and inexpensive urinary dipstick is a useful screening tool to identify patients with rapid kidney function decline (RKFD).

In a study of 2,574 subjects followed for a median time of 7 years, use of the urinary dipstick to identify proteinuria "correctly identified progression status for 90.8 % of patients, mislabeled 1.5 % as RKFD, and missed 7.7 % with eventual RKFD" [1].

1. Clark WF. Dipstick proteinuria as a screening strategy to identify rapid renal decline. J Am Soc Nephrol. 2011;22:1729.

Diseases of the Prostate

In a setting of lower urinary tract symptoms (LUTS), a patient with benign prostatic hyperplasia (BPH) may have an elevated prostatic specific antigen (PSA) level and an elevated free PSA level.

The total PSA, a biomarker associated with prostate cancer, can be elevated in patients with BPH [1]. In this setting, a prostate cancer patient may have a low free PSA level. However, based on a 9-year study of 1,709 men, Meigs et al. conclude, "Elevated free PSA levels predict clinical BPH independent of total PSA levels" [2].

In the latter cited study, high levels of physical activity and, curiously, cigarette smoking seemed to reduce the odds of developing BPH, while heart disease and use of beta-blocker medication increased the risk [2].

1. Roehrborn CG, et al. Definition of at-risk patients: baseline variables. BJU Int. 2006;97 Suppl 2:7.
2. Meigs JB, et al. Risk factors for clinical benign prostatic hyperplasia in a community-based population of healthy aging men. J Clin Epidemiol. 2001;54:935.

If acute urinary retention develops suddenly in the setting of BPH, review the patient's medication list.

A recent study demonstrated a risk of acute urinary retention in patients taking both short- and long-acting inhaled anticholinergic medications [1]. Other drugs that can precipitate acute urinary retention in the BPH patient include medications taken for allergic rhinitis and colds: ephedrine, pseudoephedrine, phenylpropanolamine, and antihistamines such as chlorpheniramine and diphenhydramine [2].

1. Stephenson A, et al. Inhaled anticholinergic drug therapy and the risk of acute urinary retention in chronic obstructive pulmonary disease: a population-based study. Arch Intern Med. 2011;23:914.
2. Lehman JM, et al. Pharmacotherapy of allergic rhinitis. Allergy Front. 2010;5:19.

Advising patients about decisions regarding PSA testing requires up-to-date information and clear communication.

With dueling guidelines and the specter of missing a cancer diagnosis versus the hazards of overtreatment of prostate tumors, how to advise patients is less than

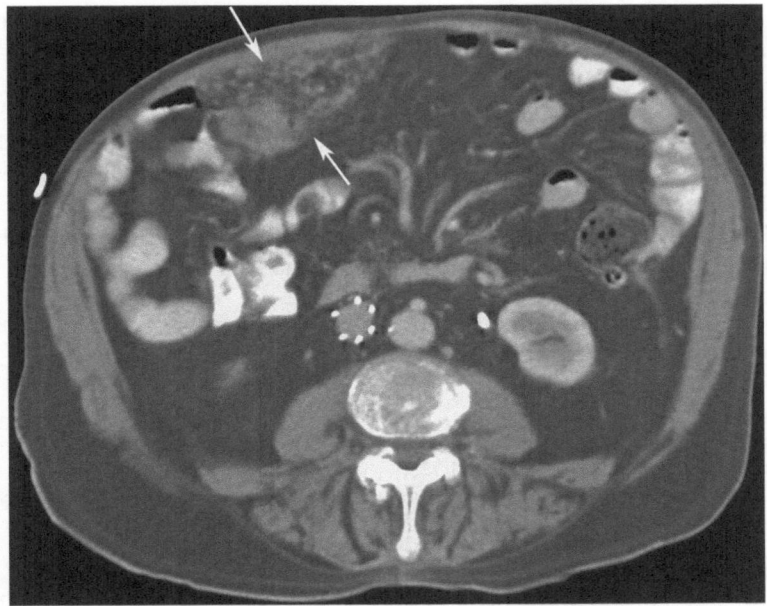

Fig. 9.3 Prostate cancer in a 75-year-old man. CT image demonstrates omental infiltration (*arrows*) seen in the absence of ascites or other signs of peritoneal carcinomatosis. Note the presence of an inferior vena cava filter

crystal clear. See Fig. 9.3. Although I am sure that things will change before the ink is dry on this page of the book, here are some facts that may prove helpful:

European Randomized Study of Screening for Prostate Cancer (ERSPC) trial: The ERSPC trial, aka the Göteborg study, involved 20,000 men, half invited for PSA testing every 2 years beginning in 1995 and up to the median age of 69 and half not invited. At the end of 14 years, prostate cancer mortality was reduced almost by half in those screened with PSA, in the face of a substantial risk of overdiagnosis [1].

National Health Interview Survey (NHIS) study: In this study, authors found PSA testing performed on 30.7 % of elderly men with low life expectancy, strongly suggesting over- testing [2].

Use of a single PSA screen suggested: Lilja et al. collected blood from 21,277 men and followed them more a median of 23 years. They suggest: "A single PSA determination at or before age 50 predicts advanced prostate cancer diagnosed up to 30 years later" [3].

Lower PSA threshold proposed: Presenting at a 2011 Genitourinary Cancers Symposium, Bul reported on 15,758 screened men 55–74 years old with an initial PSA level below 3.0 ng/mL. When this cohort was followed over up to 11 years, there were 23 cancer- related deaths. Among these 23 men, "an initial PSA level of 2.0–2.9 ng/mL was 7.6 times more likely to result in death than an initial level below 1.0 ng/mL, and was 4 times more likely to result in death than an initial level of 1.0–1.9 ng/mL." In addition, the suggestion is made that men with initial PSA levels below 1.0 ng/mL (45 % of the sample) might need screening at longer intervals than currently recommended by some guidelines, perhaps up to every 8 years [4].

The conclusion from all of this is: Decisions regarding PSA screening should be personalized, with the patient involved in informed decision-making.

1. Hugosson J, et al. Mortality results from the Göteborg randomized population-based prostate-cancer screening trial. Lancet. 2010;11:725.
2. Drazer MW, et al. Population-based patterns and predictors of prostate-specific antigen screening among older men in the United States. J Clin Oncol. 2011;29:1736.
3. Lilja H, et al. Prediction of significant prostate cancer diagnosed 20 to 30 years later with a single measure of prostate-specific antigen at or before age 50. Cancer. 2011;15:1210.
4. Bul M. Oral abstract. Presented at 2011 genitourinary cancers symposium, Orlando, Feb 2011.

Digital rectal examination (DRE) causes a numerically small but statistically significant rise in serum PSA levels.

I found three studies with similar results. All found "statistically significant" rises in total PSA following DRE. Here are the figures for one of them. Cevik et al. conducted a prospective study of 50 men ages 42–75 with symptoms of lower urinary tract outflow obstruction, with blood samples taken prior to, 30 min following, and 24 h following DRE. The mean PSA prior to DRE was 4.09 ± 0.67 ng/mL (range 0.2–19.47). Thirty minutes following DRE, the mean PSA value was 4.50 ± 0.63 (range 0.15–17.75). The mean 24-h PSA value was 4.28 ± 0.68 (range 0.23–24.12). For the record, the eventual diagnosis in these 50 men is: five had prostate cancer and 45 had BPH [1–3].

1. Cevik I, et al. Short-term effect of digital rectal examination on serum prostate-specific antigen levels: a prospective study. Eur Urol. 1996;29:403.
2. Collins GN, et al. The effect of digital rectal examination, flexible cystoscopy and prostatic biopsy on free and total prostatic specific antigen, and the free-to-total prostate specific antigen ratio in clinical practice. J Urol. 1997;157:1744.
3. Lechevallier E, et al. Effect of digital rectal examination on serum complexed and free prostate specific antigen and percentage of free prostate specific antigen. Urology. 1999;54:857.

Relative finger lengths suggest prostate cancer risk.

Rahman et al. studied the cancer risk versus the right-hand pattern in 1,542 men with prostate cancer, compared with 3,044 men without prostate cancer. The suggestion is that the relative lengths of digits are fixed in utero, perhaps as an indicator for intrauterine testosterone levels.

They found a reduced incidence of prostate cancer in men whose index finger was longer than the ring finger, suggesting "a protective effect with a 33 % risk reduction (OR 0.67; 95 % CI 0.57–80)" [1]. This raises the question: Shall we examine relative finger lengths in making individualized decisions about PSA testing?

1. Rahman AA, et al. Hand pattern indicates prostate cancer risk. Br J Cancer. 2011;104:175.

Disorders of the Scrotal Contents

Although we think of varicocele as classically left-sided, in some populations there is a higher incidence of right-sided and bilateral varicocele.

Varicocele occurs in up to 15 % of adolescent boys and young men and, based on physical examination reports, is considered overwhelmingly to be on the left side, owing to the anatomy of the left spermatic vein. Some patients will report aching discomfort, especially following activity. We have always taught that an isolated right-sided varicocele suggests the possible presence of some obstruction to venous return, such as a tumor or thrombosis of the renal vein. But newer imaging methods are revealing that many varicoceles are not solely left-sided.

Many men with varicoceles have impaired fertility, a problem likely to bring them to medical attention. In a study of 286, such infertile men using contact thermography, Doppler sonography, and venography, 255 (89.2 %) were found to have varicoceles. Of these, 45 occurred on the left, 4 on the right, and 206 bilaterally [1].

In a study of 354 men with a mean age of 60.7 years using physical examination, varicocele was found on the left only in 78, on the right only in 4, and bilaterally in 70 subjects examined, yielding a 42 % prevalence of varicocele in this population of older individuals. They also found that bilateral varicoceles were especially likely to be associated with softer, smaller testes, but with no direct decrease in serum testosterone levels [2].

And just to pay tribute to a zebra cause of varicoceles, Sayfan et al. report a case of right-sided varicocele as part of situs inversus [3].

1. Gat Y, et al. Varicocele: a bilateral disease. Fertil Steril. 2004;81:424.
2. Canales BK, et al. Prevalence and effect of varicoceles in an elderly population. Urology. 2005;66:627.
3. Sayfan J, et al. Right-sided varicocele associated with situs inversus. Fert Steril. 1978;30:716.

Acute scrotal pain requires urgent diagnostic attention and often surgery.

The reason for the urgency is the specter of spermatic cord torsion/testicular torsion, especially problematic because it occurs in boys and young men whose reproductive years generally are ahead of them. What is the diagnostic spectrum of acute scrotal pain? There have been a number of studies following "acute scrotum" patients to eventual diagnosis. Here is one from Finland involving 388 boys under age 17 presenting consecutively with acute scrotal pain, all of whom underwent urgent surgery to assure correct diagnosis and therapy. In this series, 174 patients (45 %) had torsion of the testicular appendage, 100 (26 %) had spermatic cord torsion, 38 (10 %) had epididymitis, 32 (8 %) had incarcerated inguinal hernias, and 44 (11 %) had other disorders. The authors note that all torsed testicles were saved if surgery was performed within 6 h, but only half were saved when pain was present more than 6 but less than 12 h [1]. See Fig. 9.4. Spermatic cord torsion and incarcerated inguinal hernia must both be listed as *must-not-miss diagnoses*.

1. Makela E, et al. A 19-year review of pediatric patients with acute scrotum. Scand J Surg. 2007;96:62.

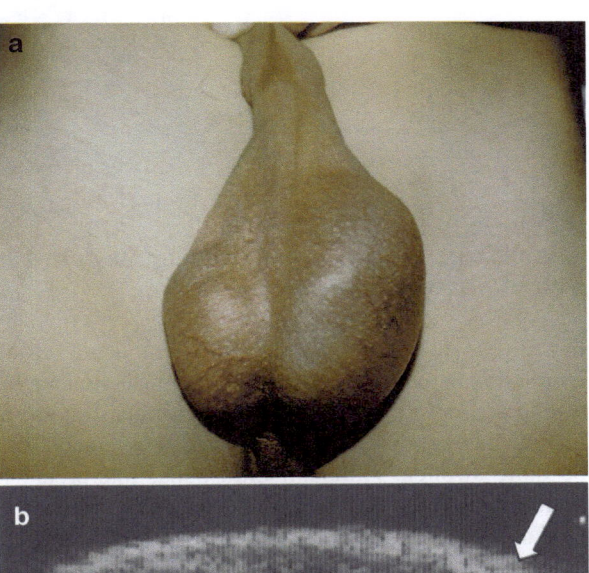

Fig. 9.4 (**a**) Torsion of the left spermatic cord in an 18-year-old boy, who reported more than 10 days of symptoms. Enlarged left hemi-scrotum and a darkish supra-testicular mass. (**b**) Thickening of the scrotal wall (*arrows*) caused by edema. (**c**) Intraoperative view showing the twisting on the spermatic cord (*arrows*) and the hemorrhagic and dark necrotic testis

Fig. 9.4 (continued)

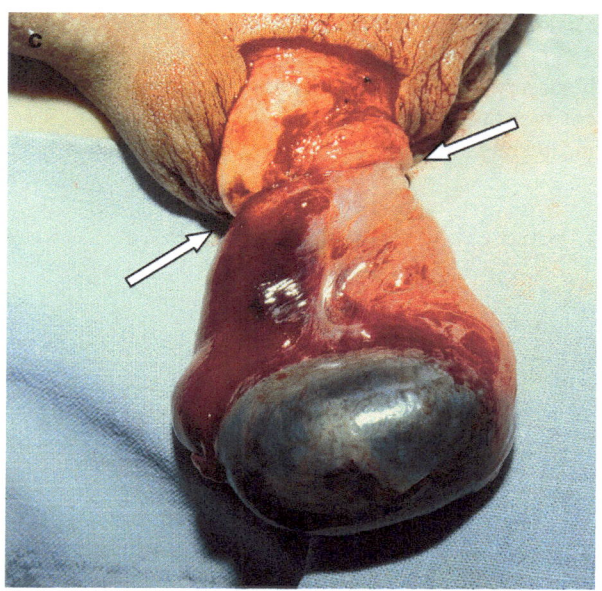

The presence of the cremasteric reflex may prove helpful in assessing the boy with suspected acute testicular torsion.

In a 7-year study involving 245 boys with acute scrotal swelling, there was 100 % correlation between the presence of the ipsilateral cremasteric reflex and absence of testicular torsion [1]. Physical findings suggesting the diagnosis of testicular torsion include the presence of a high-riding, transversely oriented testicle which may also be quite swollen. Although ultrasound, interpreted in conjunction with clinical findings, may be useful in diagnosis, you should not waste valuable time if the modality is not promptly available. In the end, a presumptive diagnosis of testicular torsion calls for immediate surgery [2].

1. Rabinowitz R. The importance of the cremasteric reflex in acute scrotal swelling in children. J Urol. 1984;132:89.
2. Yang C, et al. Testicular torsion in children: a 20-year retrospective study in a single institution. Sci World J. 2011;11:362.

Testicular cancer (TC) may present with any of several symptoms: a self-discovered painless mass, heaviness in the scrotum, or localized aching or pain.

The most common malignancy of men age 20–35 years; TC has a remarkable cure rate, nearly 99 %, if diagnosed early, making it another urologic *must-not-miss diagnosis* [1]. Risk factors that, if present, support a suspicion that a patient with scrotal symptoms has a tumor include a family history of TC, a history of cryptorchidism or a contralateral tumor, Klinefelter syndrome, infertility, tobacco use, and white race [1, 2]. In almost all cases, the next diagnostic step should be ultrasonography [2, 3].

1. Shaw J. Diagnosis and treatment of testicular cancer. Am Fam Physician. 2008;77:469.
2. Albers P, et al. Guidelines on testicular cancer. Eur Urol. 2008;53:478.
3. Winter T. There is a mass in the scrotum—what does it mean? Evaluation of the scrotal mass. Ultrasound Quarterly. 2009;25:195.

Cryptorchidism, testicular trauma, orchitis (including mumps orchitis), and orchiectomy are all risk factors for male breast cancer.

Male breast cancer accounts for about 1 % of all breast cancers in either gender and about 1 % of all cancers of any type in men. Risk factors include a family history of breast cancer, Klinefelter syndrome, and radiation exposure [1, 2]. The classic presentation of male breast cancer is a painless lump, with bloody nipple discharge noted in 75 % of cases with malignancies [1].

Kijima et al. report a 64-year-old man with bilateral breast cancer following hormone therapy—androgen blockade followed by use of an antiandrogen agent for prostate cancer [3].

1. Sani MI, et al. Male breast cancer: a case report. Internet J Surg. 2009;21(2). Available at: http://www.ispub.com/journal/the_internet_journal_of_surgery/volume_21_number_2_1/article/male-breast-cancer-a-case-report.html.
2. Weiss JR, et al. Epidemiology of male breast cancer. Cancer Epidemiol Biomarkers Prev. 2005;14:20.
3. Kijima Y, et al. Synchronous bilateral breast cancer in a male patient following hormone therapy for breast cancer. Int J Clin Oncol. 2009;14:253.

Progressive necrosis of the skin and subcutaneous tissues of the scrotum and perineum describes Fournier syndrome.

A rare, but potentially lethal polymicrobial necrotizing soft tissue infection, Fournier syndrome is chiefly a disease of men and is sometimes called idiopathic scrotal gangrene [1]. In one series 21 % of cases involved the female perineum [2]. Prompt diagnosis is followed by antibiotic therapy and robust debridement [3].

1. Rudolph R, et al. Fournier's syndrome: synergistic gangrene of the scrotum. Am J Surg. 1975;5:591.
2. Norton KS, et al. Management of Fournier's gangrene: an eleven year retrospective analysis of early recognition, diagnosis, and treatment. Am Surg. 2002;68:709.
3. Oo A, et al. Use of adjunctive treatments in improving patient outcome in Fournier's gangrene. Singapore Med. 2011;52:194.

Diseases Affecting the Penis

Many, perhaps even most, dermatoses that involve other areas can affect the skin of the penis.

There is a wide variety in the types of penile dermatoses. Here are some of them [1–3]:

Contact dermatitis: Those of us who have practiced in the Eastern US are well familiar with the painful blistering that can result when the poison ivy allergen is transferred from hands to penis.

Secondary syphilis: Syphilis, an old disease making a comeback, can cause penile lesions loaded with infectious spirochetes.

Psoriasis: Probably the most common inflammatory disorder of the penis, psoriasis causes scaly, erythematous plaques [2].

Herpes simplex virus: Look for clusters of vesicles on an erythematous base.

Condyloma acuminata: Also known as venereal warts, these infectious viral lesions are characterized by villous projections. See Fig. 9.5.

Scabies: The skin of the penis and scrotum offers a hospitable environment for *Sarcoptes scabiei*, aka the itch mite.

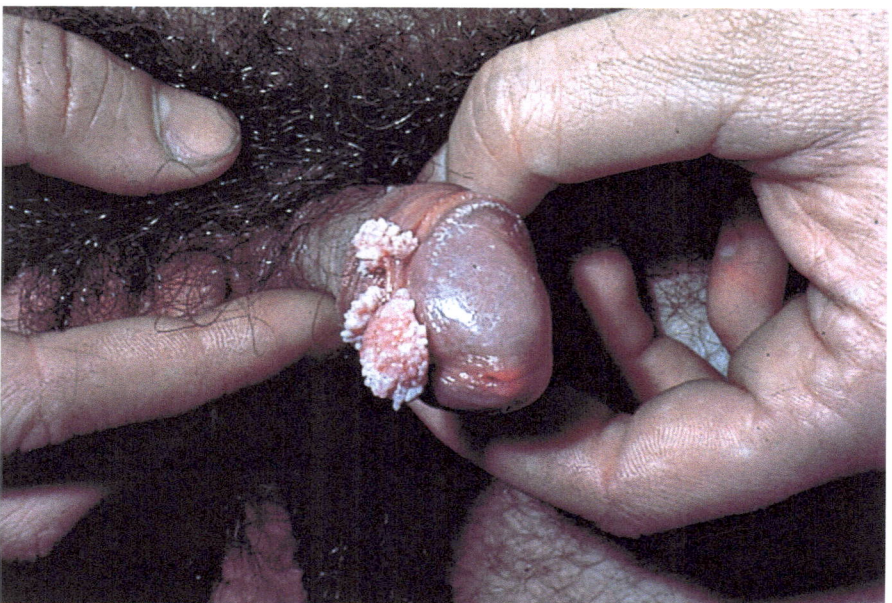

Fig. 9.5 Condyloma acuminata

Several of the diseases mentioned here highlight the need for gloved hands during the examination.

1. Buechner SA. Common skin disorders of the penis. BJU Int. 2002;90:498.
2. Goldman BD. Common dermatoses of the male genitalia. Postgrad Med J. 2000;108:89.
3. Nash E. Conditions affecting the penis. InnovAiT. 2010;3:38.

Squamous cell carcinoma in situ of the penis—erythroplasia of Queyrat and Bowen disease—cannot be excluded on physical examination alone.

The apparently benign appearance of squamous cell carcinoma in situ can lead to long delays in diagnosis as the disease progresses and until a biopsy is finally attained. The astute clinician will be highly suspicious of velvety red or keratotic plaques of the penis. With Bowen disease, there may be crusting and drainage. Prompt biopsy is indicated, even though lichen planus or psoriasis can have a similar appearance [1–3].

1. Duncan KO, et al. Epithelial precancerous lesions. Access Med. Available at: http://www.accessmedicine.com/content.aspx?aID=2981564.
2. Teichman JM, et al. Noninfectious penile lesions. Am Fam Physician. 2010;81:167.
3. Brown PB. Erythroplasia of Queyrat. Br J Plast Surg. 1966;19:378.

Routine physical examination may miss the presence of phimosis.

Phimosis, a condition in which the distal foreskin of the penis cannot be retracted over the glans, is physiologic in early childhood and absent in 99 % of young men age 17 and older. But that means that one in a hundred men have this problem, which would probably not be identified in the usual screening physical examination.

Phimosis is not an emergency, but paraphimosis is. Paraphimosis describes the condition when the foreskin is retracted proximal to the glans penis and cannot be returned to its normal position. Those men at greatest risk have a partial phimosis, setting the stage for entrapment. Causes include scarring following the trauma of forced foreskin retraction, piercing with various jewelry or other objects, crushing injuries, and balanoposthitis (inflammation of the glans and prepuce). In infants,

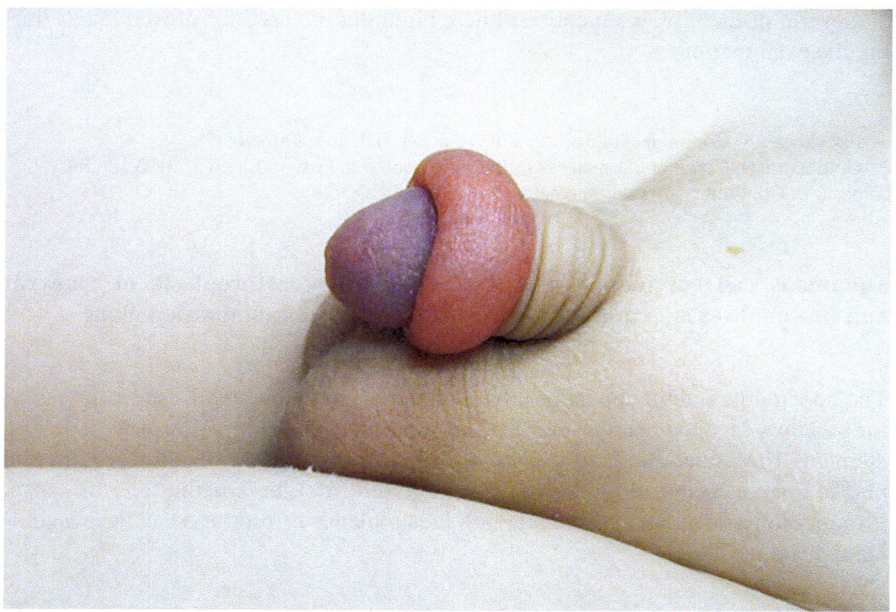

Fig. 9.6 Paraphimosis results when a tight foreskin is trapped in the retracted position and edema ensues

paraphimosis is most likely to occur as a caregiver retracts the foreskin to clean the glans penis. Because penile necrosis and autoamputation have been reported, urgent urologic referral of these patients is mandatory [1]. See Fig. 9.6.

1. Wiler J. Symptoms: dysuria. Emerg Med News. 2010;32:10.
2. Little B, et al. Treatment options for paraphimosis. Int J Clin Pract. 2005;59:591.
3. Raman SR, et al. Coital paraphimosis causing penile necrosis. Emerg Med J. 2008;25:454.

Selected Problems of the Kidney and Male Genitourinary System

Patients with lower urinary tract symptoms (LUTS)—frequency, nocturia, dysuria, and so forth—have a high incidence of erectile dysfunction (ED).

Erectile dysfunction, the inability to attain or maintain a penile erection of sufficient quality to permit satisfactory sexual intercourse, accounted for 25 % of male sexual problems reported in a study by Laumann et al. involving 1,491 patients [1, 2]. Patients, however, may hesitate to mention the problem: In the Laumann et al. study, less than one-quarter of patients with sexual problems had sought medical help [2].

Clinicians should be especially diligent in asking patients with LUTS about ED. A study of 1,274 men with LUTS revealed that 62 % of these individuals had erectile dysfunction [3]. In another study involving 17,068 men responding to the American Urological Association Symptom Index and queries about ED, Mondul et al. found an increased risk of ED with increasing severity of LUTS [4].

1. McVay KT. Erectile dysfunction. N Engl J Med. 2007;357:2472.
2. Laumann EO, et al. A population-based survey of sexual activity, sexual problems and associated help-seeking behavior patterns in mature adults in the United States of America. Int J Impotence Res. 2009;21:171.
3. Vallancien G, et al. Sexual dysfunction in 1274 European men suffering from lower urinary tract symptoms. J Urol. 2003;169:2257.
4. Mondul AM, et al. A prospective study of lower urinary tract symptoms and erectile dysfunction. J Urol. 2008;179:2231.

Making the diagnosis of ED may be important because of the company it keeps.

ED is considered a vascular disorder and suggests a risk of cardiovascular disease, especially in diabetic men. In a study of 2,306 type 2 diabetic subjects ages 54.2 ± 12.7 years followed for 1.7–7.1 years, the investigators found: "The incidence of CHD events was higher in men with ED than those without (19.7/1,000 person-years, 95 % CI 14.3–25.2 person-years vs. 9.5/1,000 person-years, 95 % CI 7.4–11.7 person-years)" [1].

A study in Belgium found hyperlipidemia common in ED patients and suggests that ED "might therefore serve as a sentinel event for coronary heart disease" [2].

ED is common in men with both hypothyroidism and hyperthyroidism, according to a study of 56 men with thyroid dysfunction, with the suggestion that the thyroid dysfunction might be the cause of the ED [3].

In a study involving 23,119 men, there was a higher likelihood of ED in men with restless leg syndrome, with more severe ED problems associated with higher frequency of nocturnal leg restless episodes [4].

In older men, ED may indicate the presence of testosterone deficiency, especially if they fail to respond to the use of phosphodiesterase (PDE) type 5 inhibitors [5, 6]. These testosterone-deficient ED patients may find that their ED responds to administration of testosterone, reported in one study to "convert over half of these men into phosphodiesterase type 5 responders" [6].

1. Ma RC, et al. Erectile dysfunction predicts coronary heart disease in type 2 diabetes. J Am Coll Cardiol. 2008;51:2045.
2. Roumeguere T, et al. Erectile dysfunction is associated with a high prevalence of hyperlipidemia and coronary heart disease risk. Eur Urol. 2033;44:355.
3. Krassas GE, et al. Erectile dysfunction in patients with hyper- and hypothyroidism: how common and should we treat? Endocrine Care. 2008;93:1815.
4. Gao X, et al. Restless leg syndrome and erectile dysfunction. Sleep. 2010;33:75.
5. Caretta N, et al. Erectile dysfunction in aging men: testosterone role in therapeutic protocols. J Endocrinol Invest. 2005;28:108.
6. Blute M, et al. Erectile dysfunction and testosterone deficiency. Front Horm Res. 2009;37:108.

An etiologic diagnosis can be made in approximately 40% of cases of priapism.

Priapism, generally described as a penile erection persisting for four or more hours in the absence of sexual stimulation, is often of unknown cause. You should, however, consider causes such as penile or perineal trauma, spinal cord trauma, sickle cell disease, pelvic infection, pelvic tumor, leukemia, and medication use [1]. Suspect medications include PDE type 5 inhibitors, as well as trazodone (Desyrel), which has been dubbed on the street "traz-erect" [1, 2]. A case of glucose-6-phosphate dehydrogenase deficiency-associated priapism has been reported [3].

There is urgency to the diagnosis of priapism, requiring identification of underlying hemodynamics [4]. Specifically, there are two types of priapism: nonischemic and ischemic. The former, often related to trauma, occurs less commonly than the ischemic type and is usually treated conservatively. Ischemic priapism, the more commonly occurring type, is likely to be painful and it carries a risk of ongoing ED. This type typically necessitates active procedural intervention [5].

1. Tanagho E, et al., editors. Smith's general urology. 17th ed. New York: McGraw Hill; 2007.
2. King SH, et al. Tadalafil-associated priapism. Urology. 2005;66:432.
3. Burnett AL, et al. Glucose-6-phosphate dehydrogenase deficiency: an etiology for idiopathic priapism? J Sex Med. 2008;5:237.
4. Broderick GA, et al. Priapism: pathogenesis, epidemiology, and management. J Sex Med. 2010;7:476.
5. Huang YC, et al. Evaluation and management of priapism: 2009 update. Nat Rev Urol. 2009;6:262.

Symptom patterns can suggest causative organisms in men with urethral discharge.

Urethritis causes various symptoms, such as itching, tingling, and dysuria. In a study of 154 men with urethritis, the men with gonococcal urethritis had more severe symptoms—especially heavy urethral discharge and cloudy, purulent discharge—than those with other types of urethritis: chlamydial urethritis, nongonococcal, and non-chlamydial. The diagnosis in all of these subjects was confirmed by the nucleic acid amplification test [1].

1. Takahashi S, et al. Analysis of clinical manifestations of male patients with urethritis. J Infect Chemother. 2006;12:283.

Urine color can provide important diagnostic clues.

Urochrome is the pigment that gives urine its characteristic pale yellow to honey-colored hue. But the presence of other substances can cause some very interesting urine colors:

Blue-green urine: When a patient has blue-green urine, think first of drugs. One offender is methylene blue, found in several urinary antispasmodic products such as Prosed-DS and the discontinued product Urised [1]. Methylene blue may also be found in traditional Chinese medicine [2]. Blue-green urine has also been reported in patients taking metoclopramide (Reglan) [3], amitriptyline (Elavil) [4], and the inorganic herbicides mefenacet and imazosulfuron [5]. Other possible causes of blue-green urine include triamterene (Dyrenium), cimetidine (Tagamet), promethazine (Phenergan), and indomethacin [6].

Orange urine: Think again of drugs, especially the urinary tract anesthetics phenazopyridine (Pyridium) and ethoxazene (Serenium) and the antibiotic rifampin (Rifadin), sometimes prescribed as meningitis prophylaxis to exposed individuals. Dark-yellow urine bordering on orange can also follow ingestion of large amounts carrots or vitamins B2 (riboflavin) or C [6, 7].

Pink-red urine: Think first of blood in the urine, one of the alarm symptoms mentioned above. Once the presence of blood has been excluded, the search for other causes can begin. Ask about the consumption of beets, blackberries, or rhubarb [6, 8]. Drugs that can cause pink-red urine include phenytoin (Dilantin); phenothiazines; phenolphthalein, the active ingredient in Ex-Lax; and the hypnotic agent propofol (Diprivan), which achieved notoriety as the probable cause of death of singer Michael Jackson [6, 7, 9].

Brown-black urine: I think first of the possibility of bilirubin or myoglobin in the urine. Porphyria cutanea tarda must be considered [10]. Medication culprits that have been linked to dark urine include methyldopa (Aldomet), nitrofurantoin (Furadantin), methocarbamol (Robaxin), furazolidone (Furoxone), antimalarials primaquine and chloroquine, and laxatives containing senna and cascara. Foods have also been implicated in dark brown urine, specifically the robust consumption of fava beans or rhubarb (6, 7, 11).

1. Cotton SW, et al. The case of the blue-green urine. Clin Chem. 2011;57:4.
2. Lam CW, et al. A case of green urine due to a traditional Chinese medicine containing methylene blue. N Z Med J. 2010;123:71
3. Pak F. Green urine: an association with metoclopramide. Nephrol Dial Transplant. 2004;19:2677.
4. Greenberg M. Verdoglobinuria. Clin Toxicol. 2008;46:485.
5. Shim YS, et al. A case of green urine after ingestion of herbicides. Korean J Intern Med. 2008;23:42.
6. Slawson M. Thirty-three drugs that can discolor urine and/or stools. RN. 1980;43:40.
7. Raymond JR, et al. Abnormal urine color: differential diagnosis. South Med J. 1988;81:837.
8. Saran R, et al. An unusual cause of pink urine. Nephrol Dial Transplant. 1998;13:1579.
9. Rosenberg JW. Phenytoin and red urine. JAMA. 1983;250:1842.
10. Rich MW. Porphyria cutanea tarda: don't forget to look at the urine. Postgrad Med. 1999;105:208.
11. Noll WW, et al. Causes of dark urine. JAMA. 1980;243:2398.

Chapter 10
The Female Reproductive System

*The surgical cycle in woman: Appendix removed, right kidney
hooked up, gallbladder taken out, gastroenterostomy, clean
sweep of the uterus and adnexa.*

Sir William Osler (1849–1919) [1]

Contents

R.B. Taylor, *Diagnostic Principles and Applications*,
DOI 10.1007/978-1-4614-1111-6_10, © Springer Science+Business Media, LLC 2013

The Osler quote above seems both humorous and just a little cynical. Sir William had a rich sense of humor; he was the man who once published a totally fanciful case report of "penis captivus" under the pseudonym Egerton Yorrik Davis [2]. As to invasive procedures inflicted upon our female patients, today Osler might add breast augmentation, Botox injections, and facelift. Of course, Osler was a "medical doctor," and not a surgeon.

1. Osler W. Quoted in: Sir William Osler: aphorisms from his bedside teachings and writings. Bean WB, editor. New York: Henry Schuman; 1950.
2. Taylor RB. White coat tales: medicine's heroes, heritage, and misadventures. New York: Springer; 2008. p. 25.

Vaginitis

The cause of vaginitis can be suggested using readily available clinical methods.

Vaginitis—inflammation of the vagina and related structures—is a manifestation and not a diagnosis until the specific cause is determined. Although causes can include foreign body reaction, contact dermatitis/vaginitis, atrophic vaginitis, cervicitis, and desquamative inflammatory dermatitis, the three most common infectious causes are bacterial vaginosis (BV), trichomoniasis, and vulvovaginal candidiasis (VVC) [1, 2].

An early question must be asked: Is this simply a normal, physiologic discharge, generally described as clear or white, lacking offensive characteristics, and varying with the menstrual cycle? [3]. Or is it something else?

Although symptoms alone cannot distinguish among possible causes of vaginitis, here are some diagnostic pearls that might be provided by the history and physical examination, based on a structured literature review [4]:

Perceived odor: The absence of a perceived odor makes the diagnosis of BV unlikely (LR 0.07; 95 % CI 0.01–0.51).

Itching: The patient's lack of itching makes the diagnosis of VVC less likely (range of LRs 0.18 (95 % CI 0.05–0.70) to 0.79 (95 % CI 0.72–0.87)).

Inflammatory signs: The presence of local inflammatory signs makes the diagnosis of VVC more likely (range of LRs 2.1 (95 % CI 1.5–2.8) to 8.4 (95 % CI 2.3–3.1)).

Presence of odor on examination: The presence of a pungent "high cheese" aroma on examination suggests the presence of BV (LR 3.2; 95 % CI 2.1–4.7).

Absence of odor on examination: This suggests the diagnosis of VVC (LR 2.9; 95 % CI 2.4–5.0).

Adding the whiff test (sniffing a fishy odor released when potassium hydroxide [KOH] is added to the vaginal discharge), determination of the vaginal pH using a pH strip, and office microscopy provides even more diagnostic clues.

Positive whiff test: A positive whiff test has a sensitivity of 94.1 % and specificity of 87.5 % in the diagnosis of BV [5].

Vaginal pH: A pH < 4.5 and a positive or negative whiff had a sensitivity of 83.7 % in the diagnosis of VVC [5].

Positive whiff test and vaginal pH > 5.4: This combination points to a diagnosis of trichomoniasis, confirmed by finding motile trichomonads on microscopy [2].

1. Quan M. Vaginitis: diagnosis and management. Postgrad Med. 2010;122:117.
2. Hainer BL, et al. Vaginitis: diagnosis and treatment. Am Fam Phys. 2011;83:807.
3. Spence D, et al. Vaginal discharge. BMJ. 2007;335:1147.
4. Anderson MR, et al. Evaluation of vaginal complaints. JAMA. 2004;291:1368.
5. Thulkar J, et al. Utility of pH test and whiff test in syndromic approach to abnormal vaginal discharge. Indian J Med Res. 2010;131:445.

Abnormal Uterine Bleeding

Up to half of all women with menorrhagia may have bleeding disorders.

Menorrhagia—menstrual flow exceeding 7 days and/or total blood loss >80 mL—affects about 5 % of women of reproductive age in Western countries each year [1]. What's more, 30 % of US women receive a hysterectomy before age 60, and the presenting complaint in 50–70 % of these women is menorrhagia [2]. But not all abnormal uterine bleeding is caused by fibroids.

In the half or more of menorrhagic women without coagulopathy or systemic disease, the leading diagnoses are uterine fibroids (especially in women under age 40), endometrial polyps (in women over age 40), and dysfunctional uterine bleeding (indicating that no identifiable cause of menorrhagia could be found.) [1]

However, in a study of 115 adolescent and perimenopausal women with menorrhagia, 47 % were found to have hemostatic abnormalities including platelet dysfunction, von Willebrand disease, and coagulation factor deficiencies [3]. Other non-gynecologic causes of menorrhagia to be considered include anticoagulant use, hypothyroidism, and severe liver disease. Of course, gynecologic and non-gynecologic diseases can coexist. And there is always the possibility of a complication of early pregnancy.

1. Hurskainen R, et al. Diagnosis and treatment of menorrhagia. Acta Obstet Gynecol Scand. 2007;86:749.
2. El-hemaidi I, et al. Menorrhagia and bleeding disorders. Curr Opin Obstet Gynecol. 2007;19:513.
3. Philipp CS, et al. Age and the prevalence of bleeding disorders in women with menorrhagia. Obstet Gynecol. 2005;105:61.

In patients describing prolonged and/or heavy menstrual flow, the patient's estimate of blood loss may be more helpful than some believe.

In their review article, Hurskainen et al. assert, "The subject's own assessment of the amount of menstrual blood loss does not generally reflect the true amount" [1]. However, Heath et al. used a menstrual recall method to estimate the extent of menstrual loss compared to a weighted reference method. They found that their menstrual recall method could differentiate between low and high levels of menstrual blood loss in the 29 young adult women studied [2].

1. Hurskainen R, et al. Diagnosis and treatment of menorrhagia. Acta Obstet Gynecol Scand. 2007;86:749.
2. Heath AL, et al. Validation of a questionnaire method for estimating the extent of menstrual blood loss in young adult women. J Trace Elem Med Biol. 1999;12:231.

Amenorrhea

Look for the presence of a genetic or anatomic abnormality in girls with primary amenorrhea.

Here I will discuss two such disorders: Müllerian agenesis and the Kallmann syndrome. Müllerian agenesis, aka uterovaginal atresia, the Mayer–Rokitansky–Küster–Hauser syndrome, or simply the Rokitansky syndrome, is the second most common cause of primary amenorrhea, trailing only gonadal dysgenesis, including Turner syndrome. These girls, who are chromosomally 46,XX develop normal secondary sexual characteristics, but fail to menstruate owing to absence of a uterus and a shortened vagina ending in a blind pouch [1]. See Fig. 10.1.

The Kallmann syndrome, which can occur in both sexes, combines hypogonadotropic hypogonadism and anosmia or hyposmia. Hearing loss may also occur, as

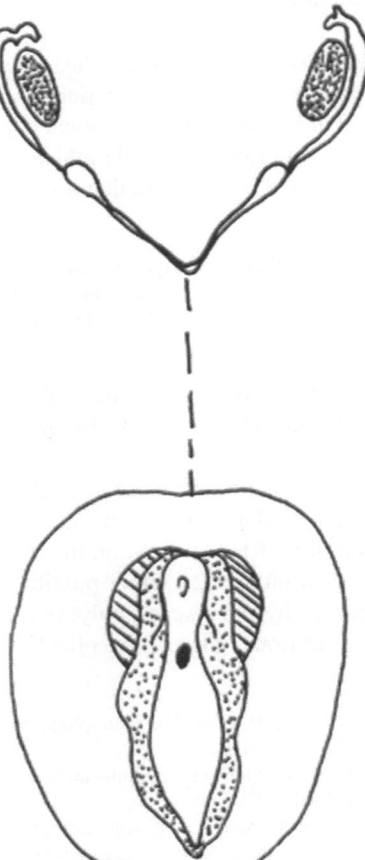

Fig. 10.1 Schematic representation of genital anomalies encountered in Mayer–Rokitansky–Küster–Hauser syndrome. The rudimentary uterine horn consists of muscle bundles and some endometrial tissue. The tubes and ovaries are normally displayed. The perineal anatomy shows a female phenotype but no vaginal opening

described in Chap. 5. Primary amenorrhea and delayed or underdeveloped secondary sexual characteristics prompt evaluation at the time of expected puberty. Curiously, the patient, having never had a normal sense of smell, may be unaware of her (or his) anosmia or hyposmia [2, 3].

Other structural causes of primary amenorrhea include an imperforate hymen and transverse vaginal septum, both likely to cause increasing pain at the time menstrual flow from the uterus begins.

1. Carranza-Lira S, et al. Rokitansky syndrome and MURCS association—clinical features and basis for diagnosis. Int J Fertil Women's Med. 1999;44:250.
2. Kaplan JD, et al. Clues to an early diagnosis of Kallman syndrome. Am J Med Gen. 2010;152A:2796.
3. Dodé C, et al. Kallman syndrome. Eur J Hum Genetics. 2009;17:139.

Adolescent athletes and dancers may experience delayed menarche and/or amenorrhea.

Exercise-induced amenorrhea in young female athletes is well recognized. This syndrome has also been reported in ballet dancers, who engage in vigorous activity and in whom thinness is valued [1]. Amenorrhea, eating disorders, and bone density loss comprise the female athlete triad, which Warren et al. propose are related to nutritional issues more than to hypoestrogenism [2].

1. Frisch RE, et al. Delayed menarche and amenorrhea in ballet dancers. N Engl J Med. 1980;303:17.
2. Warren MP, et al. Exercise-induced amenorrhea and bone health in the adolescent athlete. Ann New York Acad Sci. 2008;1135:244.

Hypothalamic amenorrhea—absence of menses owing to eating disorders, athletics, or chronic illness—heads the list of causes of secondary amenorrhea.

The above, of course, assumes that the possibility of pregnancy has been excluded. In hypothalamic amenorrhea, energy deficits cause suppressed hypothalamic secretion of GnRH [1]. Next on the list of suspected causes are hyperprolactinemia and ovarian failure [2]. Other possibilities include Sheehan syndrome, Asherman syndrome, thyroid disease, polycystic ovary syndrome, and inappropriate use of androgens or oral contraceptive pills [2, 3].

1. Golden NH, et al. The pathophysiology of amenorrhea in the adolescent. Ann N Y Acad Sci. 2008;1135:163.
2. Reindollar RH, et al. Adult-onset amenorrhea: a study of 262 patients. Am J Obstet Gynecol. 1986;155:531.
3. Master-Hunter T, et al. Amenorrhea: evaluation and treatment. Am Fam Phys. 2006;73:1374.
4. Stein IF, et al. Amenorrhea associated with bilateral polycystic ovaries. Am J Obstet Gynecol. 1935;29:181.

Pelvic Pain

If estimates are true, at least one of the next ten women of reproductive age seen in your office will report chronic pelvic pain (CPP), if only you ask.

Pelvic pain, acute or chronic, is a very common clinical problem, which occurs in a variety of diseases, including interstitial cystitis, pelvic inflammatory disease (PID), and ovarian torsion, to name just a few. Chronic pelvic pain—noncyclic pain present for 6 months or longer and severe enough to prompt medical care or cause disability—has an estimated 15 % prevalence in women of childbearing age [1]. Based on a sample of women undergoing laparoscopy for non-pain-related reasons, Zondervan estimated a 39 % prevalence of CPP [2]. Risk factors for CPP include pelvic inflammatory disease, previous cesarean section, sexual abuse, heavy menstrual flow, drug or alcohol misuse, and psychological disorders [3].

Pelvic congestion syndrome, related to pelvic vein varices, has been reported as a not-uncommon cause of CPP. The usual diagnostic tools such as B-mode ultrasound and laparoscopy are likely to be unhelpful, and newer methods, such as time resolved magnetic resonance imaging (MRI), are being used increasingly [4, 5].

In a review paper from authors at the European Training Center for Gynecologic Endoscopy and Gynecologic Surgery, two authors state, regarding women with CPP undiagnosed following a general gynecologic examination: "As in nearly one-third of the cases the reason for the (chronic pelvic) pain is an endometriosis, and in another third, adhesions are responsible for the pain, the biggest part can be diagnosed and treated by laparoscopy. If laparoscopically no reason can be found, it is advisable to send the patient to a psychosomatic physician, who can then start a correspondingly differentiated diagnosis and therapy" [6]. I have concerns about these statements. Let's see: two-thirds of all patients with previously undiagnosed CPP have the two diseases mentioned, both of which conveniently can serve as indications for laparoscopy. Is this a case of "if the only tool you have is a hammer, everything you see looks like a nail?" I recall the Oslerism: "Adhesions are the last refuge of the diagnostically destitute." And finally, if the patient does not have one of the two procedurally oriented diagnoses, then off the patient goes into the psychosomatic neverland. Interesting paper.

1. Meltzer-Brody S, et al. Psychiatric comorbidity in women with chronic pelvic pain. CNS Spectr. 2011;16:29.
2. Zondervan KT, et al. The prevalence of chronic pelvic pain in women in the United Kingdom: a systematic review. Br J Obstet Gynecol. 1998;105:93.
3. Latthe P, et al. Factors predisposing women to chronic pelvic pain: systematic review. BMJ. 2006;332:749.
4. Liddle AD, et al. Pelvic congestion syndrome: chronic pelvic pain caused by ovarian and internal iliac varices. Phlebology. 2007;22:100.
5. Pandey T, et al. Use of time resolved magnetic resonance imaging in the diagnosis of pelvic congestion syndrome. J Mag Res Imaging. 2010;32:700.
6. Neis KJ, et al. Chronic pelvic pain: cause, diagnosis and therapy from a gynecologist's and an endoscopist's point of view. Gynecol Endocrinol. 2009;25:757.

Consider interstitial cystitis (IC) in the differential diagnosis of CPP.

In fact, one (urologist) author holds that "in the significant majority of gynecologic patients, chronic pelvic pain has its origin in the bladder in the chronic disease process known as interstitial cystitis" [1]. I suspect that this paper is another example of believing what one sees often is actually quite common, and I also believe that the prevalence of IC is not nearly as high as suggested. Nevertheless, the diagnosis of IC must be considered when CPP is accompanied by urinary symptoms such as dysuria (see Chap. 9), frequency, and urgency.

1. Parsons CL. Diagnosing chronic pelvic pain of bladder origin. J Reprod Med. 2004;49:235.

The symptoms of pelvic inflammatory disease (PID) can be varied and may not suggest pelvic disease at all.

Pelvic inflammatory disease can be manifested as nonspecific symptoms such as fever, nausea, vomiting, and low back or abdominal pain, as well as the more "gynecologic" complaints of vaginal discharge, intermenstrual bleeding, postcoital bleeding, and, of course, ongoing pelvic pain. Making the diagnosis and instituting prompt therapy is important because PID can lead to ectopic pregnancy or tubal-related infertility [1]. The diagnosis of PID is challenging, and one study of 23 experienced clinicians examining patients with PID revealed a curious and significant difference in the proportion of women diagnosed as having PID (0–5.7 %) [2]. One clinical sign found not to be especially helpful in the diagnosis of PID was the presence or absence of white blood cells in vaginal or cervical discharge [3].

1. Jaiyeoba O, et al. A practical approach to the diagnosis of pelvic inflammatory disease. Inf Dis Obstet Gynecol. 2011. doi:10:1155/2011.753037.
2. Doxanakis A, et al. Missing pelvic inflammatory disease? Substantial differences in the rate at which doctors diagnose PID. Sex Transm Infect. 2008;84:518.
3. Risser JMH, et al. Purulent vaginal and cervical discharge in the diagnosis of pelvic inflammatory disease. Int J STD AIDS. 2009;20:73.

With sudden, nocturnal onset of stabbing one-sided abdominal pain associated with vomiting, think of ovarian torsion.

Investigators studied 78 women who underwent laparoscopy for suspected ovarian torsion, a *must-not-miss diagnosis*. They found the following to be predictive of ovarian torsion: vomiting (OR 5.67, 95 % CI 1.69–19.0, $p = 0.005$); duration of pain less than a day (OR 3.74, 95 % CI 1.24–11.3, $p = 0.02$); and sudden/nocturnal onset

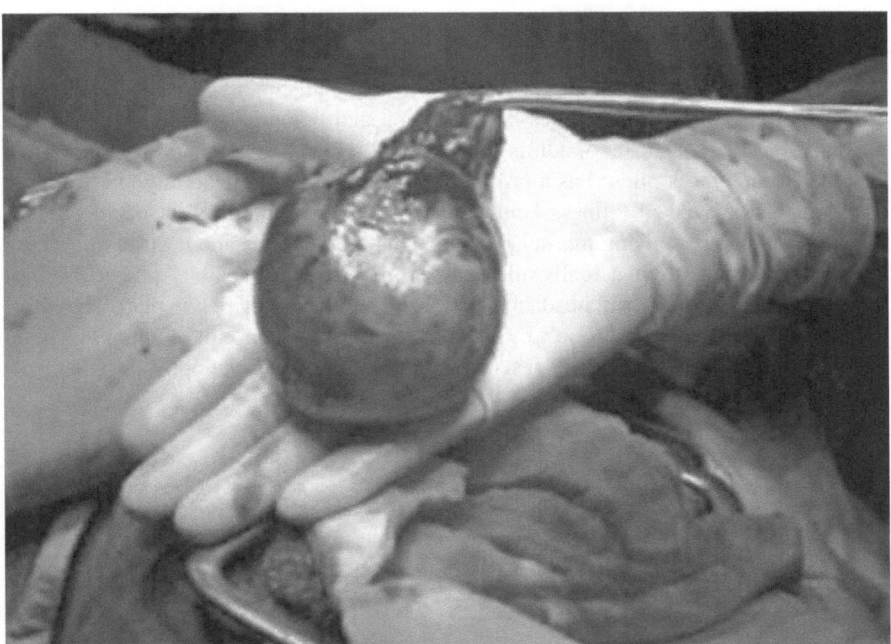

Fig. 10.2 An ovarian cyst removed after torsion

of pain (OR 4.13, 95 % CI 1.19–14.3, $p=0.02$) [1]. The pain, often described as "stabbing," may radiate to the back or groin. See Fig. 10.2.

An interesting case report describes intermittent ovarian torsion in a 12-year-old girl following use of a trampoline [2].

1. Mashiach R, et al. Sudden/nocturnal onset of acute abdominal pain, lasting less than a day and accompanied by vomiting: a telltale sign of ovarian torsion. Gyn Surg. 2010;7:297.
2. Yancey LM. Intermittent torsion of a normal ovary in a child associated with use of a trampoline. J Emerg Med. 2012;42:409.

Patients with a history of sexual abuse have an increased incidence of chronic pelvic pain.

A systematic review and meta-analysis of ten studies revealed a significant association between a history of sexual abuse and CPP (OR, 2.73; 95 % CI, 1.73–4.30) [1]. The numbers become more compelling when we consider that 25 % of US women and 16 % of men are adult survivors of childhood sexual abuse [2].

1. Paras ML, et al. Sexual abuse and lifetime diagnosis of somatic disorders: a systematic review and meta-analysis. JAMA. 2009;302:550.
2. Dube SR, et al. Long-term consequences of childhood sexual abuse by gender of victim. Am J Prev Med. 2005;28:430.

Chronic pelvic pain can be a "ticket of admission" to care.

Despite my cynicism regarding the "psychosomatic" banishment described in the Neis article above, CPP can sometimes be a sentinel, and potentially misleading, clinical presentation called a "ticket of admission." A symptom is a ticket of admission when a physical complaint is offered as a proxy for some underlying, generally psychosocial problem. It is a type of "illness behavior" [1–3]. An example might occur when a young woman experiencing marital problems, and yet anxious about discussing these with her physician, might actually offer a more "medically acceptable" physical symptom such as abdominal pain, headache, anorgasmia, or ongoing pelvic pain. The offering of the "ticket of admission" by the patient may be conscious, but often is an unconscious way to "medicalize" a sensitive problem or is a psychophysiologic manifestation of stress.

1. Black JS. Chronic pelvic pain without pathology. Available at: http://www.wasvisual.com/images/journalarticles/P-65a.pdf.
2. Craig DG. Time and the consultation in general practice. BMJ. 1978;12:1572.
3. Black JS. Sexual dysfunction and dyspareunia in the otherwise normal pelvis. Sex Marital Ther. 1988;3:213.

Ovarian Cancer

Most women with ovarian cancer have symptoms for months before the diagnosis is made.

Ovarian cancer, as the most lethal of the gynecologic cancers, is not, in fact, the "silent killer" we have long believed. Investigators in an interview study of women with invasive (616) and borderline epithelial ovarian tumors found that most (90 %) had symptoms, with a median duration of 4 months [1]. See Fig. 10.3. Bankhead et al., in a study of 124 women with suspected ovarian cancer, found as follows: "Multivariate analysis revealed persistent abdominal distension (OR 5.2, 95 % CI 1.3–20.5), postmenopausal bleeding (OR 9.2, 95 % CI 1.1–76.1), appetite loss (OR 3.2, 95 % CI 1.1–9.2), early satiety (OR 5.0, 95 % CI 1.6–15.7) and progressive symptoms (OR 3.6, 95 % CI 1.3–9.8) as independent, statistically significant variables associated with ovarian cancer" [2]. Other studies add urinary frequency, abnormal bleeding, and genital organ pain to the list [3, 4]. According to Ryerson, women with ovarian cancer presenting with gastrointestinal symptoms tend to have later diagnostic evaluation and more advanced tumors than those presenting with gynecologic complaints [4].

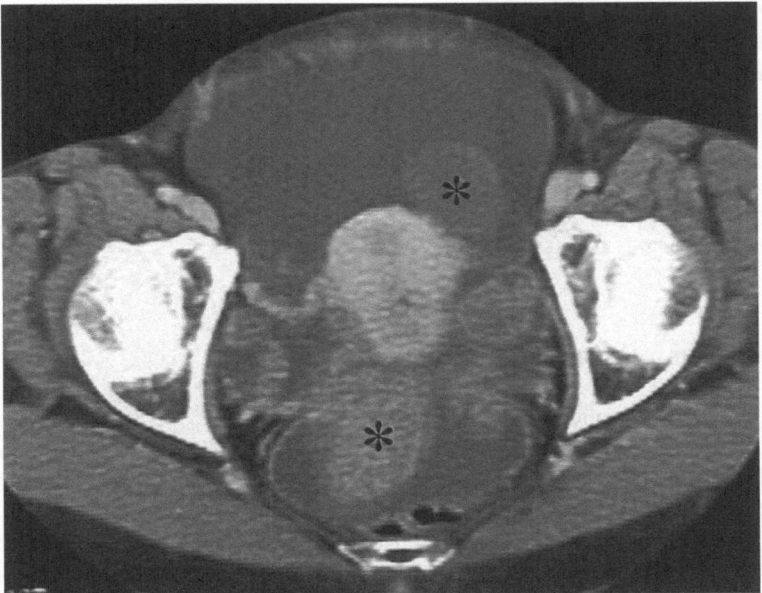

Fig. 10.3 CT scan of advanced ovarian cancer. Numerous peritoneal implants (*asterisks*) are seen in the pelvis of this patient with stage III epithelial ovarian cancer. The largest implant is present in the pouch of Douglas

1. Vine MF, et al. Types and duration of symptoms prior to diagnosis of invasive or borderline ovarian cancer. Gynecol Oncol. 2001;83:466.
2. Bankhead CR, et al. Indentifying symptoms of ovarian cancer: a qualitative and quantitative study. BJOG. 2008;115:1008.
3. Devlin SM, et al. Identification of ovarian cancer symptoms in health insurance claims data. J Womens Health. 2010;19:381.
4. Ryerson AB, et al. Symptoms, diagnoses, and time to key diagnostic procedures among older US women with ovarian cancer. Obstet Gyn. 2007;109:1053.

Unfortunately, the very symptoms that might be clues to ovarian cancer occur commonly in persons without cancer.

In a cohort of 2,235 women ages 18–70 who did not have ovarian cancer, Pitts et al. found the following symptom prevalence: abdominal bloating, 52 %; abdominal pain, 37 %; increased abdominal size, 30 %; pelvic pain, 29 %; early satiety, 18 %; and unable to eat normally, 15 % [1]. A study of symptoms often associated with ovarian cancer in 212 women with ovarian cancer compared to 1,060 matched controls led researchers to conclude that, except for abdominal distension, all had predictive values below 1 %, reflecting the common occurrence of nonspecific gastrointestinal and gynecologic complaints and the relatively low incidence of ovarian cancer. Of all the possible clues and as mentioned in Chap. 8, abdominal distension, with a 2.5 % risk of ovarian cancer, "clearly warrants investigation" [2].

1. Pitts MK, et al. High prevalence of symptoms associated with ovarian cancer among Australian women. Aust N Z J Obstet Gynecol. 2011;51:71.
2. Hamilton W, et al. Risk of ovarian cancer in women with symptoms in primary care: population based case-control study. BMJ. 2009;339:b2998.

Screening for ovarian cancer has not proved useful.

In a long-term controlled randomized trial involving 78,216 US women ages 55–74 years, ovarian cancer screening was performed annually with CA-125 and transvaginal ultrasound. The investigators found that, compared to usual care, screening did not reduce ovarian cancer mortality, but did result in a number of complications resulting from diagnostic adventures following false-positive tests [1].

1. Buys SS, et al. Effect of screening on ovarian cancer mortality: the Prostate, Lung, Colorectal and Ovarian (PLCO) Cancer Screening Randomized Controlled Trial. JAMA 2011;305:2295.

Sexual Problems

The odds are high that the woman with distressing sexual problems will not seek medical care.

In a study of 3,239 women with self-reported sexual problems plus sexually related personal distress, only about one-third sought care from a physician, and only 6 % of these women seeking advice scheduled a visit with sexual dysfunction as the chief complaint [1].

Sexual problems are common in women; in one study of 31,581 respondents, the age-adjusted point prevalence of any sexual problem was 43.1 and 22.2 % for sexually related personal distress [2]. Knoepp et al. report that in a study of 305 women, those with distressing sexual problems described decreased arousal (56.8 %), infrequent orgasm (54 %), and dyspareunia (39.7 %) as the leading manifestations [3].

1. Shifren JL, et al. Help-seeking behavior of women with self-reported distressing sexual problems. J Womens Health. 2009;18:461.
2. Shifren JL, et al. Sexual problems and distress in United States women: prevalence and correlates. Obstet Gynecol. 2008;112:970.
3. Knoepp LR, et al. Sexual complaints, pelvic floor symptoms, and sexual distress in women. J Sex Med. 2010;7:3675.

Sexual pain disorders in women can include vaginismus, vulvitis, and superficial or deep dyspareunia:

Female sexual pain can have varied causes, and a first step is to ascertain the type of discomfort.

- *Vaginismus* has been described as persistence of recurrent difficulty of the woman to permit entry of any object, such as a penis or even a finger, into the vagina, even though she expressly desires to do so. The word "spasm" is often used, and the presence of pain is not essential for the diagnosis [1]. Vaginismus has been characterized as having "a psychosexual etiology with a variable myogenic component" [2].
- *Vulvar pain*, reported to affect up to 16 % of women, can have many causes. Consider such diverse problems as candidal vulvovaginitis, allergic vulvitis, vulvar atrophy, lichen planus, lichen sclerosis, or vulvar intraepithelial neoplasia [3].
- *Dyspareunia* may be related to vaginitis of various types described above, vaginal dryness, recurrent cystitis, obstructive constipation, and even myalgia of the levator ani muscle [2]. If the patient describes deep dyspareunia, think of pelvic congestion syndrome (discussed above), endometriosis, and interstitial cystitis [4].

In a sample of adolescent girls, Landry et al. found sexual abuse, fear of sexual abuse, and trait anxiety to be noteworthy correlates of dyspareunia [5].

1. Crowley T, et al. Diagnosing and managing vaginismus. BMJ. 2009;339:25.
2. Graziottin A. Dyspareunia and vaginismus. Curr Sex Health Rep. 2008;5:43.
3. Danby CS, et al. Approach to the diagnosis and treatment of vulvar pain. Derm Ther. 2010;23:485.
4. Ferrero S, et al. Deep dyspareunia: causes, treatments, and results. Curr Opin Obstet Gynecol. 2008;20:394.
5. Landry T, et al. Biopsychosocial factors associated with dyspareunia in a community sample of adolescent girls. Arch Sex Behav. 2011;40:877.

The woman with a distressing sexual problem has a reasonable chance of having concurrent depression.

Johannes et al. studied data from the Prevalence of Female Sexual Problems Associated with Distress and Determinants of Treatment Seeking (PRESIDE) study. They found concurrent depression in approximately 40 % of women with sexual disorders of desire, arousal, or orgasm [1].

1. Johannes CB, et al. Distressing sexual problems in United States women revisited: prevalence after accounting for depression. J Clin Psychiatry. 2009;70:1698.

Problems of Pregnancy

If you ask, you will find that one of every ten pregnant women smokes cigarettes or drinks alcohol, or both.

Based on data from the Centers for Disease Control and Prevention (CDC), Carl et al. report that 11 % of US women smoke during pregnancy and 10 % drink alcohol. Furthermore, more than two-thirds do not take folate supplements when pregnant, and 3 % take medications or supplements that are recognized teratogens [1].

1. Carl J, et al. Preconception counseling: make it part of your annual exam. J Fam Pract. 2009;58:307.

Elevated serum urate levels are associated with preeclampsia, but may be poor predictors of maternal and fetal complications in women with preeclampsia.

Preeclampsia, affecting one in 20 otherwise normal pregnancies, can cause maternal and fetal morbidity and mortality. Hyperuricemia is often seen in preeclampsia. For example, in one study 72 subjects with severe preeclampsia had markedly elevated serum urate levels not found in 50 subjects with normal pregnancies [1]. But what about sequelae associated with preeclampsia? Following a systematic review of 18 articles involving 3,913 pregnant women and the incidence of complications such as fetal stillbirth, intrauterine demise, and neonatal death, investigators concluded: "Serum uric acid is a poor predictor of maternal and fetal complications in women with pre-eclampsia" [2].

1. Sagan N, et al. Serum urate as a predictor of fetal outcome in severe pre-eclampsia. Acta Obstet Gyn Scand. 1984;63:71.
2. Thangaratinam S, et al. Accuracy of serum uric acid in predicting complications of pre-eclampsia: a systematic review. BJOG. 2006;113:369.

Not all cases of preeclampsia match the textbook description of hypertension and proteinuria at >20 weeks gestation and <48 h postpartum.

Be alert for manifestations occurring outside of the usual time parameters or for gestational hypertension accompanied by abdominal pain, neurologic symptoms such as headache or blurred vision, or thrombocytopenia, in the absence of proteinuria. Atypical preeclampsia is important because maternal and fetal sequelae are similar to those seen with textbook preeclampsia [1, 2]. This is a setting in which serum urate level may be helpful in clarifying the diagnosis.

1. Stella CL, et al. Preeclampsia: diagnosis and management of the atypical presentation. J Maternal Fetal Neonatal Med. 2006;19:381.
2. Baumwell S, et al. Pre-eclampsia: clinical manifestations and molecular mechanisms. Nephron Clin Pract. 2007;106:c72.

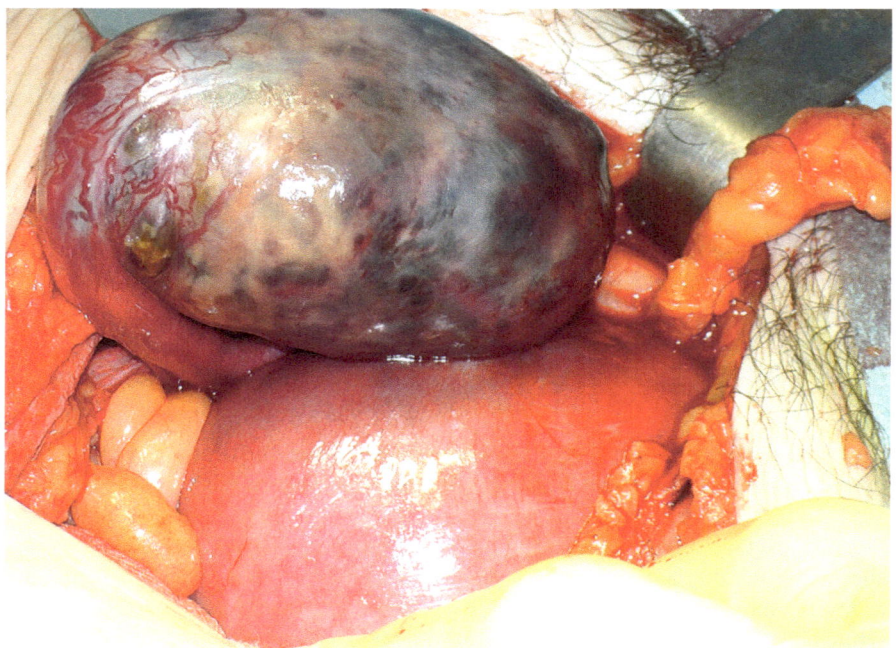

Fig. 10.4 Ectopic tubal pregnancy: laparoscopic view

In a female patient of childbearing age who mentions lateral abdominal pain in the setting of amenorrhea, think first of ectopic pregnancy (EP).

The classical triad of ectopic pregnancy is amenorrhea, abdominal pain, and vaginal bleeding, although vaginal bleeding is not always found. Worrisome risk factors for EP include previous EP or tubal surgery, known tubal pathology, intrauterine device use, infertility, or in utero diethylstilbestrol (DES) exposure [1, 2]. EP is more likely if the patient has pain characterized as severe, sharp, and/or one-sided. Physical findings increasing the likelihood of EP are cervical motion tenderness, peritoneal signs, or lateral or bilateral abdominal or pelvic tenderness to palpation [2]. See Fig. 10.4.

Be alert for the atypical EP, with implantation occurring in the abdomen, ovary, interstitial portion of the Fallopian tube, or even in a cesarean section scar. Kurt et al. report that although these uncommon types of EP occur in less than 10 % of cases, mortality in patients who suffer them is high [3].

1. Ankum WM, et al. Risk factors for ectopic pregnancy: a meta-analysis. Fertil Steril. 1996;65:1093.
2. Dart RG, et al. Predictive value of history and physical examination in patients with suspected ectopic pregnancy. Ann Emerg Med. 1999;33:283.
3. Kurt T, et al. Ectopic pregnancy. N Engl J Med. 2009;361:379.

Be alert for four risk factors that may herald rupture of an ectopic pregnancy, one of which is induction of ovulation.

In a study of 849 women with tubal ectopic pregnancies, rupture occurred in 18 %. Four factors increased the risk of rupture: never having used contraceptives (OR 1.7 [1.0–3.3]), history of tubal pathology plus infertility (OR 1.6 [0.9–2.7]), induction of ovulation (OR 2.5 [1.1–5.6]), and high level of beta-human HCG when EP is suspected (2.9 [1.5–5.6]) [1].

1. Job-Spira N, et al. Ruptured tubal pregnancy: risk factors and reproductive outcome: results of a population-based study in France. Ann J Obstet Gynecol. 1999;180:938.

Indicator clues may help identify pregnant women subjected to physical abuse.

In a study of 548 pregnant women, 60 (10.9 %) reported physical abuse prior to the current pregnancy and 36 (6.6 %) described physical abuse during the current pregnancy. The authors of the study identified three clusters of indicators that might suggest physical abuse in the setting of pregnancy [1]:

Social instability: Factors include unplanned pregnancy, low age, being unmarried, low educational attainment, and unemployment.
Unhealthy lifestyle: Think of poor diet, use of alcohol and drugs, and emotional problems.
Physical health problems: These include physical disease and prescription drug use.

Of the 24 pregnant women receiving medical treatment for the abuse, only one told her prenatal care clinician about the abuse.

1. Stewart DE, et al. Physical abuse in pregnancy. Can Med Assoc J. 1993;149:1257.

Breast Symptoms and Signs

Breast pain may be the presenting symptom of breast cancer, certainly a *must-not-miss diagnosis*.

Although the usual initial sign of breast cancer is a painless lump, up to 5 % of patients with breast cancer present with pain [1]. In a study of 106 somewhat youthful patients (mean age $27.6 \pm SD\ 10.5$ years) with mastalgia, breast cancer was found in 1.9 % [2]. In another study of 175 subjects with breast pain, imaging showed suspicious findings in four (2.2 %) and cancer in two subjects (1.1 %) [2].

Investigators in France suggest that cyclic mastalgia may be an independent and useful clinical marker of increased breast cancer risk. In their study of 247 women with cyclic mastalgia receiving no hormone therapy, 22 breast cancers were detected over a mean follow-up of 16 ± 5 years. They found the relative risk of breast cancer increased with the duration of cyclic mastalgia, and for 37 months of cyclic mastalgia was 5.1 (95 % CI 1.92–14.74) [3].

1. Golshan M. Breast pain. In: Millikan JA, et al., editors. Common surgical diseases. New York: Springer; 2008. p. 85.
2. Chowdhury RA, et al. Analysis of breast pain: a study of 110 cases. J Medicine. 2009;10:77.
3. Plu-Bureau G, et al. Cyclical mastalgia and breast cancer risk: results of a French cohort study. Cancer Epidemiol Biomarkers Prev. 2006;15:1229.

Bloody nipple discharge (ND) is an alarm finding suggesting malignant disease of the breast.

In a study of female patients with ND as their only symptom, cancer was found in 100 of 330 (30.3 %) patients with bloody ND and in 42/239 (17.6 %) of those with serous discharge [1]. In another study of nipple discharge, pathologic disease was associated with bloody ND (adjusted OR 3.7) and spontaneous ND (adjusted OR 3.2) [2].

There is controversy regarding the utility of cytologic examination of the discharge itself. I found one somewhat favorable paper reporting data regarding 1,530 women which yielded 22 results described as suspicious and 67 as malignant. Of the 22 "suspicious" cases, 18 were found to have biopsy-proven carcinoma, while cancer was found in 65 of the 67 cases in which cytologic examination of the discharge was reported as "malignant" [3]. See Fig. 10.5.

1. Montroni I, et al. Nipple discharge: Is its significance as a risk factor for breast cancer fully understood? Observational study including 915 consecutive patients who underwent selective duct excision. Breast Cancer Res Treat. 2010;123:895.
2. Morrogh M, et al. Lessons learned from 416 cases of nipple discharge of the breast. Am J Surg. 2010;200:73.
3. Gupta RK, et al. The role of nipple discharge cytology in the diagnosis of breast disease: a study of nipple discharge from 1530 patients. Cytopathology. 2004;15:326.

Fig. 10.5 (**a**) Nipple discharge cytology showing benign ductal cells and proteinaceous material. (**b**) Nipple discharge cytology showing malignant cells

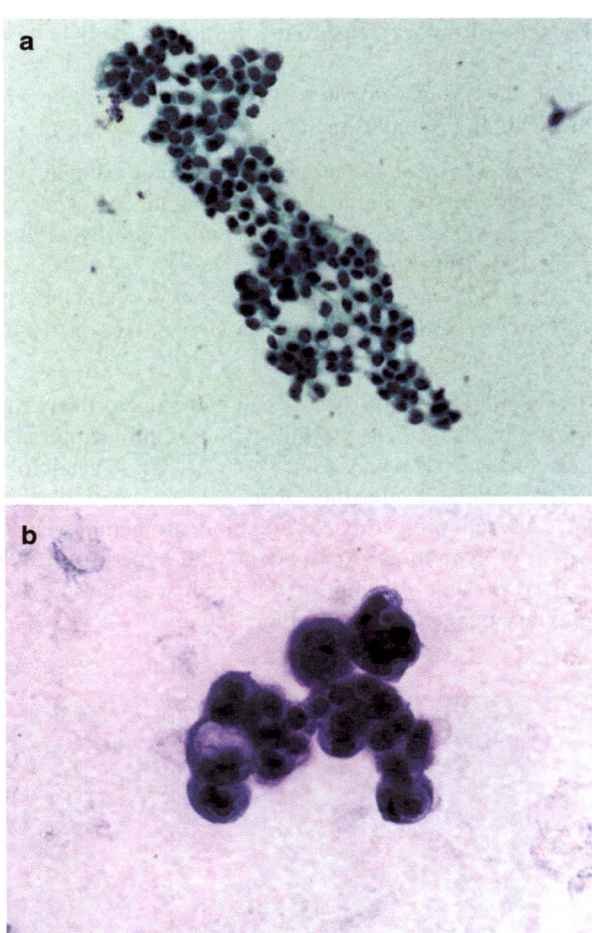

In the male patient, any sort of breast discharge is especially ominous.

Although a palpable mass is the classic presentation of male breast cancer, a few tumors will present first with nipple discharge. In a study of 14 male patients with a chief complaint of ND, eight (57 %) were found to have malignant disease [1].

1. Morrogh M, et al. The significance of nipple discharge of the male breast. Breast J. 2009;15:632.

Galactorrhea not related to medications is likely to be caused by a pituitary tumor.

The leading cause of galactorrhea seen following the neonatal period is prescription medication. Examples include [1]:

Dopamine receptor blockers: Examples include phenothiazines, selective serotonin reuptake inhibitors, metoclopramide (Reglan), and tricyclic antidepressants.
Dopamine-depleting agents: Think of antihypertensives methyldopa (Aldomet) and reserpine (Serpasil).
Drugs that inhibit dopamine release: Codeine, morphine, and heroin.
Others: These include oral contraceptives, verapamil (Calan), and cimetidine (Tagamet).

The most common disease cause of galactorrhea is hyperprolactinemia, typically caused by the secretory pituitary tumor, prolactinoma. These patients tend to have galactorrhea, seen in about 80 % of cases, accompanied by oligomenorrhea or amenorrhea and infertility. Although patients with this symptom complex should have a serum prolactin determination, prolactin levels do not correlate well with the extent of symptoms. Any patient with hyperprolactinemia should then have magnetic resonance imaging of the head, with the use of contrast material and with pituitary images [3, 4]. See Fig. 10.6.

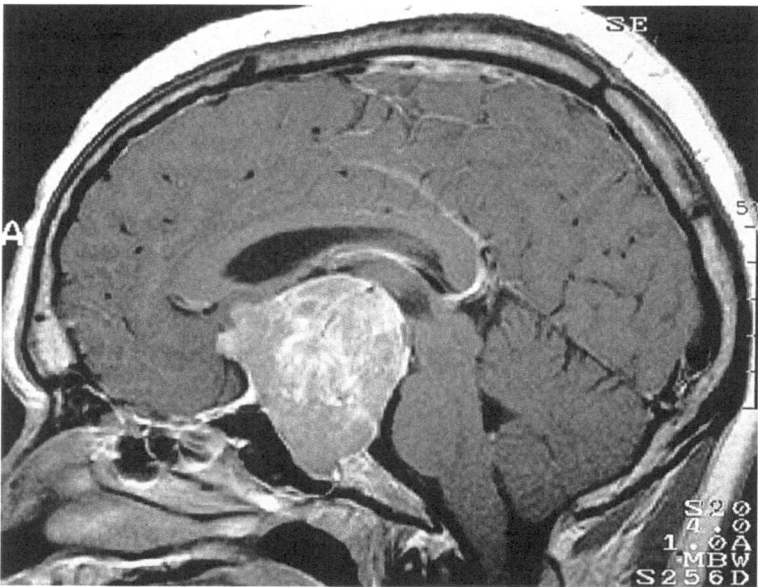

Fig. 10.6 Large pituitary adenoma

Other causes of galactorrhea include thyroid disorders, renal failure, encephalitis, and chorioepithelioma of the testis [2]. Also, don't overlook mechanical stimulation. I once encountered a young woman who had begun lactation in the wake of an abortion. I saw her 6 months later, still with galactorrhea. As it turned out, she was distressed by the leakage, and so while in her daily shower, she emptied the breasts manually, thereby unwittingly continuing her galactorrhea.

1. Luciano AA. Clinical presentation of hyperprolactinemia. J Reprod Med. 1999;44:1085.
2. Leung AKC, et al. Diagnosis and management of galactorrhea. Am Fam Phys. 2004;70:543.
3. Schlechte JA. Prolactinoma. N Engl J Med. 2003;349:2035.
4. Klibanski A. Prolactinomas. N Engl J Med. 2010;362:1219.

There are three features of the patient scenario in which a diagnosis of breast cancer is missed—a younger woman, with a chief complaint of a self-discovered mass, in whom the mammogram is read as normal or equivocal.

This cluster of breast cancer red flags was identified by our colleagues in the liability insurance industry, based on malpractice claims related to *failure to diagnose*. The authors of the report suggest that clinicians went astray in two ways: First, they were unimpressed with the physical examination of the breast. And, second, the clinicians failed to follow up with the patient after the initial consultation [1].

One facet of this problem may be the greater density of breast tissue in some younger women, which can impair the sensitivity of mammography and give rise to false-negative results [2]. In fact, according to Boyd et al., "Extensive breast density is strongly associated with the risk of breast cancer detected by screening or between screening tests" [3].

1. The Physician Insurers Association of America Breast Cancer Study. Lawrenceville, NJ: PIAA,1995.
2. Ponsky RW, et al. Mammographic breast density: effect on imaging and breast cancer risk. Natl Compr Canc Netw. 2010;8:1157.
3. Boyd NF, et al. Mammographic density and the risk and detection of breast cancer. N Engl J Med. 2007;356:227.

Despite the merits of mammography, clinical breast examination (CBE) and breast self-examination (BSE) may still be valuable in the detection of breast cancer.

A study in Canada involved 57,715 women screened using only mammography compared with 232,515 women screened with both mammography and CBE. The investigators found 5.4 cancers per 1,000 women screened with mammography alone, compared with 7.5 cancers detected when both modalities were used, although the combination screening yielded a higher number of false-positive results [1].

Breast self-examination can also play a useful role. Weiss reports, "Most studies have found that breast cancers detected by BSE are smaller than those detected without screening (i.e., BSE) and are more likely to be confined to the breast; furthermore, survival after a diagnosis of breast cancer tends to be longer among women who practice BSE than among women who do not" [2].

1. Chirally AM, et al. The contribution of clinical breast examination to the accuracy of breast screening. J Natl Cancer Inst. 2009;101:1236.
2. Weiss NS. Breast cancer mortality in relation to clinical breast examination and breast self-examination. Breast J. 2003;9:S86.

Curiously, several studies suggest that cosmetic breast implants not only do not increase breast cancer risk; they may actually have a protective effect.

One meta-analysis of epidemiologic studies conclude that the relative risk of breast cancer with breast implants was 0.72 (95 % CI 0.61–0.85) [1]. In a review of published studies, Deapen found reports describing "lower than expected risk, some with statistically significant reductions" [2].

1. Hoshaw SJ, et al. Breast implants and cancer: causation, delayed detection, and survival. Plast Reconstr Surg. 2001;107:1393.
2. Deapen DM, et al. Are breast implants anticarcinogenic? A 14-year follow-up of the Los Angeles Study. Plast Reconstr Surg. 1997;99:1346.

Selected Problems of the Female Reproductive System

Urinary symptoms suggesting cystitis may be reported during the month following a routine pelvic examination.

In a study, 63 sexually active women ages 18–40 who underwent routine pelvic examination were compared with 87 control subjects who did not have pelvic examinations. Here is what the investigators report about the study subjects: "More subjects had days with dysuria (17 % vs. 7 %, $p < .01$), days with frequency (27 % vs. 14 %, $p < .01$), days with both dysuria and frequency (13 % vs. 3 %, $p < .01$), and days with either dysuria or frequency (32 % vs. 17 %, $p < .01$)" [1]. Recognition of this tendency of pelvic examination to be associated with urinary symptoms in the following month may avoid unnecessary diagnostic investigations and even unwarranted empiric therapy.

1. Tiemstra JD, et al. Urinary symptoms after a routine pelvic exam. J Am Board Fam Med. 2011;24:290.

The classic presentation of polycystic ovary syndrome (PCOS) is evidence of hyperandrogenism and infrequent ovulation.

These features of PCOS, the most common endocrinopathy of women during the reproductive years, may include hirsutism, acne, and oligomenorrhea or amenorrhea. The diagnosis is strengthened by finding signs of polycystic ovarian morphology [1, 2]. But be alert for other clinical manifestations such as sleep apnea, metabolic syndrome, and coronary artery disease. See Fig. 10.7.

Our concerns about PCOS include the company it keeps. Women with PCOS have been reported to have an increased risk of hypercholesterolemia (OR 3.2 [1.7–6.0]), diabetes (OR 2.2 [0.9–5.2]), and hypertension (OR 1.4 [0.9–2–0]) [3]. A study in Sweden found that, when compared with control subjects, women with PCOS had a relative risk of 7.4 of developing myocardial infarction [4].

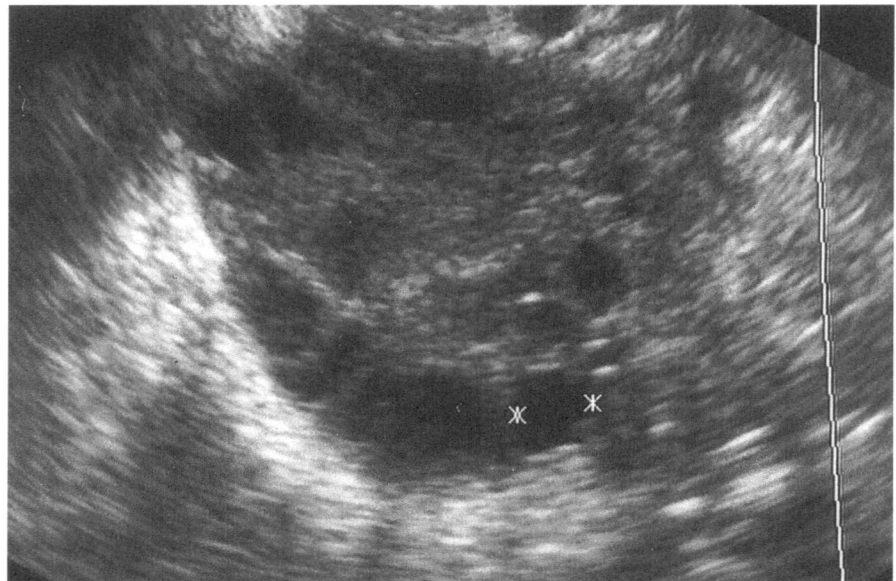

Fig. 10.7 Polycystic ovary syndrome. Ultrasound image of ovary with classic features of polycystic ovary syndrome. Note the increased stromal volume with multiple cysts arrayed at the periphery

1. Goodarzi MO, et al. Polycystic ovary syndrome: etiology, pathogenesis and diagnosis. Nat Rev Endocrin. 2011;7:219.
2. Setji TL, et al. Polycystic ovary syndrome: diagnosis and treatment. Am J Med. 2007;120:128.
3. Wild S, et al. Cardiovascular disease in women with polycystic ovary syndrome at long-term follow-up: a retrospective cohort study. Clin Endocrin. 2000;52:595.
4. Dahlgren E, et al. Polycystic ovary syndrome and risk for myocardial infarction: evaluated from a risk factor model based on a prospective population study of women. Acta Obstet Gynecol Scand. 1992;71:599.

Flushing reported by the menopausal woman may be caused by something other than fluctuating hormonal levels.

Think about the possibility of carcinoid syndrome and other causes described in Chap. 1 [1].

1. van der Lely AJ, et al. Carcinoid syndrome: diagnosis and medical management. Arq Bras Endocrinol Metabol. 2005;49:850.

Chapter 11
The Musculoskeletal System

> *The rheumatism is a common name for many aches and pains,*
> *which have yet got no peculiar appellation, though owing to*
> *very different causes.*
> English physician William Heberden (1710–1801) [1]

Contents

R.B. Taylor, *Diagnostic Principles and Applications*,
DOI 10.1007/978-1-4614-1111-6_11, © Springer Science+Business Media, LLC 2013

Dr. Heberden, remembered by the eponymous name of osteophytic spurs involving the distal interphalangeal joints often seen in patients with degenerative joint disease, lamented the lack of specificity in describing various sorts of musculoskeletal diseases. What would he have thought of aromatase inhibitor-induced arthralgia, statin-associated myalgia, cell phone thumb, and wiiitis?

1. Heberden W. Commentaries on the history and cure of diseases. 4th ed. London: Payne & Foss; 1816:chapter 79.

Symptoms can provide important clues to the etiologic diagnosis of back pain, and are more clinically useful than routine imaging.

The world's leading cause of occupational disability, back pain, has an estimated point prevalence of 15–30 %, an annual prevalence of 20–60 %, and a lifetime prevalence of 60–80 % [1]. Few disorders can claim such a widespread influence on humanity. Back pain can be conveniently classified under three categories: (1) lumbar strain/sprain (70 %); degenerative disc disease, including herniated lumbar disc disease and spinal stenosis (10 %); and everything else, including osteoporotic fracture, infection, spondylolisthesis, and trauma. A careful history is important in coming to a diagnosis.

When the pain arises in the spine or supporting structures, the patient often uses the descriptive term "aching," while radicular pain resulting from discopathy is like to be characterized as "shooting" or "stabbing." Pain from the spinous structures may be also felt in the buttocks or thighs, but pain extending to the lower leg is more likely to be radicular. When the pain is relieved by inactivity and worsened by movement, think of back strain. When prolonged sitting or leaning forward relieves the pain, the diagnosis of nerve root pressure is more likely [3].

1. O'Shea FD, et al. Inflammatory and degenerative sacroiliac joint disease in a primary back pain cohort. Arthritis Care Res. 2010;62:447.
2. Smith SW. Acute low back pain in the workplace. Evid Based Pract. 2011;14:11.
3. Cohen SP, et al. Management of low back pain. BMJ. 2008;337:a2718.

Low back pain with radicular symptoms that improve with forward flexion of the spine suggests the diagnosis of lumbar spinal stenosis (LSS).

Lumbar spinal stenosis, spinal canal narrowing that causes nerve root impingement with radicular pain, has become a common indication for lumbar spine surgery [1]. Once considered a disease of older individuals, LSS is now being seen in sports medicine clinics [2]. A helpful clue to the diagnosis is a decrease in pain with "delordosis"—forward flexion of the spine [3]. This means that LSS patients may report pain regression with climbing stairs, walking uphill, and riding a bicycle. In addition, patients often describe the discomfort as having "heavy legs" [1] (see Fig. 11.1).

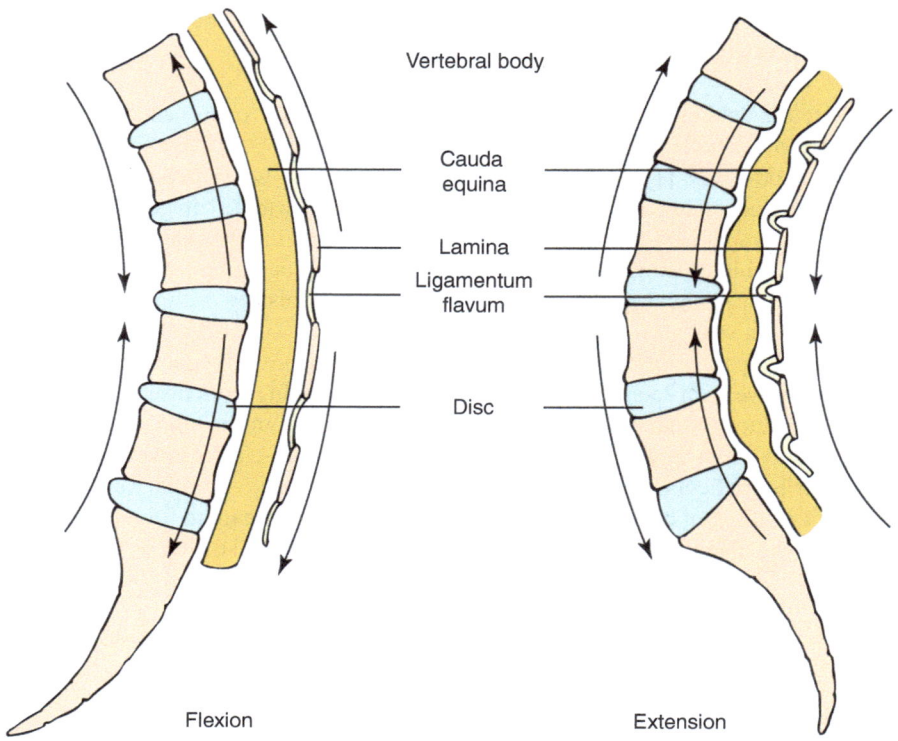

Vertebral body

Cauda
equina

Lamina
Ligamentum
flavum

Disc

Flexion   Extension

Fig. 11.1 Spinal stenosis is a condition in which the vertebral canal is narrowed in a concentric fashion, producing impingement upon the entire cauda equina and the spinal cord at higher levels. The pain may be relieved by forward flexion of the vertebral column, which creates a more capacious canal

1. Siebert E, et al. Lumbar spinal stenosis: syndrome, diagnostics and treatment. Nat Rev Neurol. 2009;5:392.
2. Englund J. Lumbar spinal stenosis. Curr Sports Med Rep. 2007;6:50.
3. Chad DA. Lumbar spinal stenosis. Neurol Clin. 2007;25:407.

While history offers numerous clues to the origin of back pain, only the straight-leg raising (SLR) test is consistently sensitive for sciatica due to lumbar disc herniation.

This conclusion followed a systematic review of the literature and added the qualification that, while the SLR test was sensitive, it had a low specificity. That is, it was often also positive in patients with low back strain [1]. Of course, finding neurologic evidence of motor or sensory loss in the lower extremities adds specificity in the diagnosis of lumbar discopathy.

In another study, investigators found that when a patient can point to (or within 2 cm of) the posterior–superior iliac spine as the source of back pain, the origin of the pain is likely to be the sacroiliac joint, and a positive response to a periarticular sacroiliac joint block is likely. The authors call this the "one-finger test" [2].

1. Rubenstein SM. A best-evidence review of diagnostic procedures for neck and low-back pain. Best Pract Res Clin Rheum. 2008;22:471.
2. Murakami E, et al. Diagram specific to sacroiliac joint pain site indicated by one-finger test. J Orthop Sci. 2008;13:492.

While "routine" lumbar spine radiography enhances patient satisfaction in patients with low back pain, it does not improve outcomes.

Numerous studies have documented the futility of imaging spines without clinical evidence suggesting serious pathology [1, 2, 3]. However, a study of 421 primary care low back pain patients randomized to lumbar spine radiography versus usual care without radiography found the following: "Participants receiving x-rays are more satisfied with their care, but are not less worried or more reassured about serious disease causing their low back pain." I find it noteworthy that no serious pathology was detected in either the imaged or the usual care group [4].

1. Chou R, et al. Imaging strategies for low-back pain: systematic review and meta-analysis. Lancet. 2009;373:463.
2. Chou R, et al. Diagnosis and treatment of low back pain: a joint clinical practice guideline from the American College of Physicians and the American Pain Society. Ann Intern Med. 2007; 147:478.
3. Bhatia NN, et al. Diagnostic modalities for the evaluation of pediatric back pain: a prospective study. J Pediatr Orthop. 2008;28:230.
4. Kendrick D, et al. The role of radiography in primary care patients with low back pain of at least six weeks duration: a randomized (unblended) controlled trial. Health Technol Assess. 2001;5:1.

Don't overlook infection as a cause of back pain.

Pyogenic vertebral osteomyelitis, an admittedly uncommon entity, is often the result of nosocomial bacteremia. Back pain is typical, but some patients present without fever [1]. Characteristic radiographic findings may be seen only late in the course of the disease [2].

Spinal epidural abscess has a classic triad—spinal pain, fever, and neurologic deficit. As might be expected, all three features may not be present. This rare disease is often associated with adjacent vertebral osteomyelitis and *Staphylococcus aureus* is the likely etiologic agent [3]. Be especially suspicious of this diagnosis when back pain and fever occur in three clinical settings: the patient who abuses intravenous drugs, the patient with bacterial endocarditis, and the patient receiving hemodialysis [4–6]. Both pyogenic vertebral osteomyelitis and spinal epidural abscess must be considered *must-not-miss diagnoses*.

1. Torda AJ, et al. Pyogenic vertebral osteomyelitis: analysis of 20 cases and review. Clin Infect Dis. 1995;2:320.
2. Fernandez M, et al. Discitis and vertebral osteomyelitis in children: an 18-year review. Pediatrics. 2000;105:1299.
3. Wong D, et al. Spinal epidural abscess. N Z Med J. 1998;11:345.
4. Curry WT, et al. Spinal epidural abscess: clinical presentation, management, and outcome. Surg Neurol. 2005;63:364.

5. Chen WC, et al. Spinal epidural abscess due to Staphylococcus aureus: clinical manifestations and outcomes. J Microbiol Immunol Infect. 2008;41:215.
6. Wong SS, et al. Spinal epidural abscess in hemodialysis patients: a case series and review. Clin J Am Soc Nephrol. 2011;6:1495.

The child with back pain can present a challenging differential diagnosis.

Here are three possible causes of back pain in children:

Scheuermann disease: Epiphyseal osteonecrosis of adjacent vertebral bodies in the thoracic spine is the cause of Scheuermann disease, aka juvenile kyphosis, the most common cause of hyperkyphosis in adolescence [1] (see Fig. 11.2).

Spondylolysis: This is a stress fracture of the pars interarticularis that may be seen in young athletes. Spondylolysis may be diagnosed by finding a feature on oblique radiographic views described as a "Scotty dog with a collar." This disease must be differentiated from spondylolisthesis, forward anterior displacement of one vertebral body on another, which, in fact, may follow an episode of spondylolysis [2].

Backpack back pain: Most US schoolchildren carry backpacks filled with books and other items amounting to 10–22 % of their body weight. One study used

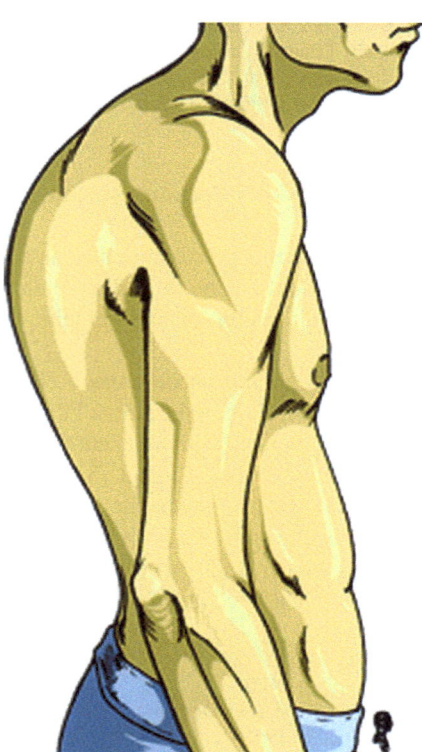

Fig. 11.2 Thoracic kyphosis in a young patient with Scheuermann disease

magnetic resonance imaging to examine the spines of children carrying backpacks. The investigators found: "Increasing backpack loads significantly compressed lumbar disc heights measured in the midline sagittal plane ($p<0.05$, repeated-measures analysis of variance [ANOVA])" [3].

1. Lowe TG, et al. Evidence based medicine: analysis of Scheuermann disease. Spine. 2007; 32:s115.
2. Cassas KJ, et al. Childhood and adolescent sports-related overuse injuries. Am Fam Physician. 2006;73:1014.
3. Neuschwander TB, et al. The effect of backpacks on the lumbar spine in children: a standing magnetic resonance imaging study. Spine. 2010;35:83.

Upper Extremity Problems

The clinical characteristics of chronic shoulder pain can help clarify the cause.

A patient with shoulder pain lasting 6 months or more often has findings that suggest the etiologic diagnosis [1]:

Adhesive capsulitis (AC): Look for diffuse pain with restricted passive motion. Be especially suspicious of this diagnosis in patients with thyroid disease and diabetes mellitus.

Rotator cuff tear: A typical scenario is a patient with pain when engaged in overhead activity and weakness on external rotation.

Acromioclavicular arthritis: These patients may describe superior shoulder pain and exhibit pain on a cross-body adduction test plus tenderness of the acromioclavicular joint.

Glenohumeral arthritis: Often seen in older patients, this disorder is characterized by a slow but progressive development of shoulder pain and restricted motion.

Subacromial/subdeltoid bursitis: Check for telltale point tenderness over the bursa.

Of course, not all shoulder pain is caused by the common disorders mentioned above. Bilateral subacromial/subdeltoid bursitis is often seen in patients with polymyalgia rheumatica [2]. And shoulder pain has been described as the presenting symptom of what later turned out to be Parkinson disease, preceding the onset of motor symptoms [3].

1. Burbank KM, et al. Chronic shoulder pain: evaluation and diagnosis. Am Fam Physician. 2008;77:453.
2. Nissen MJ, et al. Polymyalgia rheumatica and giant cell arthritis: what's new? Rev Med Suisse. 2010;17:575.
3. Stamey W, et al. Shoulder pain: a presenting symptom of Parkinson disease. J Clin Rheumatol. 2008;14:253.

Competitive swimmers often have shoulder pain, chiefly caused by supraspinatus tendinopathy.

Most (73 of 80; 91 %) of elite swimmers 13–25 years of age in a study by Sein et al. reported shoulder pain, and 84 % of these subjects had a positive impingement sign. Of those examined with magnetic resonance imaging (MRI), most (69 %) were found to have supraspinatus tendinopathy [1].

1. Sein ML, et al. Shoulder pain in elite swimmers: primarily due to swim-volume-induced supraspinatus tendinopathy. Br J Sports Med. 2010;44:105.

Most "tennis elbow" cases are not caused by playing tennis.

Up to 3 % of the population has or will have tennis elbow, properly called lateral epicondylitis. Although classically considered to be caused by playing tennis, especially using the backhand stroke, lateral epicondylitis can be caused by many other activities [1]. I have personally suffered lateral elbow pain after carrying heavy luggage, although the introduction of wheeled suitcases has helped reduce the incidence of "suitcase elbow." I have diagnosed the disorder in carpenters, auto mechanics, butchers, and one laundry worker using an overhead press.

1. Bisset L, et al. Tennis elbow. Clin Evid. 2011;20:1117.

The hand elevation test has been reported to be superior to the Tinel and Phalen tests in the diagnosis of carpal tunnel syndrome (CTS).

The carpal tunnel syndrome, the most common peripheral nerve entrapment syndrome, often leads to invasive therapy, and thus accurate diagnosis is imperative. Ahn studied 200 hands in 118 patients diagnosed with CTS, comparing the time-honored Phalen and Tinel tests with a very simple test—sustained elevation of the hand. Here is what was found [1]:

Test	Sensitivity (%)	Specificity (%)
Hand elevation	75.5	98.5
Phalen	67.5	91.0
Tinel	67.5	90.0

Based on a study of 70 patients with CTS, Amirfeyz et al. concur: "The hand elevation test may be used in isolation and is superior to questionnaires and other physical signs in the clinical diagnosis of carpal tunnel syndrome" [2] (see Fig. 11.3).

Fig. 11.3 The hand elevation test for carpal tunnel syndrome. The patient elevates the hand above the head for 1 min

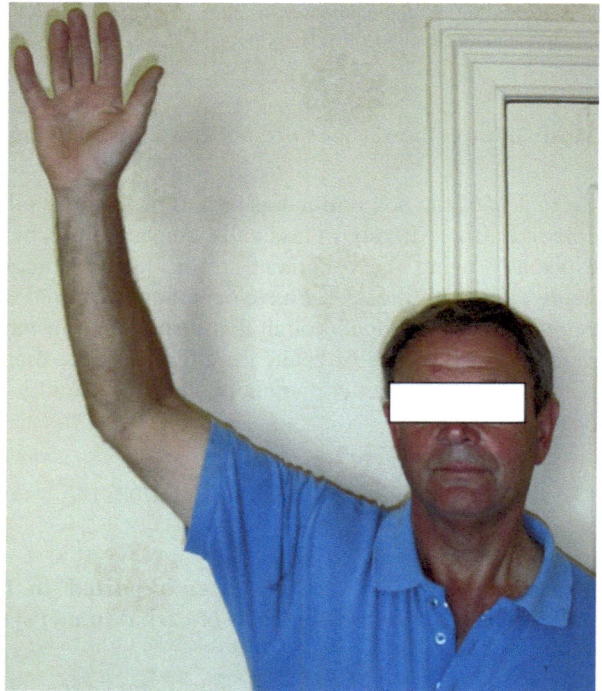

1. Ahn DS. Hand elevation: a new test for carpal tunnel syndrome. Ann Plast Surg. 2001;46:120.
2. Amirfeyz R, et al. Clinical tests for carpal tunnel syndrome in contemporary practice. Orthop Surg. 2011;131:471.

The scaphoid compression test—pushing the thumb proximally to apply pressure to the carpal navicular bone—is not a reliable diagnostic maneuver in the evaluation of a scaphoid fracture.

In a setting when a fracture is often not visible on initial x-rays, clinical signs can be especially valuable. The carpal compression test seems attractive because it is readily performed and requires no special equipment. It can even be performed with a cast in place. Esberger studied the scaphoid compression test in 99 patients with suspected scaphoid fractures. They found the test to have 70.5 % sensitivity, 21.8 % specificity, and a predictive value of only 41.9 %.

1. Esberger DA. What value the scaphoid compression test? J Hand Surg Br. 1994;19:748.

Game technology and cell phones have brought us a new host of overuse injuries.

The first report of this type of injury was a letter to the editor, published in the New England Journal of Medicine in 1990, describing thumb pain related to exuberant use of a new Nintendo brand video game. The author of the letter proposed naming the new injury "Nintendinitis" [1].

With the explosion in the use of text-enabled cell phones, we have seen an epidemic of "cell phone thumb." Karim insightfully points out that the thumb, least dexterous of all our fingers, is not engineered for repetitive movements needed for extensive use of a cell phone keypad [2].

Now we are expanding our horizons in game-related repetitive strain injuries. The latest disorder is "wiiitis," related to the use of Nintendo's fourth-generation gaming device (and incidentally for word lovers, wiiitis is the only word I know with the letter "i" occurring three times in a row). The Wii and similar motion-controlled games have brought us tendinitis, epicondylitis, enthesitis, and even cartilage injury, patellar dislocation, fractures, and lacerations [3].

1. Brasington R. Nintendinitis. N Engl J Med. 1990;322:1473.
2. Karim SA. From "playstation thumb" to "cellphone thumb": the new epidemic in teenagers. S Afr Med J. 2009;99:161.
3. Sparks DA, et al. Did too much Wii cause your patient's injury? J Fam Pract. 2011;60:404.

Lower Extremity Problems

Not all hip pain is osteoarthritis.

Here are some examples of non-arthritic hip pain:

Trochanteric bursitis: The patient with greater trochanteric bursitis describes lateral hip pain, and physician examination typically reveals tenderness over this area [1, 2].

Fatigue fracture: The femoral neck was the site of 50 % of fatigue fractures of the femur in a study of 170 patients with 185 fatigue fractures [3]. Remember that occult fractures of the hip may appear radiographically normal.

Metastatic cancer: Do not overlook the possibility that hip pain may be an early sign of cancer spread from prostate, lung, breast, or other site [1].

Other causes of hip pain include labral tears, femoroacetabular impingement, iliopsoas pathology, sacroiliac joint disease, lumbar radiculopathy, metastatic cancer, and even, rarely, early symptoms of herpes zoster infection [1].

1. Tibor LM, et al. Differential diagnosis of pain around the hip joint. Arthroscopy. 2008;24:1407.
2. Jones DL, et al. Diagnosis of trochanteric bursitis versus femoral neck stress fracture. Phys Ther. 1997;77:58.
3. Niva MH, et al. Fatigue fractures of the femur. J Bone Joint Surg. 2005;87:1385.

Some diagnostic pearls may help differentiate the various causes of knee pain.

Think of the following possibilities when you encounter a patient, especially a young patient, with knee pain:

Pain at the lateral femoral condyle: Pain in this area, sometimes described as burning in nature, is typical of the iliotibial band friction syndrome, seem chiefly in runners [1].

Medial knee pain over the upper tibia: Think of inflammation of the pes anserine bursa, located 5–6 cm distal to the joint line. Granted, medial knee joint pain is the most common type of knee pain, commonly seen in osteoarthritis, ligamentous strains, and meniscal tears. What distinguishes pes anserine bursitis is tenderness below the knee joint line combined with a painless valgus stress maneuver (i.e., the medial collateral ligament has not been torn). The patient often describes nocturnal discomfort in the involved area [2, 3] (see Fig. 11.4).

Knee pain localized to the inferior pole of the patella: This suggests patellar tendinopathy, sometimes called "jumper's knee," seen chiefly in those engaged in sports involving jumping, such as basketball [4].

Knee pain localized to the anterior tibial tubercle: In a young person, this strongly suggests Osgood–Schlatter disease, an epiphysitis of immature bony growth centers [5].

Fig. 11.4 Pes anserine bursitis

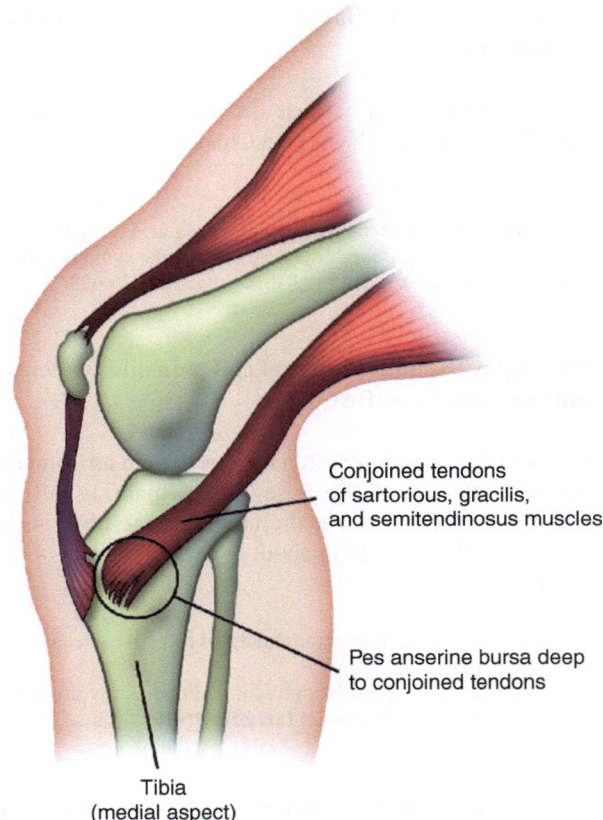

Conjoined tendons of sartorious, gracilis, and semitendinosus muscles

Pes anserine bursa deep to conjoined tendons

Tibia
(medial aspect)

Pain on repeated flexion in a younger person not explained by some more definitive pathology: This symptom pattern characterizes the patellofemoral pain syndrome, also called chondromalacia patellae, a disorder more common in women than in men. The most common site of pain is the patella during anterior–posterior compression [6, 7].

Hemarthrosis: The most likely diagnosis is an anterior cruciate ligament injury, seen in 70 % of patients with acute hemarthrosis of the knee [8].

1. Messier SP, et al. Etiology of iliotibial band friction syndrome in distance runners. Med Sci Sports Exerc. 1995;27:951.
2. Larsson LG, et al. The syndrome of anserine bursitis: an overlooked diagnosis. Arthritis Rheum. 1985;28:1062.
3. Schraeder TL, et al. Clinical evaluation of the knee. N Engl J Med 2010;363:e5.
4. Koen HE, et al. Patellar tendinopathy in athletes: current diagnostic and therapeutic recommendations. Sports Med. 2005;35:71.
5. Weiler R, et al. Osgood-Schlatter disease. BMJ. 2011;343:d4534.
6. Yates C, et al. Patellofemoral pain: a prospective study. Orthopedics. 1986;9:663.
7. Gerbino PG II, et al. Patellofemoral pain syndrome: evaluation of location and intensity of pain. Clin J Pain. 2006;22:154.
8. Ramjug S, et al. Isolated anterior cruciate ligament deficiency: knee scores and function. Acta Orthop Belg. 2008;74:643.

A popliteal cyst, aka Baker cyst, can rupture, causing swelling of the posterior calf muscles.

This fact is important because the posterior calf swelling can be misdiagnosed as acute deep vein thrombosis (see Chap. 6) [1, 2].

1. Bekou V, et al. Unilateral leg swelling: deep vein thrombosis? Phlebology. 2011;26:8.
2. Langsfeld M, et al. Baker's cysts mimicking the symptoms of deep vein thrombosis: diagnosis with venous duplex scanning. J Vasc Surg. 1997;25:658.

The child with sudden onset of calf pain and tenderness may have benign acute childhood myositis (BACM).

This disorder, seen more often in boys than in girls, tends to follow a viral infection, typically influenza. There is severe calf pain, usually bilateral, causing difficulty walking. Finding an elevated creatine kinase level is characteristic of the disease. BACM usually subsides in about a week [1, 2].

1. Mackay MT, et al. Benign acute childhood myositis: laboratory and clinical features. Neurology. 1999;53:2127.
2. Koliou M, et al. A case of benign acute childhood myositis associated with influenza A (H1N1) virus infection. Clin Microbiol Inf. 2010;16:193.

The childhood athlete with gradual onset of posterior heel pain may have calcaneal apophysitis, aka Sever disease.

This overuse disorder, more common in boys, is most likely to occur in those who engage in "running" sports, such as track, soccer, and basketball. Many of these youngsters have flat or "rigid" feet. A useful diagnostic maneuver is the calcaneal compression test, squeezing the heel from the sides to see if the pressure elicits pain.

1. Micheli LJ, et al. Prevention and management of calcaneal apophysitis in children: an overuse syndrome. J Pediatr Ortho. 1987;7:34.
2. Hendrix CL. Calcaneal apophysitis (Sever disease). Clin Pod Med Surg. 2005;22:55.

Heel pain occurring acutely upon arising from bed and improving as the day goes on is typical of plantar fasciitis.

Being on one's feet leads to micro-tears at the calcaneal origin of the plantar tendon. Some degree of healing occurs overnight, with the feet typically extended,

Fig. 11.5 Location of
common unilateral foot pain
syndromes. *M* Morton
neuroma, *P* plantar fasciitis,
T tarsal tunnel syndrome

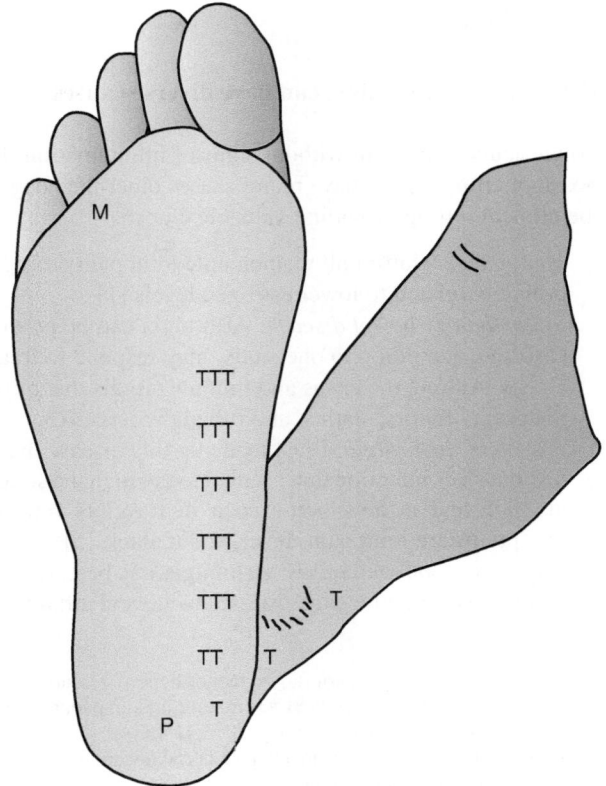

and then tearing occurs each morning upon standing. Patients thus typically exhibit pain on dorsiflexion of the foot. Imaging may be helpful but is generally unnecessary [1, 2]. Other causes of foot pain are Morton neuroma and tarsal tunnel syndrome (see Fig. 11.5).

1. Neufeld SK, et al. Plantar fasciitis: evaluation and treatment. J Am Acad Ortho Surg. 2008;16:338.
2. Goff JD, et al. Diagnosis and treatment of plantar fasciitis. Am Fam Physician. 2011;84:676.

Joint Pain

Polyarticular arthralgia can have diverse causes.

Polyarticular joint pain without signs of inflammation (heat, swelling, redness, and possibly effusion) can have many causes other than degenerative joint disease, with the clinical setting providing valuable clues:

Menopause: Half of all women note joint pain during the menopausal transition, probably related to lower estrogen levels [1].

Inflammatory bowel disease: Arthralgia can be part of inflammatory bowel disease and, according to one study, may respond to treatment with probiotics [2].

Drugs: Among the drugs and immunizations that might cause arthralgia are aromatase inhibitors, statins, and rubella vaccines [3, 4].

Travelers' arthralgia: I just made up this disease name to identify Chikungunya fever, a virus infection that seemed to begin in the southwest Indian Ocean islands in 2005 and is now being seen in travelers returning from Southeast Asia. Symptoms are joint pain, fever, and malaise [5].

Some less common causes: Arthralgia has been reported in patients with hemochromatosis, acromegaly, osteomalacia, and atrial myxoma [6].

1. Jagliano M. Menopausal arthralgia: fact or fiction? Maturitas. 2010;67:29.
2. Karimi O, et al. Probiotics (VSL#3) in arthralgia in patients with ulcerative colitis and Crohn's disease: a pilot study. Drugs Today. 2005;41:453.
3. Horimoto Y, et al. Arthralgia in 329 patients taking aromatase inhibitors. Breast Care. 2009;4:319.
4. Campion J, et al. Statins and joint pain. Brit J Clin Pharmacol. 2008;66:570.
5. Taubitz W, et al. Chikungunya fever in travelers: clinical presentation and course. Clin Inf Dis. 2007;41:e1.
6. Praitano ML, et al. Recurrent transitory ischemic attacks with skin lesions, arthralgia and myalgia should prompt suspicion of atrial myxoma. J Neurol Neurosurg Psychiatry. 2010;81:302.

The patient with episodic pain in one or more joints alternating with symptom-free intervals of weeks to months may have palindromic rheumatism (PR).

Up to two-thirds of patients with PR will eventually develop rheumatoid arthritis [1]. Some of them will have positive tests for inflammatory arthritis—anticitrullinated protein/peptide antibodies and rheumatoid factors [2]. Parenthetically, I have puzzled over this disease name: The word "palindrome" refers to a word or phrase that means the same read in either direction. For example, the words *civic* and *racecar* are palindromes. Perhaps the term refers to the recurring nature of the arthritic symptoms.

1. Koskinen E, et al. Palindromic rheumatism: long-term outcomes of 60 patients diagnosed in 1967–84. J Rheumatol. 2009;36:1873.
2. Rantapää-Dahlqvist S. What happens before the onset of rheumatoid arthritis? Curr Opin Rheumatol. 2009;21:272.

Fig. 11.6 Dactylitis of the hand in a patient with psoriatic arthritis

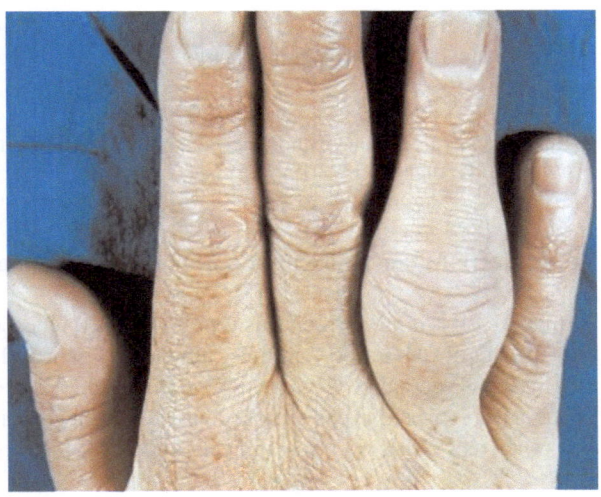

Dactylitis and/or enthesitis suggest the possibility of psoriatic arthritis (PsA).

Dactylitis describes a "sausage-like" swelling of fingers or even toes, caused by inflammation of both joints and soft tissues, with flexor tenosynovitis commonly found in these digits [1] (see Fig. 11.6). Enthesitis is inflammation of the insertion of tendon into bone; a common site of enthesitis in these patients is the insertion of the Achilles tendon into the calcaneus [2, 3].

Why might these facts be important? First, the incidence of PsA in persons over age 30 seems to be rising, if only because of increased recognition of the disease [4]. Second, not all patients with PsA have skin manifestations. About 20 % of patients with PsA have "psoriatic arthritis sine psoriasis," with joint manifestations occurring some time before skin lesions develop. A family history of psoriasis helps identify these patients [5].

1. Kane D, et al. Ultrasonography in the diagnosis and management of psoriatic dactylitis. J Rheumatol. 1999;26:1746.
2. Gisondi P, et al. Lower limb enthesopathy in patients with psoriasis without clinical signs of arthropathy: a hospital-based case-control study. Ann Rheum Dis. 2008;67:26.
3. De Simone C, et al. Achilles tendinitis in psoriasis: clinical and sonographic findings. J Am Acad Dermatol. 2003;49:217.
4. Wilson FC, et al. Time trends in epidemiology and characteristics of psoriatic arthritis over 3 decades: a population-based study. J Rheumatol. 2009;36:361.
5. Olivieri I, et al. Psoriatic arthritis sine psoriasis. J Rheumatol Suppl. 2009;83:28.

When compared with patients with PsA, patients with rheumatoid arthritis (RA) exhibit more tenderness in various locations.

In a study of 50 PsA patients compared with 51 RA patients, investigators used a dolorimeter to assess tenderness at a variety of sites. They found greater tenderness in RA subjects than in PsA subjects when they tested actively inflamed joints, fibrositic sites, and control nonarticular sites [1].

1. Buskila D, et al. Patients with rheumatoid arthritis are more tender than those with psoriatic arthritis. J Rheumatol. 1992;19:1115.

Viral infections can cause joint pathology resembling rheumatoid arthritis.

Human T-cell lymphotropic virus type 1 (HTLV-1) has been found to cause destructive arthritis in laboratory animals. Other causes of inflammatory arthritis include rubella virus, hepatitis C virus, alphaviruses such as Ross River virus, varicella, Epstein-Barr virus, herpes simplex virus, cytomegalovirus, and enterovirus infections such as Coxsackie virus and echovirus [1–4].

1. Palazzi C, et al. Hepatitis C virus-related arthritis. Autoimmunity Rev. 2008;8:48.
2. Toivanen A. Alphaviruses: an emerging cause of arthritis? Curr Opin Rheumatol. 2008;20:486.
3. Toussirot E, et al. Pathophysiological links between rheumatoid arthritis and the Epstein-Barr virus: an update. Joint Bone Spine. 2007;74:418.
4. Calabrese LH, et al. Viral arthritis. Infect Dis North Am. 2005;19:963.

Muscle Pain

The patient with polymyalgia rheumatica may have a normal erythrocyte sedimentation rate (ESR).

Polymyalgia rheumatica is an inflammatory condition of older individuals that tends to begin with muscular aches and stiffness in the shoulders and pelvic girdle and that is closely related to giant-cell arteritis. This latter disease, a vasculitis that can involve large-to-medium-sized arteries, is dangerous because it can result in permanent visual loss [1].

An elevated sedimentation rate has classically been a cornerstone of the diagnosis of polymyalgia rheumatica/giant-cell arteritis. Yet, several studies have shown that the ESR is normal at the time of presentation in about 20 % of patients [2, 3].

1. Salvarani C, et al. Polymyalgia rheumatica and giant-cell arteritis. Lancet. 2008;372:234.
2. Ellis ME, et al. The ESR in the diagnosis and management of the polymyalgia rheumatica/giant cell arteritis syndrome. Ann Rheum Dis. 1983;42:168.
3. Helfgott SM, et al. Polymyalgia rheumatica in patients with a normal erythrocyte sedimentation rate. Arthritis Rheum. 1996;39:304.

There is no gold standard for the diagnosis of fibromyalgia.

This statement—almost word for word—appears in two papers on fibromyalgia, a disorder characterized by chronic somatic pain accompanied by stiffness, fatigue, impaired sleep, depressed mood, and, sometimes, cognitive dysfunction [1, 2]. The disease is diagnosed three to six times more often in women than in men [3].

Katz et al. studied 206 patients using tender point examination, American College of Rheumatology (ACR) survey criteria, and clinical diagnosis. The ACR tender point findings were not a factor in clinical and survey criteria but were considered useful in clinical diagnosis of fibromyalgia. The investigators report that ACR survey criteria and clinical diagnosis were moderately concordant (72–75 %) [2].

1. Goldenberg DL. Diagnosis and differential diagnosis of fibromyalgia. Am J Med. 2009;122:s14.
2. Katz RS, et al. Fibromyalgia diagnosis a comparison of clinical survey, and American College of Rheumatology criteria. Arthritis Rheum. 2006;54:169.
3. Marcus DA. Fibromyalgia: diagnosis and treatment options. Gender Med. 2009;6:139.

Muscle pain causes include some drugs we use.

Myalgia has been reported associated the use of statins [1], ciprofloxacin (Cipro) [2], and mesalazine (Lialda and others), the latter reported following its use to treat a child with Crohn disease [3].

1. Jacobson TA. Toward pain-free statin prescribing: clinical algorithm for diagnosis and management of myalgia. Mayo Clin Proc. 2008;83:687.
2. Eisele S, et al. Ciprofloxacin-related severe acute myalgia necessitating emergency care treatment: a case report and review of the literature. Int J Clin Pharmacol Ther. 2009;47:165.
3. Persic M, et al. Severe myalgia associated with mesalazine treatment in a child with Crohn's disease. Eur J Clin Pharmacol. 2007;63:315.

In addition to the better known causes described above, myalgia can be associated with some uncommon conditions.

Here are three, admittedly unlikely, causes of muscle pain:

Trichinellosis, aka trichinosis: This parasitic disease, contracted by ingestion of the encysted larvae of *Trichinella* species in undercooked meat, causes myalgia, fever, abdominal pain, periorbital edema, and eosinophilia [1, 2].
Lead poisoning: A case report describes a 35-year-old man whose lead poisoning presented as severe, progressive myalgia [3].
McArdle disease: This rare glycogen storage disease causes muscle pain, sometimes associated with myoglobinuria triggered by exercise [4, 5].

1. Taylor WR, et al. Acute febrile myalgia in Vietnam due to trichinellosis following the consumption of raw pork. Clin Infect Dis. 2009;49:e79.
2. Kennedy ED, et al. Trichinellosis surveillance: United States, 2002–2007. MMWR Surveill Summ. 2009;58:1.
3. Petterson T, et al. Lead poisoning presenting as acute severe myalgia. Acute Med. 2010;9:24.
4. Schmidt B, et al. McArdle's disease in two generations: autosomal recessive transmission with manifesting heterozygote. Neurology. 1987;37:1558.
5. Lucia A, et al. McArdle disease: what do neurologists need to know? Nature Clin Pract Neurology. 2008;4:568.

Muscle Weakness

Ocular muscle weakness may be the first symptom of myasthenia gravis (MG).

Ptosis and/or diplopia, caused by weakness of voluntary muscles related to the eye, are present at the onset of myasthenia gravis in half or more of all patients. The ptosis of MG is elicited by brief opposition to closure of the lids, followed by the eyes opening widely with scleral exposure, a phenomenon termed the "peek sign" [1]. One observer found ocular symptoms present at onset in 65 % of 432 patients with the disease [2].

In a systematic review of 15 studies, Scherer et al. found that the presence of the "peek sign" increased the likelihood of MG by a remarkable ratio of 30.0 (95 % CI 3.2–278.0). These investigators also found another useful key to the diagnosis of MG: a history of "speech becoming unintelligible during prolonged speaking" (LR 4.5, CI 1.2–17.0) [3].

1. Osher RH, et al. Orbicularis fatigue: the "peek sign" of myasthenia gravis. Clin Sci. 1979;97:677.
2. Oosterhuis HJGH. The ocular signs and symptoms of myasthenia gravis. Arch Ophthalmol. 1982;52:363.
3. Scherer K, et al. Does this patient have myasthenia gravis? JAMA. 2005;293:1906.

Muscle weakness closing the jaw is more likely than jaw-opening weakness to point to the diagnosis of MG.

In a study of 46 patients with flaccid quadriplegia with various etiologies, investigators found jaw-closing weakness in 88.8 % of nine patients with MG. In contrast, jaw-opening weakness was more common among patients with polymyositis/dermatomyositis (71.4 % of seven patients), hypokalemic periodic paralysis (83.3 % of six patients), and Guillain–Barré syndrome (4.1 % of 24 patients) [1].

1. Pal S, et al. Jaw muscle weakness: a differential indicator of neuromuscular weakness: preliminary observations. Muscle Nerve. 2011:43;807.

The patient with hyperthyroidism who suddenly develops flaccid paralysis especially affecting the proximal muscles may have thyrotoxic hypokalemic periodic paralysis.

The sudden onset of this disorder may take the patient to the emergency department, where finding a low serum potassium level and elevated thyroxine and triiodothyronine levels points to the diagnosis of thyrotoxic hypokalemic periodic paralysis [1]. There is also a familial type of hypokalemic periodic paralysis that is transmitted as an autosomal dominant disease [2].

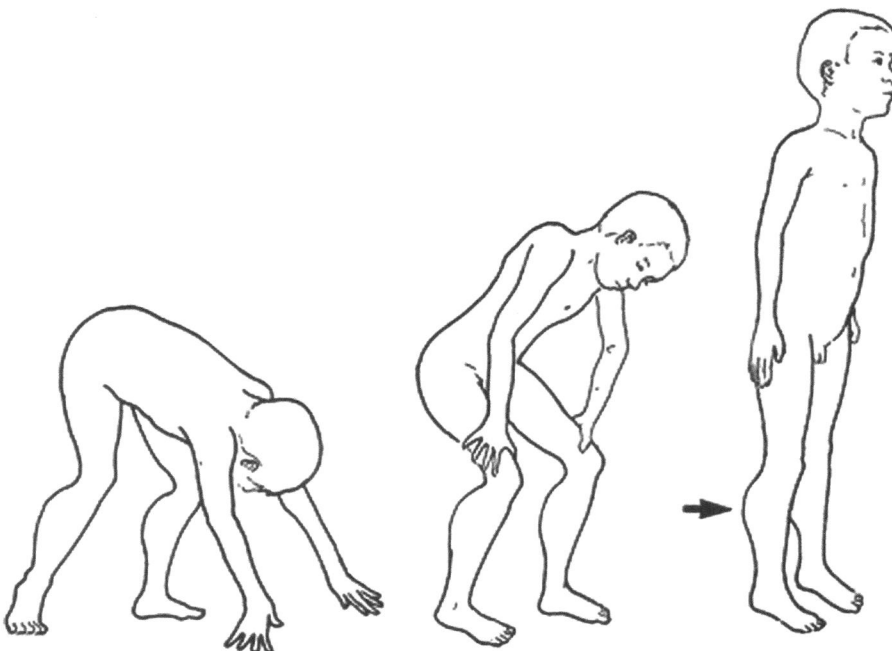

Fig. 11.7 Gower sign

1. Pothiwala P, et al. Thyrotoxic periodic paralysis: a review. J Intens Care Med. 2010;25:71.
2. Da Silva MR, et al. A mutation in the KCNE3 potassium channel gene is associated with thyro-toxic hypokalemic periodic paralysis. J Clin Endo Metab. 2002;87:4881.

The young child exhibiting "difficulty" with large muscle skills, such as climbing and running, may have Duchenne muscular dystrophy (MD).

Duchenne MD typically presents in males during early childhood, often at age two or three, with an insidious development of muscular weakness, especially in the lower extremities. The patient may exhibit Gower sign, described as "climbing up the legs" when arising from the floor (see Fig. 11.7). Other motor manifestations may include a lumbar lordosis and a waddling gait. Calf enlargement (pseudohyper-trophy) is commonly noted [1, 2]. Cardiomyopathy is part of the disease pattern, and, in one study of 328 patients with Duchenne MD, cardiac disease was present in all by age 18 [3]. Cognitive impairment may also be noted.

Patients with Becker MD, which begins later in life, will also show pseudohyper-trophy of the calf muscles. These patients tend to have slower progression of muscle impairment compared to those with Duchenne MD, but cardiac disease may be a prominent finding [4, 5].

1. Beggs AH, et al. Improved diagnosis of Duchenne/Becker muscular dystrophy. J Clin Invest. 1990;85:613.
2. Kohler M, et al. Disability and survival in Duchenne muscular dystrophy. J Neurol Neurosurg Psychiatry. 2009;80:320.
3. Nigro G, et al. The incidence and evolution of cardiomyopathy in Duchenne muscular dystrophy. Int J Cardiol. 1990;26:271.
4. Yazawa M, et al. A family of Becker's progressive muscular dystrophy with severe cardiomyopathy. Eur Neurol. 1987;27:13.
5. Saito M, et al. Cardiac dysfunction with Becker muscular dystrophy. Am Heart J. 1996;132:642.

Selected Problems of the Musculoskeletal System

The patient with a painful extremity that exhibits vasomotor changes, trophic skin manifestations, and eventual bone demineralization has the classic symptoms and signs of the complex regional pain syndrome (CRPS).

Previously called reflex sympathetic dystrophy or Sudeck atrophy, the CRPS may follow a minor injury, fracture, surgery, a stroke or heart attack, or no report of any apparent precipitating event. A typical patient may present with neuropathic pain in a cool, pale or a warm, red extremity. There may also be edema or abnormal sweating and eventually even loss of joint mobility [1, 2].

1. Birklein F. Complex regional pain syndrome. J Neurol. 2005;252:131.
2. Atkins RM. Complex regional pain syndrome. J Bone Joint Surg. 2003;85:1100.

The use of ultrasound may prove helpful in detecting fractures in children.

In a study of 25 occult fractures involving various bones and joints in 25 children, average age 7.7 years, the use of routine radiography was compared to ultrasonography. Routine x-rays failed to demonstrate fractures in 13 subjects. On balance, ultrasound detected cortical discontinuity, a sign of fracture, in 23 children and was suspicious in the other two [1].

Of course, radiography and ultrasonography are not always available. In a pinch, a stethoscope and tuning fork can help diagnose fractures in long bones, according to Weiss. As an example, he describes assessment of a suspected tibial fracture: "Take your tuning fork and bang it and put it on the proximal tibia. Take your stethoscope and listen over the medial malleolus, the distal tibia. Then compare it to the other side. Even if there is a nondisplaced linear fracture through that bone, that sound will be dampened significantly so that you will be able to tell the difference." Weiss reports 99 % sensitivity in tests of 100 patients [2].

1. Cho KH, et al. Ultrasound diagnosis of either an occult or missed fracture of an extremity in pediatric-aged children. Korean J Radiol. 2010;11:84.
2. Weiss EA. Quoted in: London S. When improvised case is the name of the game. Fam Pract News. 2010:97.

Pain, tenderness, swelling, and warmth persisting, even increasing, following a soft tissue injury is the classic presentation of myositis ossificans (MO).

The x-ray will reveal heterotropic bone formation, with flocculent densities resembling bony callus, often with periosteal reactive changes [1]. Not all cases follow trauma; one study of 15 subjects with MO revealed two instances of recent surgery and five patients with no trauma history at all [2].

Fig. 11.8 Osteoid osteoma with central nidus in the left femur

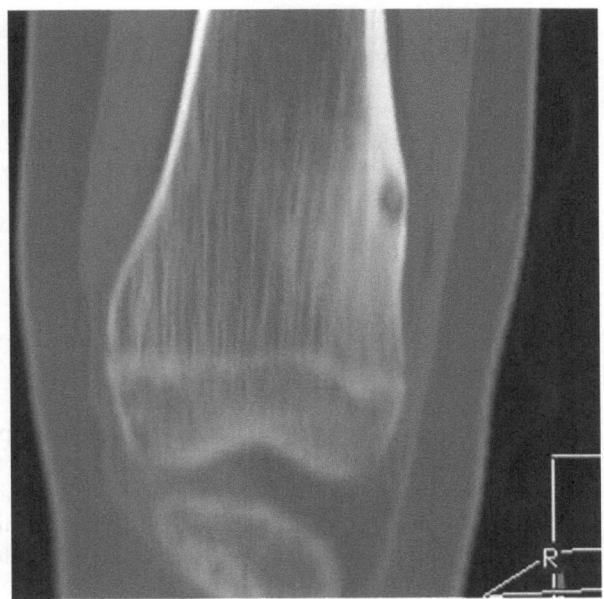

On radiologic examination, MO can be confused with osteogenic sarcoma. Two facts can be helpful in distinguishing the two entities: In long bones, osteogenic sarcoma is generally found in the metaphysis, while MO is more likely to be located in the area of the diaphysis. Secondly, on close examination of the roentgenograms, osteogenic sarcoma is likely to be seen disrupting the cortex, while with MO the bony cortex remains intact [3, 4]. In the end, biopsy may be needed, although Martin advises, "Early biopsy is not recommended because of the difficulty in distinguishing the formation from cancer" [1].

1. Martin DM, et al. Myositis ossificans. N Engl J Med. 2011;364:378.
2. Meng SQ, et al. Myositis ossificans: a clinicopathologic analysis of 15 cases. Zhonghua Bing Li Xue Za Zhi. 2008;37:665.
3. Muñoz-Mahamud E, et al. Myositis ossificans mimicking parosteal osteosarcoma: a case report and literature review. Acta Orthop Belg. 2011;77:274.
4. Tyler P, et al. The imaging of myositis ossificans. Semin Musculoskel Radiol. 2010;14:201.

A young adult patient with severe bone pain dramatically relieved by aspirin or other nonsteroidal anti-inflammatory drugs (NSAIDs) may have osteoid osteoma.

Many patients report that the intense pain is nocturnal [1]. The tumor is likely to occur in the long bones or spine, although radicular pain has been reported [2]. The typical radiologic appearance is a small radiolucent area in a sclerotic region termed a nidus (see Fig. 11.8). Most cases of osteoid osteoma heal spontaneously, and recovery may be hastened by the use of NSAIDs, although some of these tumors are excised for definitive diagnosis or for pain relief [3].

1. Kitsoulis P, et al. Osteoid osteoma. Acta Orthop Belg. 2006;72:119.
2. Ebrahimzadeh MH, et al. Osteoid osteoma: a diagnosis for radicular pain of extremities. Orthopedics. 2009;32:821.
3. Goto T, et al. Administration of nonsteroidal anti-inflammatory drugs accelerates spontaneous healing of osteoid osteoma. Arch Orthop Trauma Surg. 2011;131:619.

Osteopenia and osteoporosis have some diverse origins other than the usual risk factors.

We think of the classic presentation of osteopenia/osteoporosis as a disease of post-menopausal, thin, white women, who may smoke cigarettes, have a history of low calcium intake, and/or exhibit low serum levels of vitamin D [1]. Osteopenia/osteoporosis should also be suspected in patients with chronic obstructive lung disease (COPD) [2], multiple sclerosis [3], thalassemia [4], sickle-cell anemia [5], and even idiopathic adolescent scoliosis [6].

1. Karaguzel G, et al. Diagnosis and treatment of osteopenia. Rev Endocr Metab Disord. 2010;11:237.
2. Ferguson GT, et al. Prevalence and progression of osteoporosis in patients with COPD. Chest. 2009;136:1456.
3. Kampman MT, et al. Multiple sclerosis, a cause of secondary osteoporosis? Acta Neurologica Scand. 2010;124:44.
4. Chatterjee R, et al. Osteopenia-osteoporosis syndrome in patients with thalassemia: understanding of type of bone disease and response to treatment. Hemoglobin. 2009;33:S136.
5. Miller RG, et al. Prevalence and progression of osteoporosis in patients with COPD. Am J Hematol. 2006;81:236.
6. Sadat-Ali M, et al. Does scoliosis cause low bone mass? A comparative study between siblings. Eur Spine J. 2008;17:944.

Examining the "thumb in a clenched fist" can be a useful screening test for Marfan syndrome.

Steinberg describes the test as "having the patient make a fist over the thumb. When positive the thumb clearly extended beyond the confines of the fist." The phenomenon occurs because of the long, spidery digits and joint laxity seen in the Marfan syndrome. The author cautions against forcing or stretching the thumb, and he reports that in a series of "several hundred" patients, only three had a positive test in the absence of other signs of Marfan syndrome [1].

1. Steinberg I. A simple screening test for the Marfan syndrome. Am J Roentgenol. 1966;97:118.

Chapter 12
The Skin and Subcutaneous Tissues

The power of making a correct diagnosis is the key to all success in the treatment of skin diseases; without this faculty, the physician can never be a thorough dermatologist, and therapeutics at once cease to hold their proper position, and become empirical.
American dermatologist Louis A. Duhring (1845–1913) [1]

Contents

R.B. Taylor, *Diagnostic Principles and Applications*,
DOI 10.1007/978-1-4614-1111-6_12, © Springer Science+Business Media, LLC 2013

Louis A. Duhring was professor of dermatology at the University of Pennsylvania in the 1880s and a pioneer in dermatology, now remembered with the eponymous disease name, Duhring disease, aka dermatitis herpetiformis. This quotation, published in 1871 in the *American Journal of Syphilography and Dermatology*, must spark some nostalgic reflection for clinicians. First, note the name of the journal. In Duhring's time, the study of syphilis was a prominent concern of those who specialized in diseases of the skin. The original name of the specialty board was the American Board of Dermatology and Syphilology, with the name changed to the American Board of Dermatology as recently as 1955. And I applaud Duhring's quest for the correct diagnosis. Yet, while Duhring decries empirical treatment of skin disease, he and his colleagues had few remedies we would today consider to be of much benefit no matter what the diagnosis. The development of Salvarsan for syphilis, antibiotics to treat infections, and steroids for almost everything dermatologic was still decades away.

1. Duhring LA. Diagnosis of skin diseases. Am J Syphilography Dermatol. 1871;2:104.

Macules, Papules, and Plaques

In a patient with a maculopapular rash, think first of a viral exanthema or drug reaction.

After all, the most common things occur most commonly. In a young person, and especially if fever is present, think of a viral exanthema as a cause of a maculopapular rash. The common viral exanthemas have some telltale signs that, since some of these diseases may be seen less commonly today, merit brief review [1]:

Viral disease	Classic sign that may be present
Measles	Koplik spots in the oral mucosa
Rubella	Retroauricular lymphadenopathy
Roseola	The rash occurs as the fever subsides
Erythema infectiosum (fifth disease)	Erythematous ("slapped") cheeks
Infectious mononucleosis	Hepatosplenomegaly

Although not a viral infection, scarlet fever may also cause a maculopapular rash, with circumoral pallor, a "strawberry" tongue, and prominence of the rash in the skin folds (Pastia sign) [1].

When it comes to drugs, a maculopapular rash can complicate the use of virtually any medication. Think about a penicillin derivative, cephalosporin, nonsteroidal anti-inflammatory agent (NSAID), or radiocontrast agent [2]. Remember also that a high percentage of patients with infectious mononucleosis who take ampicillin will develop a maculopapular rash [1].

Less common causes of a maculopapular rash that I encountered in my research are acute brucellosis [3], cutaneous Hodgkin disease [4], and adult-onset Still disease [5]. In toxic shock syndrome, a macular or maculopapular rash may occur, followed by desquamation [6].

1. Garcia JJG. Differential diagnosis of viral exanthemas. Open Vaccine J. 2010;3:65.
2. Schnyder B. Approach to the patient with drug allergy. Med Clin N Am. 2010;94:665.
3. Omidi A, et al. Acute brucellosis with pancytopenia and maculopapular rash. Iran J Path. 2009;4:133.
4. Rho YK, et al. A case of cutaneous Hodgkin's disease presented with a maculopapular rash. Korean J Dermatol. 2008;46:1262.
5. Freund V, et al. A 39-year old patient with maculopapular rash, recurrent fever, and arthralgia. Der Hautartz. 2009;60:578.
6. Andrews MM, et al. Recurrent non-menstrual toxic shock syndrome: clinical manifestations, diagnosis, and treatment. Clin Infect Dis. 2001;32:1470.

Erythematous plaques with silvery scales occurring on the scalp and extensor surfaces of the back, elbows, and knee describe the classical presentation of psoriasis (see Fig. 12.1).

The nails are often involved, with pitting and loosening of the nail plate sometimes noted [1]. Sometimes the ear canals are affected. The disease is not uncommon, affecting 2.5 % of white patients and 1.3 % of African Americans [2]. Psoriasis is significant not only for its impact on the quality of life but also for the risks it seems to bring. In a study of 3,236 patients with psoriasis compared with 2,500 controls, investigators found that the psoriasis cohort had a higher prevalence of diabetes mellitus, hypertension, and dyslipidemia. They report: "After controlling for these variables, we found a higher prevalence not only of ischemic heart disease (odds ratio [OR] 1.78; 95 % confidence interval [CI], 1.51–2.11) but also of cerebrovascular (OR 1.70; 95 % CI 1.33–2.17) and peripheral vascular (OR 1.98; 95 % CI 1.32–2.82) diseases in patients with psoriasis compared with controls." Psoriasis was also found to be an independent risk factor for mortality (OR 1.86; 95 % CI 1.56–2.21) [3]. The cardiovascular risk findings were confirmed by a recently published systematic review of the literature [4]. Pearce et al. also report a series of documented deaths attributable to psoriasis [5].

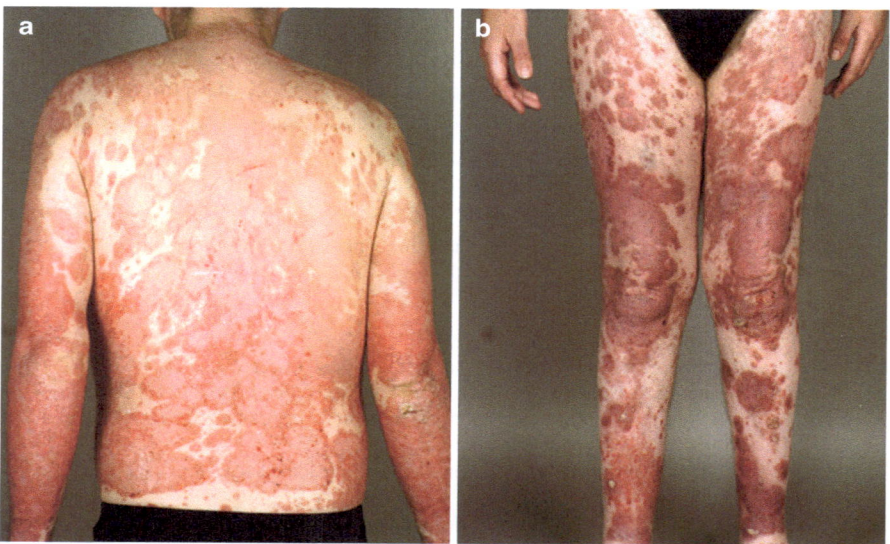

Fig. 12.1   A patient with severe psoriasis showing lesions of the back (**a**) and legs (**b**)

1. Jiaravuthisan MM, et al. Psoriasis of the nail: anatomy, pathology, clinical presentation, and a review of literature on therapy. J Am Acad Dermatol. 2007;57:1.
2. Gelfand JM, et al. The prevalence of psoriasis in African Americans: results from a population-based study. J Am Acad Dermatol. 2005;52:23.
3. Prodanovich S, et al. Association of psoriasis with coronary artery, cerebrovascular, and peripheral vascular diseases and mortality. Arch Dermatol. 2009;145:700.
4. Patel RV, et al. Psoriasis and vascular disease-risk factors and outcomes: a systematic review of the literature. J Gen Intern Med. 2011;26:1036.
5. Pearce DJ, et al. Death from psoriasis: representative US data. J Dermatol Treat. 2006;17:302.

Pityriasis rosea (PR) sometimes does not present with the typical "Christmas tree" pattern rash.

Atypical PR may be confused with secondary syphilis, nummular eczema, guttate psoriasis, cutaneous lupus erythematosus, pityriasis versicolor, and cutaneous T cell lymphoma [1]. The well-demarcated, pink "herald patch" occurring as the early manifestation of PR could be misdiagnosed (and erroneously treated) as a dermatophytosis. A child with PR may have an "inverse rash." While the patches of adults (generally young adults) are typically on the chest, neck, back, and upper arms, the rash in children may spare these areas and instead involve the face, distal extremities, or the axillary and inguinal regions [2].

An interesting possibility to watch is described in reports that the H1N1 virus may be a cause of PR, adding one more question to ask in taking a diagnostic history of patients with puzzling skin patches [3, 4]. Or will this turn out to be one more instance of simple lowered resistance to concurrent disease associated with the flu?

1. Browning JC. An update on pityriasis rosea and other similar childhood exanthems. Curr Opin Pediatr. 2009;21:481.
2. Trager JD. Scaly pubic plaques in a 2-year-old girl—or an "inverse" rash. J Pediatr Adolesc Gynecol. 2007;20:109.
3. Kwon NH, et al. A novel influenza A (H1N1) virus as a possible cause of pityriasis rosea? J Eur Acad Dermatol Venereol. 2011;25:368.
4. Mubki TF, et al. A case of pityriasis rosea concurrent with the novel influenza A (H1N1) virus. Pediatr Dermatol. 2001;28:341.

The rash of secondary syphilis, although typically maculopapular, is best described as (almost) pleomorphic—and potentially infectious.

In a study of 105 persons with secondary syphilis, the distribution of skin lesions was as follows: maculopapular, 73 subjects; papular, 13; macular, 10; annular papular, six; papulopustular, two; and psoriasiform papular, one [1]. But about the adjective "pleomorphic," note the absence of vesicular lesions on this list. A helpful diagnostic clue to the diagnosis of secondary syphilis is finding lesions on the palms and soles, although this manifestation may also be seen in Rocky Mountain spotted fever. The lesions of secondary syphilis can be confused with pityriasis rosea (see Fig. 12.2).

Fig. 12.2 Pityriasis
rosea-like lesions of
secondary syphilis involving
the chest

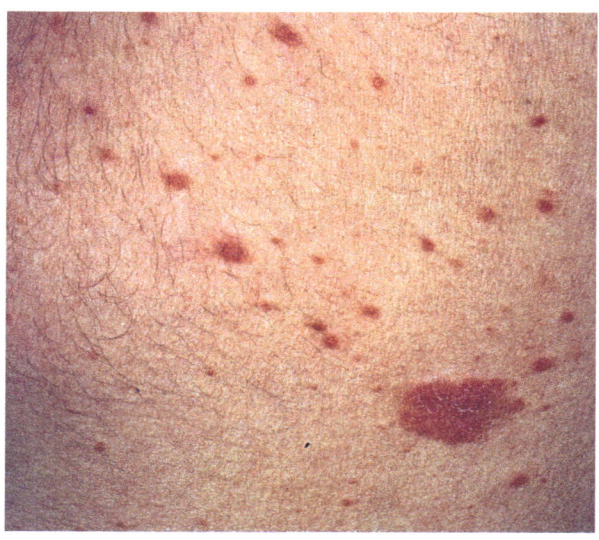

1. Chapel TA. The signs and symptoms of secondary syphilis. Sex Transm Dis. 1980;7:161.

Other, less commonly occurring, diseases that may manifest maculopapular or plaque-like lesions are lichen planus (LP), sarcoidosis, and Hansen disease (HD).

Here is what we might find with these three diverse clinical entities:

Lichen planus: The classic lesion of LP is a polygonal, flat, pruritic, violaceous papule or plaque, often found on the flexor surfaces of the wrists [1]. Oral lesions are common, and pain in the oral mucosa or gingiva is a common complaint [2]. The surfaces of both cutaneous and oral lesions may exhibit Wickham striae, reticulated white lines [1]. A rare variant is esophageal lichen planus, most likely to present with the symptom of dysphagia [3].

Sarcoidosis: A "great imitator" like syphilis, sarcoidosis can involve a variety of organ systems, including the skin, where the disease can cause macules, patches, papules, ulcers, granulomas, and alopecia [4].

Hansen disease/leprosy: Skin manifestations of this slowly evolving infectious disease include erythematous macules, papules, nodules, and plaques, which may be hypopigmented [5, 6]. A key to the diagnosis may be finding anesthetic skin lesions, reminding us that, according to Wilder-Smith, "Leprosy is the most common treatable peripheral nerve disorder worldwide" [6]. Curiously, there have been recent reports linking Hansen disease to armadillos in the southern United States [7] (see Fig. 12.3).

Fig. 12.3 Multiple anesthetic
erythematous lesions of
borderline tuberculoid
leprosy

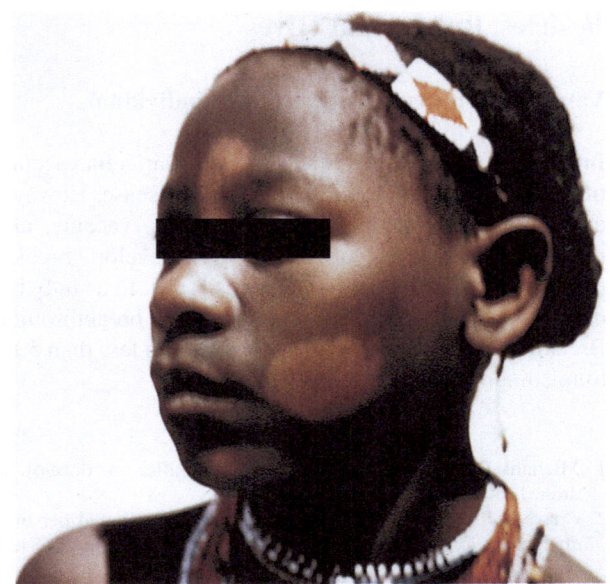

1. Lehman JS, et al. Lichen planus. Int J Dermatol. 2009;48:682.
2. Ingafou M, et al. Oral lichen planus: a retrospective study of 690 British patients. Oral Dis. 2006;12:463.
3. Fox LP, et al. Lichen planus of the esophagus: what dermatologists need to know. J Am Acad Dermatol. 2011;65:175.
4. Kang MJ, et al. Cutaneous sarcoidosis presenting as multiple erythematous macules and patches. Ann Dermatol. 2009;21:168.
5. Becker L, et al. Nonpruritic plaques. J Fam Pract. 2009;58:657.
6. Wilder-Smith EP, et al. Nerve damage leprosy and its management. Nat Clin Pract Neurol. 2008;4:656.
7. Abide JM, et al. Three indigenous cases of leprosy in the Mississippi delta. South Med J. 2008;101:635.

Vesicles, Bullae, and Hives

Varicella can occur in a vaccinated individual.

Introduced to the United States in 1995, varicella vaccine has reduced the incidence of chicken pox and mortality due to the disease. However, not all have received the currently recommended two doses of the vaccine, and among individuals who received a single dose, up to 20 % will develop "breakthrough disease" following exposure to the varicella zoster virus [1, 2]. In a study by Kuter et al. of 1,102 children receiving two injections, the rate of breakthrough disease was only 1.5 %. Breakthrough disease tends to be mild, with less than 50 lesions, and may be subject to misdiagnosis [3].

1. Michalik DE, et al. Primary vaccine failure after one dose of varicella vaccine in healthy children. J Infect Dis. 2008;197:944.
2. Chaves SS, et al. Varicella disease among vaccinated persons: clinical and epidemiological characteristics, 1997–2005. J Infect Dis. 2008;197 Suppl 2:S127.
3. Kuter B, et al. Are two doses of varicella vaccine more effective? Pediatr Inf Dis J. 2004;23:132.

The patient with a long-standing, intensely pruritic, blistering eruption of the skin may have dermatitis herpetiformis (DH).

Also sometimes called Duhring disease (see the quote and comments at the beginning of this chapter), DH causes papulovesicles filled with a watery fluid or plaques especially seen on the elbows, knees, and gluteal area. The eruption may look like herpes, hence the name of the disease, but the diseases are unrelated. DH is considered to be the skin manifestation of celiac disease, and recognition of the entity is easier if the patient has gastrointestinal (GI) manifestations. Even in the majority of DH cases without GI symptoms, all have a gluten-sensitive enteropathy, and the rash typically responds to gluten restriction in the diet [1–3].

1. Reunala T. Dermatitis herpetiformis: coeliac disease of the skin. Ann Med. 1998;30:416.
2. Fry L. Dermatitis herpetiformis. Balirrieres Clin Gastroenterol. 1995;9:371.
3. Ingen-Houz-Oro S. Dermatitis herpetiformis: a review. Ann Dermatol Venereol. 2011;138:221.

Flaccid bullae involving diverse areas including the oropharynx characterize pemphigus, a life-threatening, autoimmune disease.

Diagnosis can be confusing at times, because the bullae rupture easily and the skin may exhibit only erosion. Pain occurs commonly, especially after rupture of bullae. Lesions may even be seen in the ear and nose. Diagnosis is confirmed by histologic findings of epidermal acantholysis (loss of cohesion between epidermal cells) and immunologic tests—an enzyme-linked immunosorbent assay (ELISA) [1, 2].

1. Ioannides D, et al. Pemphigus. J Eur Acad Dermatol Venereol. 2008;22:1478.
2. Robati RM, et al. Mucosal manifestations of pemphigus vulgaris in the ear, nose and throat; before and after treatment. J Am Acad Dermatol. 2012;67:e249. doi:10.1016/j. jaad.2011.06.022.

A bullous eruption may occur in the lower extremities in diabetic patients.

Termed bullosis diabeticorum, the blisters have been postulated to be related to poor vascular supply to the skin in the face of venous insufficiency, leading to the characteristic blisters [1, 2].

1. Basarab T, et al. Bullosis diabeticorum: a case report and literature review. Clin Exp Dermatol. 1995;20:218.
2. Ghosh SK, et al. Bullosis diabeticorum: a distinctive blistering eruption in diabetes mellitus. Int J Diabetes Dev Countries. 2009;29:41.

A vesicular rash appearing on the sides of the fingers and perhaps in other areas such as the arms or chest may be an id reaction.

Look for a coincidental fungal infection, often on the foot [1]. My most recent case was a young woman who had recently begun Taekwondo lessons, conducted barefoot on mats shared with others. She had barely noticed her recently acquired dermatophytosis of the foot, the trigger for the id reaction.

1. Brannon H. Id reaction. About.com/Dermatology. Available at: http://dermatology.about.com/od/glossaryi/g/id_reaction.htm.

A clue to the diagnosis of urticaria is this: The lesions come and go.

"With the exception of urticarial vasculitis, urticaria typically lasts less than 24–36 h at one site. A rash that persists longer should raise the suspicion of another inflammatory process," according to Weldon [1]. Urticaria—with intensely pruritic, raised wheals—is generally self-limited but may become frustratingly chronic. Urticaria may be misdiagnosed as erythema multiforme (look for target or iris-shaped lesions, described below), atopic dermatitis (a flexor surface distribution is a clue), or Henoch–Schönlein purpura (purpuric lesions likely) [2]. Laboratory investigations are generally unproductive, and most cases of chronic urticaria are idiopathic.

Hives can, however, occur with some noteworthy diseases. Acute urticaria is commonly observed in the prodromal stage of hepatitis A and B infection and, although rarely, in hepatitis C infection [3]. Lyme disease may present as an urticarial rash [4]. In children, think of viral illness or antibiotic drug therapy [5].

In a study of 130 patients with chronic urticaria, a specific cause was found in only 58 individuals (45 %), of whom 50 were diagnosed by clinical history and the remaining 8 by standardized questionnaire. In no patient was there a benefit gained by any type of laboratory testing [6].

1. Weldon D. When your patients are itching to see you: not all hives are urticaria. Allergy Asthma Proc. 2005;26:1.
2. Schaefer P. Urticaria: evaluation and treatment. Am Fam Physician. 2011;83:1078.
3. Cribier B. Urticaria and hepatitis. Clin Rev Allergy Immunol. 2006;30:25.
4. Teere AC, et al. The early clinical manifestations of Lyme disease. Ann Intern Med. 1983;99:76.
5. Mortreaux P. Acute urticaria in infancy and early childhood: a prospective study. Arch Dermatol. 1998;134:319.
6. Kozel MM, et al. Evaluation of a clinical guideline for the diagnoses of physical and chronic urticaria and angioedema. Acta Dermatol Venereol. 2002;82:270.

Target or iris-shaped lesions with central clearing, especially found on the extremities and trunk, characterize erythema multiforme (EM).

The target lesion is identified by the concentric rings (see Fig. 12.4). Huff reports that in "most patients disease (i.e., EM) is associated with recurrent herpes simplex infections" [1]. Other important triggers are mycoplasma infections and reactions to drugs such as sulfonamides, penicillin, or phenytoin (Dilantin) [2].

1. Huff JC. Erythema multiforme. Dermatol Clin. 1985;3:141.
2. Stampien TM, et al. Erythema multiforme. Am Fam Physician. 1992;46:1171.

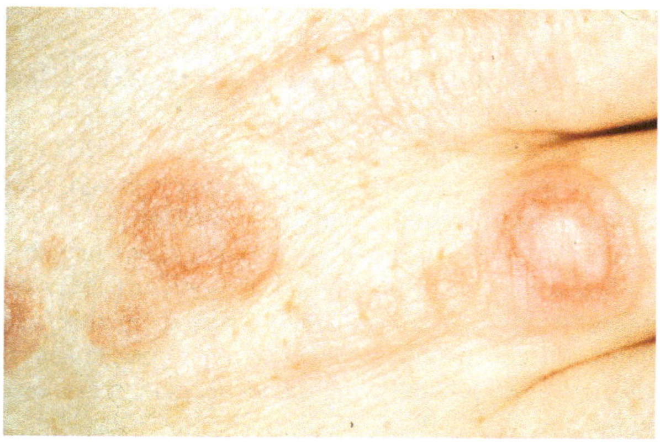

Fig. 12.4 Erythema multiforme target lesion. The typical target lesion consists of two to three concentric rings; the central one is dusky and surrounded by an erythematous ring. The outer ring is paler in color

Abnormal Pigmentation of the Skin

An abnormal yellow hue to the skin or a halo nevus may be associated with pernicious anemia (PA).

The yellow skin is due to bilirubin released during hemolysis of macrocytic red blood cells and not to anemia, which would be more likely to cause pallor. These patients with PA may also exhibit premature graying of the hair and hyperpigmentation of the nails. A significant association of pernicious anemia with a (Sutton's) halo nevus, as well as with blue eyes and blond hair, has been described [1, 2] (see Fig. 12.5).

A more or less yellow color of the skin can be caused by other entities as well. These include jaundice, myxedema, nephritic syndrome, excessive ingestion of beta-carotene in food or as a dietary supplement, and digitalis poisoning [3, 4].

1. Noppakun N, et al. Reversible hyperpigmentation of skin and nails with white hair due to vitamin B12 deficiency. Arch Dermatol. 1986;122:896.
2. Dawber RPR. Integumentary associations of pernicious anemia. Br J Dermatol. 1970;82:221.
3. Ortonne JP, et al. Latest insights into skin hyperpigmentation. J Invest Dermatol Sympos Proc. 2008;13:10.
4. Prince MR, et al. Beta-carotene accumulation in serum and skin. Am J Clin Nutr. 1993;57:175.

Skin hyperpigmentation may be the manifestation that alerts patient and clinician to the presence of hemochromatosis, aka "bronze diabetes."

Described by Cowan as a "preventable cause of liver disease," hemochromatosis is a disease with an underestimated prevalence [1]. Niederau et al. report the following

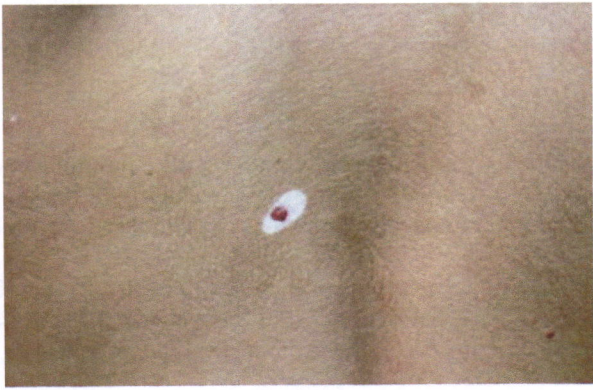

Fig. 12.5 Halo nevus

frequency of various manifestations at the time of diagnosis in 251 patients with hemochromatosis [2]:

- Abnormal liver function tests, 75 %
- Weakness and lethargy, 74 %
- Skin hyperpigmentation, 70 %
- Diabetes mellitus, 48 %
- Impotence, 45 % in males
- Arthralgia, 44 %
- ECG abnormalities, 31 %

1. Cowan ML, et al. The increasing hospital disease burden of hemochromatosis in England. Aliment Pharmacol Ther. 2010;31:247.
2. Niederau C, et al. Epidemiology, clinical spectrum and prognosis of hemochromatosis. Adv Exp Med Biol. 1994;356:293.

A patient, especially an older patient, with slate-blue skin may have argyria.

Argyria, the term coming from the ancient Greek word for silver, describes discoloration of the skin and other tissues due to the accumulation of silver compounds. The most likely source of the silver is the use of compounds containing colloidal silver [1, 2]. These were once widely used (hence, my "older patient" descriptor above) to treat upper respiratory infections and allergies, and from my own childhood, I can recall my mother earnestly "painting" my sore throat with just such a preparation. Amazingly, these preparations are still available and used today.

Localized argyria has been reported in a patient with silver earrings imbedded in the ears for several years [3]. With the current fad of body piercing with rings and studs, are we on the threshold of an epidemic of localized argyria?

1. Chang AL, et al. A case of argyria after colloidal silver ingestion. J Cutan Pathol. 2006;33:808.
2. Kim Y, et al. A case of generalized argyria after ingestion of colloidal silver solution. Am J Ind Med. 2009;52:246.
3. van den Nieuwenhuijsen IJ, et al. Localized argyria caused by silver earrings. Dermatologica. 1988;177:189.

Ashen gray macules and papules with a palpable erythematous border occurring in a symmetric and widespread distribution describe erythema dyschromicum perstans, also known as the Cinderella syndrome.

The term "Cinderella syndrome" alludes to the storybook character who swept cinders and ashes until her skin was ashen gray. The disease is rare and has chiefly been described in Latin American populations [1, 2]. The sobriquet Cinderella syndrome can be a little confusing; this same term has been used to describe the phenomenon of adoptive girls falsely claiming to be dressed in ragged clothing while being forced to do more household chores than their (allegedly more favored) biological siblings [3].

1. Schwartz RA. Erythema dyschromicum perstans: the continuing enigma of Cinderella or ashy dermatosis. Int J Dermatol. 2004;43:230.
2. Muñoz C, et al. A case of Cinderella: erythema dyschromicum perstans (ashy dermatosis or dermatosis cinecienta). Skin. 2011;9:63.
3. Goodwin J, et al. Children who simulate neglect. Am J Psychiatry. 1980;137:1223.

Consider a drug-related cause in any patient with hyperpigmented skin.

One author describes drugs as the cause of 10–20 % of cases of hyperpigmentation, especially in older individuals. The chief offenders are nonsteroidal anti-inflammatory drugs (NSAIDs), amiodarone, tetracyclines, psychotropic drugs, cytotoxic drugs, and heavy metals. Any of several mechanisms may be involved, including an accumulation of the drug itself, a photosensitizing reaction, an action of melanin, and drug-induced synthesis of pigments [1–3].

1. Dereire O. Drug-induced skin pigmentation: epidemiology, diagnosis and treatment. Am J Clin Dermatol. 2001;4:253.
2. Stahli BE, et al. Amiodarone-induced skin hyperpigmentation. QJM. 2011;104:723.
3. D'Agostine ML, et al. Imipramine-induced hyperpigmentation: a case report and review of the literature. J Cutan Path. 2009;36:799.

Hyperpigmentation of the skin is one of the manifestations of Addison disease.

Do not overlook the "muddy" hyperpigmentation of Addison disease, primary adrenal insufficiency, which in one instance included pigmentation of a scar. Other features seen may include weight loss, lethargy, and postural hypotension [1].

1. Bourke T, et al. Addison's disease, a spectrum of presentation. Pediatr Res. 2010;68:549.

Disorders of the Nails

Single, white transverse bands of the fingernails, sometimes called Mees' lines or Reil lines, can suggest a diverse list of possible causes.

Mees lines were once considered key to the diagnosis of arsenical poisoning, a problem we seldom encounter today [1]. The single white bands in the nails have subsequently been described in patients with cardiac insufficiency, pneumonia, psoriasis, sickle-cell anemia, Hodgkin disease, and thallium toxicity. When associated with infectious febrile disease, we call these Reil lines [2].

A variant is the paired, narrow, white transverse lines considered by Muehrcke to be diagnostic of hypoalbuminemia and known today as Muehrcke lines [3]. These lines have also been described in other settings, such as evidence of past acute renal failure, sickle-cell crisis, and septicemia, as well as in adults and children receiving cancer chemotherapy [4, 5].

1. Quecedo E. Mees' lines: a clue for the diagnosis of arsenic poisoning. Arch Dermatol. 1996;3:349.
2. Hudson JB. Transverse white lines in the fingernails after acute and chronic renal failure. Arch Intern Med. 1996;117:276.
3. Muehrcke RC. The fingernails in chronic hypoalbuminemia. Br Med J. 1956;1:1327.
4. Schwartz RA, et al. Muehrcke's lines of the fingernails. Arch Intern Med. 1979;139:242.
5. Chen W, et al. Nail changes associated with chemotherapy in children. J Eur Acad Dermatol Venereol. 2007;21:186.

Beau lines—transverse ridges in the nails—are generally the residue of a previous severe illness, often manifested as a high fever.

Other causes of Beau lines include trauma and even exposure to cold temperatures in patients with Raynaud disease (see Fig. 12.6).

Fig. 12.6 Fingernails left
hand: transverse ungual
grooves (Beau lines, *BL*) and
dystrophic nail changes such
as splitting and color changes
(nail dystrophy, *ND*) were
visible on all nails 6 months
after increased food intake by
nasogastric/gastrostomy tube
feeding in a malnourished
disabled child

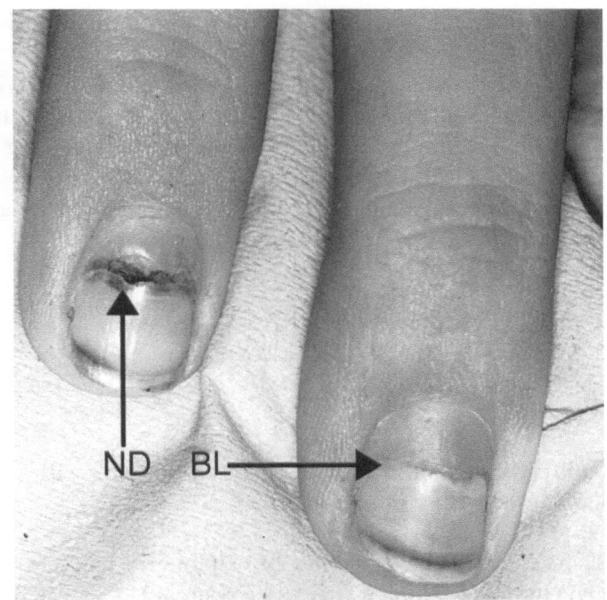

1. Richert B, et al. Nail disorders in children: diagnosis and management. Am J Clin Dermatol. 2011;12:101.
2. Fawcett RS, et al. Nail abnormalities: clue to systemic disease. Am Fam Physician. 2004;15:1417.

The "half-and-half" nail syndrome suggests the presence of renal failure with azotemia.

Lindsay describes 25 patients in whom the proximal nail bed is pale and the distal nail is pink, red, or brown, with the border sharply demarcated. Of these 25 subjects, 24 had renal disease and 21 had azotemia [1]. The half-and-half nail has also been described in four patients with Crohn disease [2].

1. Lindsay PG. The half-and-half nail. Arch Intern Med. 1967;119:583.
2. Zagoni T, et al. The half-and-half nail: a new sign of Crohn's disease? Report of four cases. Dis Colon Rect. 2006;49:1071.

Yellow nails may be a manifestation of pulmonary disease.

There is a rare syndrome—the so-called yellow nail syndrome—characterized by yellow, thickened nails, lymphedema, and respiratory tract disease. The cause is unknown [1]. In one series of 41 patients, the following respiratory manifestations were noted: pleural effusion (46 %), bronchiectasis (44 %), chronic sinusitis (41 %), and recurrent pneumonias (22 %). In the reported series, 26 patients (63 %) had lymphedema [2].

1. Maldonado F, et al. Yellow nail syndrome. Curr Opin Pulm Med. 2009;15:371.
2. Maldonado F, et al. Yellow nail syndrome: analysis of 41 consecutive patients. Chest. 2008;134:375.

Nail pitting, well known to occur in patients with psoriasis, can also be seen associated with alopecia areata.

There is a difference that may be helpful. The nail pits of psoriasis tend to be larger and fewer and exhibit no particular pattern. In contrast, the pits of alopecia areata are likely to be shallower, larger in number, and arranged in a crosshatched pattern [1].

1. Sehgal VN, et al. Nail biology, morphologic changes, and clinical ramifications, part 1. Skin. 2011;9:39.

Add human immunodeficiency virus (HIV) infection to the list of diseases that can cause digital clubbing.

Finger clubbing—so-called drumstick digits or Hippocratic fingers—can actually be a little difficult to diagnose with certainty. A useful indicator is the Schamroth sign: When the terminal phalanges of like digits are placed together, there is normally a diamond-shaped window. This window is lost in patients with clubbing, a phenomenon first described by Schamroth, who was a physician who also happened to have clubbing caused by endocarditis [1] (see Fig. 12.7).

Clubbing can be associated with panoply of cardiac, pulmonary, gastrointestinal, endocrine, and infectious diseases [2]. My first clinical case was a young woman with long-standing sarcoidosis of the pulmonary cavity. Over the past decade, we have added HIV infection to the list of clubbing causes. Zar, in South Africa, found clubbing in 20 % of 150 HIV-infected children [3], and Dever, in New Jersey, reports that of 78 HIV-infected adults studied, 36 % had the bulbous enlargement of the distal phalanges [4].

Also, just to confuse the picture a little, not all clubbing is caused by chronic disease. Primary digital clubbing, transmitted by a recessive or dominant trait, accounts for 5–10 % of cases [5].

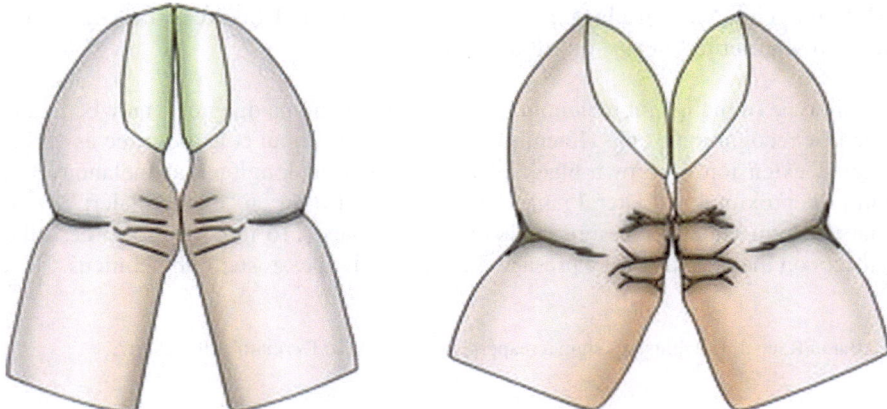

Fig. 12.7 Schamroth sign: the diamond shape window between fingers is absent

1. Cheng TO. A unique eponymous sign of finger clubbing (Schamroth sign) that is named not only after a physician who described it but also after the patient who happened to be the physician himself. Am J Cardiol. 2005;96:1614.
2. Spicknall KE, et al. Clubbing: an update on diagnosis, differential diagnosis, pathophysiology, and clinical relevance. J Am Acad Dermatol. 2005;52:1020.
3. Zar HJ, et al. Finger clubbing in children with human immunodeficiency virus infection. Ann Trop Pediatr. 2001;21:15.
4. Dever LL, et al. Digital clubbing in HIV-infected patients: an observational study. AIDS Patient Care STDS. 2009;23:19.
5. Stein RA. Digital clubbing: finally, a gene. Clin Genetics. 2009;75:119.

Koilonychia—spoon-shaped nails—may be seen in patients with hypochromic anemia and may also occur following chemical exposure.

Since the 1942 case report by Clarke, we have associated koilonychia with chronic hypochromic anemia [1]. In fact, the nail abnormality may be seen in the presence of iron deficiency either with or without anemia [2] and may also be seen in patients with hemochromatosis [3]. Occupational koilonychia has been reported in patients using organic solvents in cabinetmaking [4] and chemicals employed in hairdressing ("hairdresser's koilonychia") [5]. Familial koilonychia with an autosomal dominant pattern has also been described [2].

1. Clarke BG. Hypochromic anemia with koilonychia (spoon nails). N Engl J Med. 1942;227:338.
2. Crosby DL, et al. Familial koilonychia. Cutis. 1989;44:209.
3. Fawcett RS, et al. Nail abnormalities: clues to systemic disease. Am Fam Physician. 2004;69:1417.
4. Ancona-Alayon A. Occupational koilonychia from organic solvents. Contact Dermatitis. 2006;1:367.
5. Alanko K, et al. Hairdresser's koilonychia. Am J Contact Dermatitis. 1997;8:177.

Melanonychia, brown-black pigmentation of the nail bed, can be caused by lentigo, pigmented nevus, or subungual melanoma.

A rare type of malignant melanoma, subungual melanoma diagnosis may be facilitated by recognition of the Hutchinson sign—which Baran et al. describe as "periungual extension of brown-black pigmentation from longitudinal melanonychia onto the proximal and lateral nail folds." [1] Here I offer an "eponym alert": Note that the term Hutchinson sign is also used (see page 116 in Chap. 5) to describe blisters on the nose that may presage the onset of herpes zoster ophthalmicus.

1. Baran R, et al. Hutchinson's sign: a reappraisal. J Am Acad Dermatol. 1996;34:87.

Think of medication with patients who have hyperpigmented or otherwise discolored nails but consider other possibilities also.

Various drugs that can cause discoloration or hyperpigmentation of the nails include minocycline (Minocin), which can also discolor teeth; antimalarials; zidovudine (Retrovir); and various chemotherapeutic agents [1, 2]. Blue fingernails have been reported in black patients with pernicious anemia [3]. And white nails may be seen in patients with chronic liver disease, an association which Shearn reports has a "high specificity" [4].

1. Valeyrie-Allanore L, et al. Drug-induced skin, nail and hair disorders. Drug Safety. 2007;30:1011.
2. Tavares J, et al. Discoloration of the nail beds and skin from minocycline. CMAJ. 2011;183–224.
3. Carmel R. Hair and fingernail changes in acquired and congenital pernicious anemia. Arch Intern Med. 1985;145:484.
4. Shearn MA. Nails and systemic disease. West J Med. 1978;129:358.

Disorders of the Hair

Female patients with hirsutism are prime suspects for the diagnosis of polycystic ovary syndrome (PCOS), but don't forget about the possibility of adrenal hyperplasia (AH) caused by 21-hydroxylase deficiency.

PCOS is common in hirsute women. In one series of 350 women with hirsutism and/or androgenic alopecia, investigators found polycystic ovaries in 81 % of women with irregular menses and in 52 % of those with regular cycles [1]. Although the incidence of AH in hirsute women is low—1.2 % in one study—the clues to the diagnosis are severe hirsutism and virilization in the presence of regular menses, perhaps associated with short stature and a family history of the disease [2].

Other causes of hirsutism include Cushing syndrome, the HAIR-AN syndrome (a constellation of hyperandrogenism [HA], insulin resistance [IR], and acanthosis nigricans [AN]), use of androgenic medication, and tumors of the ovary, pituitary, or adrenal glands [3]. The Endocrine Society recommends. "We suggest testing for elevated androgen levels in women with moderate or severe hirsutism or hirsutism of any degree when it is sudden in onset, rapidly progressive, or associated with other abnormalities such as menstrual dysfunction, obesity, or clitoromegaly" [4].

1. O'Driscoll JB, et al. A prospective study of the prevalence of clear-cut endocrine disorders and polycystic ovaries in 350 patients presenting with hirsutism or androgenic alopecia. Clin Endocrinol. 1994;41:231.
2. Chetkowski RJ, et al. The incidence of late-onset congenital adrenal hyperplasia due to 21-hydroxylase deficiency among hirsute women. J Clin Endocrinol Metab. 1984;58:595.
3. Somani N, et al. The clinical evaluation of hirsutism. Dermatol Ther. 2008;21:376.
4. Martin KA, et al. Evaluation and treatment of hirsutism in premenopausal women: an Endocrine Society clinical practice guideline. J Clin Endocrinol Metab. 2008;93:1105.

Alopecia areata (AA) is an autoimmune disease that may be accompanied by various related disorders.

Chu et al. studied 4,334 patients with AA, finding significant associations with vitiligo, lupus erythematosus, atopic dermatitis, psoriasis, allergic rhinitis, and autoimmune thyroid disease. Thyroid disease was especially related to AA when the age of onset was older than 60 years (OR 2.52) [1] (see Fig. 12.8).

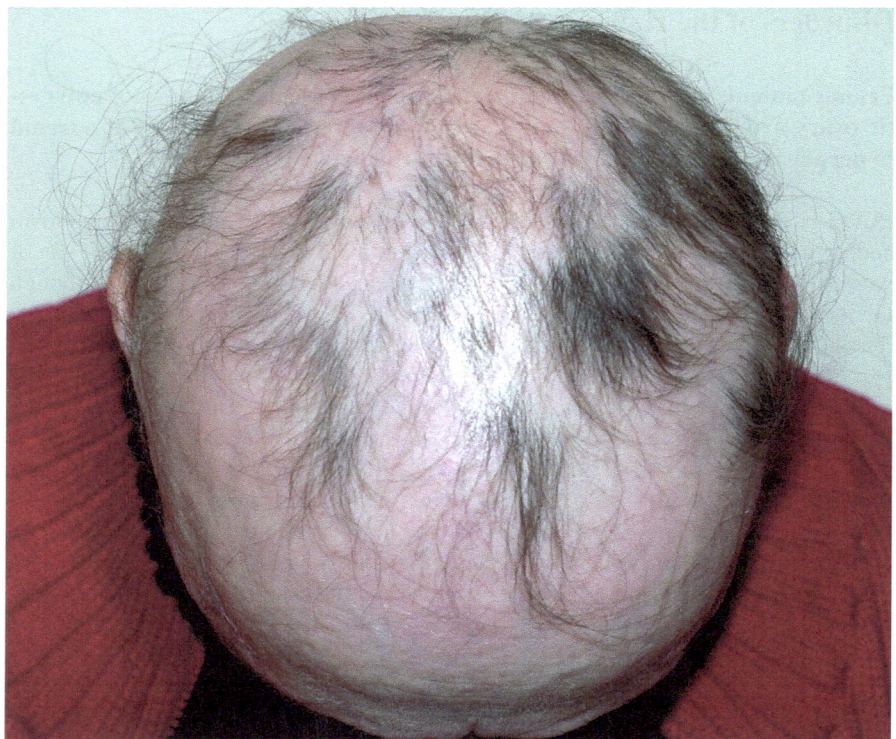

Fig. 12.8 Female patient presenting with her first episode of alopecia areata at the age of 62

1. Chu SY, et al. Comorbidity profiles among patients with alopecia areata: the importance of onset age, a nationwide population-based study. J Am Acad Dermatol. 2011;65:949.

Early androgenic alopecia (AGA)—male pattern hair loss—may signal the presence of cardiovascular disease risk factors.

One study reports a significant association between AGA and metabolic syndrome, with high-density lipoprotein (HDL) of particular importance [1]. Following a study of 80 young males with early AGA and 80 matched controls, investigators recommend assessing insulin resistance and cardiovascular-related risk factors in young males with especially prominent male pattern baldness [2].

1. Su LH, et al. Association of androgenic alopecia with metabolic syndrome in men: a community based survey. Brit J Dermatol. 2010;163:371.
2. González-González JG, et al. Androgenetic alopecia and insulin resistance in young men. Clin Endocrinol. 2009;71:494.

Hair loss can be caused by psychotropic drugs.

Possible offenders are lithium, causing alopecia in 12–19 % of long-term users; valproic acid/divalproex (Depakote), with a 12 % dose-dependent incidence of hair loss; and carbamazepine (Tegretol) with hair loss in up to 6 % of patients taking the drug [1]. Of all the many drugs that can cause hair loss, why do I emphasize the psychotropic medications? It is because hair loss in these patients might be erroneously attributed to the stress of their psychiatric illnesses.

1. Mercke Y, et al. Hair loss in psychopharmacology. Ann Clin Psych. 2000;12:35.

Hair loss can be a manifestation of secondary syphilis.

Syphilis is still with us, and one of the manifestations of the secondary stage of the disease is alopecia syphilitica, which can be in either a diffuse or moth-eaten pattern. Do not confuse this finding with alopecia areata (described above), tinea capitis, or trichotillomania [1].

1. Bi MY, et al. Alopecia syphilitica: report of a patient with secondary syphilis presenting as moth-eaten alopecia and a review of its common mimickers. Dermatol Online J. 2009;15:6.

Think of the possibility of vitamin B12 deficiency in patients with premature whitening of the hair.

Cobalamin deficiency can cause both depigmentation of the hair and hyperpigmentation of the skin [1]. An alternative possibility is substance addiction, which one author suggests as a cause of early graying of the hair [2].

1. Heath M, et al. Cutaneous manifestations of nutritional deficiency. Curr Opin Pediatr. 2006;18:417.
2. Reece AS. Hair graying in substance addiction. Arch Dermatol. 2007;143:116.

Some hair abnormalities are part of rare, but noteworthy, syndromes.

Here are some uncommon and curious causes of abnormal hair, all most likely to be encountered in infants and children:

> *Uncombable hair syndrome*: Called *cheveux incoiffables* in France and "mop hair" in Australia, the uncombable hair syndrome describes the presence of unruly, disorganized hair—what my granddaughter would call a permanent bad hair day. There are pathognomonic findings on light microscope examination of a hair shaft [1, 2].

Menkes kinky hair syndrome: This is sex-linked neurodegenerative disorder characterized by cognitive deterioration, seizures, bladder diverticula, low levels of serum copper and ceruloplasmin, and, of course, kinky hair [3, 4].

Elejalde syndrome: An autosomal recessive disease, Elejalde syndrome causes silvery hair, skin that bronzes upon sun exposure, and mental deterioration [5, 6].

Waardenburg syndrome: A piebald white forelock is seen in some patients with Waardenburg syndrome, which also is manifested as pigmentary anomalies of the iris and sensorineural deafness (see Chap. 5) [7].

1. Calderon P, et al. Uncombable hair syndrome. J Am Acad Dermatol. 2009;61:512.
2. Jarell AD, et al. Uncombable hair syndrome. Pediatr Dermatol. 2007;24:436.
3. Menkes JH. Kinky hair disease: twenty five years later. Brain Dev. 1988;10:77.
4. Cosimo QC, et al. Kinky hair, kinky vessels, and bladder diverticula in Menkes disease. J Neuroimag. 2011;21:e114.
5. Duran-McKinster C, et al. Elejalde syndrome—a melanolysosomal neurocutaneous syndrome. Arch Dermatol. 1999;135:182.
6. Inamadar AC, et al. Silvery hair with bronze-tan in a child: a case of Elejalde disease. Indian J Dermatol Venereol Leprol. 2007;73:417.
7. Dourmishev AL, et al. Waardenburg syndrome. Int J Dermatol. 1999;38:656.

Skin Manifestation of Systemic Diseases

A few days of fever and malaise followed by the appearance of erythematous macules, sometimes target shaped and with purpuric centers, suggest the early stages of Stevens–Johnson syndrome (SJS).

These early manifestations soon evolve to vesicles and bullae that slough readily. The lips are generally involved. Skin sloughing in SJS generally involves less than 10 % of the body, and if there is sloughing of more than 30 % of skin, the disease is called toxic epidermal necrolysis (TEN) [1]. SJS and TEN are listed here as systemic diseases because both are idiosyncratic responses to drugs or one of a long list of infectious agents, including *Mycoplasma pneumoniae*. Sulfonamides, penicillins, allopurinol (Zyloprim), anticonvulsants, and NSAIDs are drugs that have been implicated [2]. One study identifies allopurinol as the "most common cause" of SJS and TEN in Europe and Israel [3]. Acetaminophen (Tylenol) has been suspected as a cause [4]. In many instances, no cause can be identified.

1. Bastuji-Garin S, et al. Clinical classification of cases of toxic epidermal necrolysis, Stevens-Johnson syndrome, and erythema multiforme. Arch Dermatol. 1993;129:92.
2. Mockenhaupt M, et al. Stevens-Johnson syndrome and toxic epidermal necrolysis: assessment of medication risks with emphasis on recently marketed drugs. The EuroSCAR Study. J Invest Dermatol. 2008;128:35.
3. Halevy S, et al. Allopurinol is the most common cause of Stevens-Johnson syndrome and toxic epidermal necrolysis in Europe and Israel. J Am Acad Dermatol. 2008;58:25.
4. Levi N, et al. Medications as risk factors of Stevens-Johnson syndrome and toxic epidermal necrolysis in children: a pooled analysis. Pediatrics. 2009;123:e297.

The appearance of painful, red nodules on the shins describes the classic onset of erythema nodosum (EN).

The nodules, actually a panniculitis of the subcutaneous fat, generally occur in a symmetrical pattern. More important than the EN is the potential cause. The most likely trigger is streptococcal pharyngitis. Other possible triggers include tuberculosis, sarcoidosis, inflammatory bowel disease, cancer, viral or fungal infection, and drugs such as penicillins, sulfonamides, and oral contraceptives [1, 2]. EN is the most common nonspecific skin manifestation of sarcoidosis; its presence suggests a favorable prognosis for the systemic disease [3].

1. Schwartz RA, et al. Erythema nodosum: a sign of systemic disease. Am Fam Physician. 2007;75:695.
2. Cribier B, et al. Erythema nodosum and associated diseases: a study of 129 cases. Int Dermatol. 1998;37:667.
3. Marchall RM, et al. Cutaneous sarcoidosis. Semin Respir Crit Care Med. 2010;31:442.

Heliotropic rash and Gottron papules are (probably) pathognomonic of dermatomyositis.

An autoimmune disease characterized by microangiopathy affecting muscle and skin, dermatomyositis has two distinctive features: The heliotrope rash is violaceous to darker red, sometimes accompanied by edema, and involves the periorbital skin. Gottron papules are elevated, erythematous papules overlying bony prominences of the dorsal finger joints, knees, and elbows [1, 2]. Dermatomyositis is associated with internal malignancy in up to one-quarter of patients [3].

1. Kalakas MC, et al. Polymyositis and dermatomyositis. Lancet. 2003;362:971.
2. Neto R, et al. Juvenile dermatomyositis: review and update of the pathogenesis and treatment. Rev Bras Rheumatol. 2010;50:299.
3. Callen JP, et al. Dermatomyositis. Clin Dermatol. 2006;24:363.

Photosensitivity, Raynaud phenomenon, chronic urticaria, alopecia, and mouth ulcers can all be cutaneous manifestations of systemic lupus erythematosus (SLE).

In a study of 73 patients with SLE, Yell et al. found the following: photosensitivity in 46 subjects (63 %); Raynaud phenomenon in 44 (60 %); chronic urticaria, aggravated by sun exposure, in 32 (44 %); non-scarring alopecia in 29 (40 %); and mouth ulcers in 23 (31.5 %) [1]. There may also be erythema of the proximal nail folds and splinter hemorrhages in the fingernails [2]. The earliest manifestation is likely to be a discoid rash, occurring a mean of 1.74 years before the diagnosis of SLE in one series of 130 subjects [3].

1. Yell JA, et al. Cutaneous manifestations of systemic lupus erythematosus. Br J Dermatol. 1996;135:355.
2. Tunc SE, et al. Nail changes in connective tissue diseases: do nail changes provide clues for the diagnosis? J Eur Acad Dermatol Venereol. 2007;21:497.
3. Heinlen LD, et al. Clinical criteria for systemic lupus erythematosus precede diagnosis, and associated autoantibodies are present before clinical symptoms. Arthritis Rheum. 2007;56:2344.

Sarcoidosis, a nonspecific granulomatous multisystem disease, may cause translucent yellow-red papules of the skin.

The skin areas most commonly affected by cutaneous sarcoidosis are the head and neck. The skin lesions of sarcoidosis, which lack disease-specific histologic characteristics, can be disfiguring and resistant to treatment [1, 2].

1. Marchall RM, et al. Cutaneous sarcoidosis. Semin Respir Crit Care Med. 2010;31:442.
2. Lodha S, et al. Sarcoidosis of the skin. Chest. 2009;136:583.

Multiple café-au-lait spots can be seen in diseases other than neurofibromatosis.

The hallmarks of neurofibromatosis type 1, a common genetic disease with an autosomal dominant mode of inheritance, are multiple café-au-lait spots and cutaneous neurofibromas. However, other disorders can be associated with discrete tan-colored patches. These include McCune–Albright syndrome, Noonan syndrome, Legius syndrome, and ring chromosome syndromes [1, 2].

1. Jabbour SA, et al. Rare syndromes. Clin Dermatol. 2006;24:299.
2. Shah KN. The diagnostic and clinical significance of café-au-lait macules. Pediatr Clin NA. 2010;57:1131.

Skin lesions can offer clues to the diagnosis of some serious infectious diseases.

The following are three noteworthy diseases with characteristic skin findings:

Lyme disease (LD): Also called Lyme borreliosis, LD causes a (probably) pathognomonic expanding erythematous lesion—erythema chronicum migrans—in three-quarters of infected individuals (see Fig. 12.9). Other skin manifestations

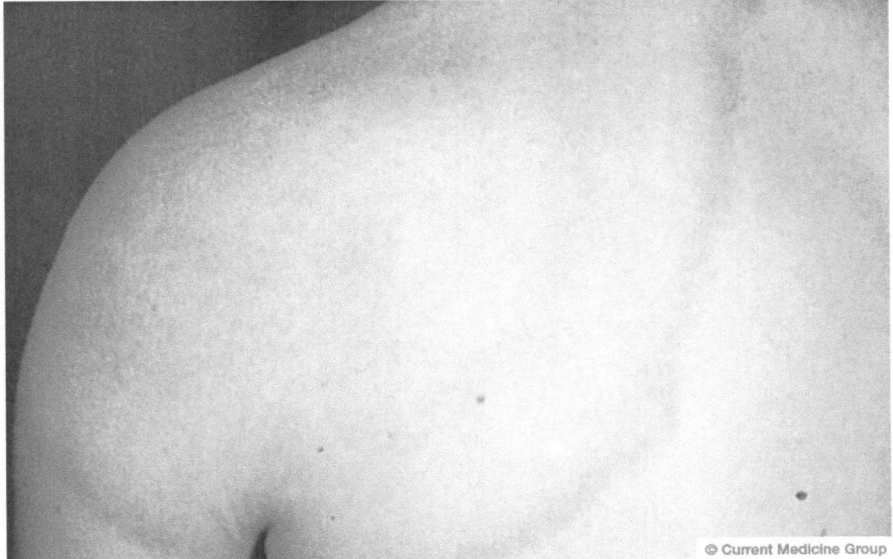

© Current Medicine Group

Fig. 12.9 Erythema chronicum migrans (ECM): the appearance of ECM is generally annular, with a sharply demarcated outer border, and it is erythematous or bluish, warm to the touch, flat, and minimally tender or nontender

that may be seen during the course of LD are erythematous atrophic plaques called acrodermatitis chronica atrophicans, morphea, lichen sclerosus et atrophicus, and cutaneous B cell lymphoma [1, 2].

HIV: Most HIV-infected patients will develop one or more skin disorders during the course of their disease. The acquired immunodeficiency syndrome (AIDS) defining skin disorder is Kaposi sarcoma, an indolent vascular tumor found chiefly on the extremities, genitalia, face, and oral mucosa. In a study of 263 HIV/AIDS patients, the most common skin problems encountered were generalized prurigo, oral candidiasis, herpes zoster, and vaginal candidiasis [3, 4].

Tuberculosis (TB): The most common presentation of cutaneous tuberculosis is lupus vulgaris—reddish-brown nodular lesions with ulcerations that are found chiefly on the face and ears [5, 6].

1. Eisendle K, et al. The expanding spectrum of cutaneous borreliosis. G Ital Dermatol Venereol. 2009;144:157.
2. Melane MS, et al. Diagnosis of Lyme disease based on dermatologic manifestations. Ann Intern Med. 1991;114:490.
3. Zancanaro PCQ, et al. Cutaneous manifestations of HIV in the era of highly active antiretroviral therapy: an institutional urban clinic experience. J Am Acad Dermatol. 2006;54:581.
4. Mbuagbaw J, et al. Patterns of skin manifestations and their relationships with CD4 counts among HIV/AIDS patients in Cameroon. Int J Dermatol. 2006;45:280.
5. Wozniacka A, et al. Lupus vulgaris: report of two cases. Int J Dermatol. 2005;44:299.
6. Wang H, et al. Cutaneous tuberculosis: a diagnostic and therapeutic study of 20 cases. J Dermatol Treat. 2011;22:310.

Premalignant and Malignant Tumors of the Skin

An enlarging growth on the sun-exposed areas of the skin of an adult may well be a basal cell carcinoma (BCC).

One fact tipping the odds toward this diagnosis is the relative frequencies of the major skin cancers. In an 18-year study of 84,836 female nurses living in the USA, there were 8,215 cases of BCC, 863 cases of squamous cell carcinoma (SCC), and 420 cases of melanoma [1]. Although BCC is usually considered slow growing, Wrone et al. found aggressive-growth BCC in 20.7 % of 432 biopsy specimens [2]. Be suspicious of BCC in patients who have had previous disease: In a 5-year study of 1,000 patients with BCC, 36 % developed a second BCC [3].

1. Qureshi AA, et al. Geographic variation and risk of skin cancer in US women. Arch Intern Med. 2008;168:501.
2. Wrone DA, et al. Increased proportion of aggressive-growth basal cell carcinoma in the Veterans Affairs population of Palo Alto, California. J Am Acad Dermatol. 1996;35:907.
3. Robinson JK. Risk of developing another basal cell carcinoma: a 5-year prospective study. Cancer. 1987;60:118.

Patients with a history of arsenic ingestion are at special risk of developing BCC.

Unlikely, you may think. But arsenic has been found in drinking water supplies in New Hampshire [1]; in many foods, with seafood having the highest concentrations [2] and with a 2011 report of arsenic in apple juice; and even medications, such as a product in Australia known as Bell's Asthma Medication [3]. In the Wild West of unregulated food supplements available today, could there be other products containing arsenic?

1. Karagas MR, et al. Design of an epidemiologic study of drinking water arsenic exposure and skin and bladder cancer risk in a US population. Environ Health Perspect. 1998;106 Suppl 4:1047.
2. Tao SS, et al. Dietary arsenic intakes in the United States: FDA Total Diet Study. Food Addit Contam. 1999;16:465.
3. Boonchai W, et al. Basal cell carcinoma in chronic arsenicism occurring in Queensland, Australia, after ingestion of an asthma medication. J Am Acad Dermatol. 2000;43:664.

Cutaneous squamous cell carcinoma can present in many forms: plaques, papules, nodules, or ulcerative lesions.

The location of the lesion can be a clue: More than half of all SCCs occur on the head and neck, probably related to the increased sun exposure in this area [1–3].

Because of the variety of presentations possible, biopsy is needed to establish (or rule out) the diagnosis of SCC [2]. Be especially suspicious in persons with freckling of the arms [3]. In dark-skinned ethnic groups, SCC, rather than BCC, is the most common cutaneous cancer [4].

1. Gurudutt VV, et al. Cutaneous squamous cell carcinoma of the head and neck. J Skin Cancer. 2011;2011:502723. Epub 21 Feb 2011.
2. Bonerandi J, et al. Guidelines for the diagnosis and treatment of cutaneous squamous cell carcinoma and precursor lesions. J Eur Acad Dermatol Venereol. 2011;25 Suppl 5:1.
3. English DR, et al. Demographic characteristics, pigmentary and cutaneous risk factors for squamous cell carcinoma of the skin: a case-control study. Int J Cancer. 1998;76:628.
4. Gloster HM Jr, et al. Skin cancer in people of color. J Am Acad Dermatol. 2006;55:741.

Be very suspicious of malignant change in ulcers occurring in traumatized skin, especially in scars following burns.

Such a lesion may be a Marjolin ulcer, a rare but aggressive cancer of the skin arising in chronic wounds, including pressure sores (see Fig. 12.10). Most of these tumors are SCCs. Marjolin ulcer malignancies can metastasize to local regional lymph nodes and can also recur locally [1, 2].

1. Esther RJ, et al. Marjolin ulcers: secondary carcinomas in chronic wounds. J South Orthop Assoc. 1999;8:181.
2. Copcu E, et al. Thirty-one cases of Marjolin ulcers. Clin Exp Dermatol. 2003;28:138.

Organ transplant patients have an increased risk of skin cancer, especially SCC.

In these patients, SCC occurs more often than BCC, the opposite of what is found in the normal population. There is also a 2–5-fold increase in the incidence of malignant melanoma in posttransplantation patients. The increased incidence in skin cancers is attributed to the postoperative use of immunosuppressive drugs [1].

1. Le Mire L, et al. Melanomas in renal transplant patients. Br J Dermatol. 2006;154:472.

A nevus that looks different than all the rest—the "ugly duckling sign"—may be a melanoma.

Scope et al. tested the "ugly duckling theory" by showing back skin images of 12 patients to various healthcare workers: 13 dermatologists, five dermatology nurses, and eight nonclinical medical staff members. These observers identified all five

Fig. 12.10 Marjolin ulcer: 15 years ago the patient had suffered a thermal burn of the heel

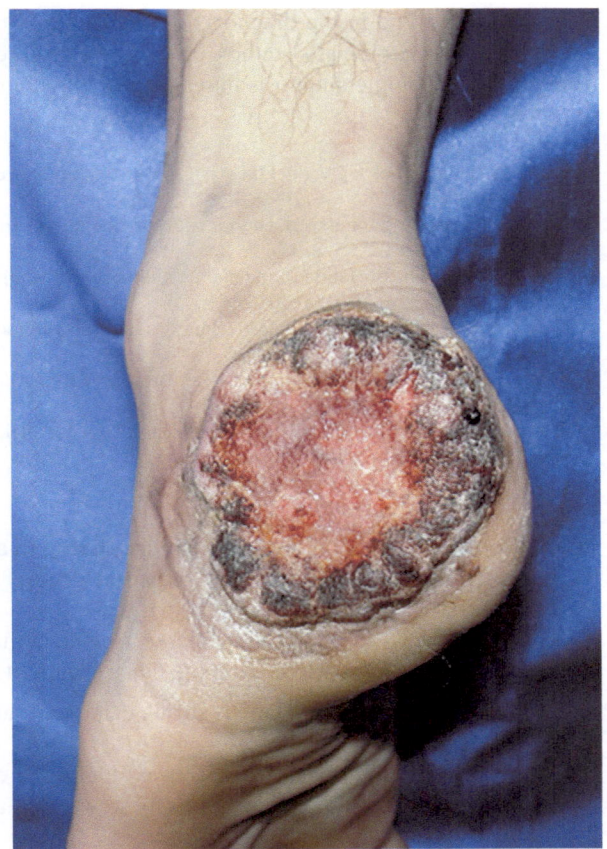

melanomas and only three of 140 benign moles as "ugly" [1]. Especially worrisome would be a pigmented tumor with a notch [2]. The incidence of melanoma has been rising faster than any other cancer, and early detection is the best way to lower mortality [3]. The "ugly duckling" sign is used in concert with the better known ABCD criteria:

- A—asymmetry of the lesion
- B—border irregularity
- C—color unevenly distributed
- D—diameter greater than 6 mm

Even with all of the above diagnostic clues, Patel et al. hold that the "diagnosis of melanoma by simple visual inspection is incorrect in almost one out of every three melanoma diagnoses" [4].

Chia et al., in Australia (where many reports on melanoma originate), found 195 melanomas in the 686 clinically suspicious lesions tumors undergoing histologic examination, yielding a number needed to treat (in this case, biopsy) of four in their study [5].

The current trend in the diagnosis of melanoma is the use of the dermoscope, termed the "dermatologist's stethoscope", as we, according to Argenziano, "move from clinicopathologic diagnosis into an era of clinicoimaging diagnosis" [6].

1. Scope A, et al. The "ugly duckling" sign: agreement between observers. Arch Dermatol. 2008;144:58.
2. Orient JM, editor. Sapira's art and science of diagnosis. 3rd ed. Philadelphia: Lippincott, Williams & Wilkins; 2005. p. 138.
3. Rigel DS, et al. The evolution of melanoma diagnosis: 25 years beyond ABCDs. CA: A cancer journal for clinicians: 2010;60:301.
4. Patel JK, et al. Newer technologies/techniques and tools in the diagnosis of melanoma. Eur J Dermatol. 2008;18:617.
5. Chia ALK, et al. Melanoma diagnosis: Australian dermatologists' number needed to treat. Australasian J Dermatol. 2008;49:12.
6. Argenziano G, et al. Dermoscopy—the ultimate tool for melanoma diagnosis. Semin Cutan Med Surg. 2009;28:142.

In addition to the dedicated sun worshipers living in a tropical climate, there is an increased risk of melanoma in some other groups as well.

Above I mentioned the increased incidence of melanoma and other skin cancers in organ transplant patients. Here are some other groups at risk:

Indoor tanning devotees: There is strong evidence that indoor tanning is carcinogenic in humans [1].

Accessibility to air travel: The increased incidence of melanoma in this group suggests that those who can afford to fly to warm beaches in the winter months put themselves at risk [2].

Insulin resistance: A 2011 report comparing 55 melanoma patients with 165 controls suggested that insulin resistance is potentially an independent risk factor for melanoma [3].

1. Lazovich D, et al. Indoor tanning and risk of melanoma: a case–control study in a highly exposed population. Cancer Epidemiol Biomarkers Prev. 2010;19:1557.
2. Agredano YZ, et al. Accessibility to air travel correlates strongly with increasing melanoma incidence. Melanoma Research. 2006;16:77.
3. Antoniadis AG, et al. Insulin resistance in relation to melanoma risk. Melanoma Res. 2011;21:541.

SCC, BCC, and melanoma are only three of the skin tumors you will see in practice.

The following are some miscellaneous facts about various other skin growths:

Cutaneous horn: This protrusion of abnormal keratinized material may be associated with a number of premalignant and malignant skin diseases. One report describes a cutaneous horn associated with Kaposi sarcoma [1].

Dermatofibroma: A common, generally benign, fibrohistiocytic tumor most often found on the extremities, dermatofibroma has been reported metastasizing to the lungs [2].

Keratoacanthoma: This keratocytic epithelial tumor, typically presenting as a dome- shaped papule with a central keratolytic plug, may be a variant of SCC. The lesion tends to grow rapidly and, in rare instances, metastasis can occur [3] (see Fig. 12.11).

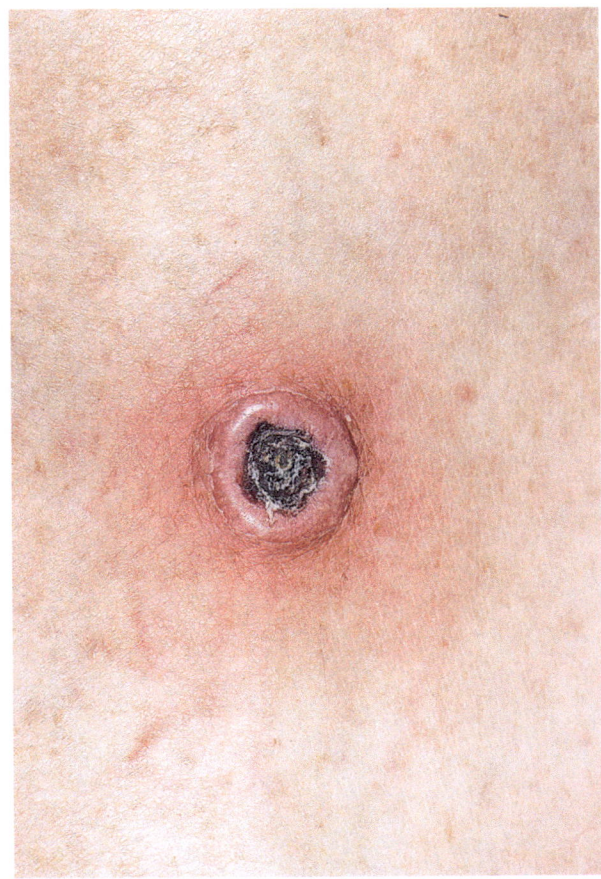

Fig. 12.11 Keratoacanthoma

Sarcoma: Sarcomas can occur on the skin, one more reason to submit all lumps removed for histologic examination [4].

1. Onak KN, et al. Cutaneous horn-related Kaposi's sarcoma: a case report. Case Report Med. 2010; doi:10.1155/2010/825949.
2. Basero EB, et al. Dermatofibroma metastasizing to the lung. Arch de Bronconeumologia. 2009;45:521.
3. Precancerous lesions and cutaneous carcinomas. In: Fitzpatrick's color Atlas and synopsis of clinical dermatology. Available at: http://accessmedicine.com/content.aspx?aID=5186972.
4. Sussman JL. Unexamined mass isn't benign at all. J Fam Pract. 2010;59:354.

Selected Problems of the Skin and Subcutaneous Tissues

Well circumscribed, waxy, glistening, atrophic plaques on the shins are likely to be necrobiosis lipoidica.

The lesions are sometimes called necrobiosis lipoidica diabeticorum because some, but not all, patients with this condition are diabetic, will become diabetic, or have a family history of diabetes [1]. Skin cancers can develop in the areas of chronic ulceration.

1. O'Toole K, et al. Necrobiosis lipoidica: only a minority of patients have diabetes mellitus. Br J Dermatol. 1999;140:283.

Weber–Christian disease (WDC) typically begins with tender subcutaneous nodules on the extremities and sometimes also on the abdomen, chest, or buttocks.

Formally known as relapsing febrile nodular nonsuppurative panniculitis, WCD is a systemic inflammatory disease of fat tissue that may also be manifested as fever, joint pain, or myalgia [1, 2].

1. Negalur VG, et al. Weber-Christian disease. J Assoc Physicians India. 2003;51:724.
2. Panush RS, et al. Weber-Christian disease: analysis of 15 cases and review of the literature. Medicine. 1985;64:181.

The "wake sign" has been described as pathognomonic of scabies.

What is the wake sign? This phenomenon is seen as the mite leaves behind a pattern resembling the wake left on the water by a moving ship. Yoshizumi et al. hold that the sign is specific for scabies and is valuable because it is visible by the naked eye and it points toward the location of the burrowing mite [1]. Of course, the classical burrow of scabies is linear or s-shaped, but the wake sign is an important clue, when present.

1. Yoshizumi J, et al. "Wake sign:" an important clue for the diagnosis of scabies. Clin Exp Dermatol. 2009;34:711.

Intertriginous xanthomas are pathognomonic of familial heterozygous hypercholesterolemia (FHC).

An autosomal dominant disorder with high serum LDL levels, FHC causes various types of xanthomas in diverse areas. The intertriginous xanthomas, although rare, are considered specific to the disease [1].

1. Pietroleonardo L, et al. Skin manifestations in familial heterozygous hypercholesterolemia. Acta Dermatovenerol Alp Panonica Adriat. 2009;18:183.

Fig. 12.12 A young boy infected with M. ulcerans has a Buruli ulcer covering a portion of his torso

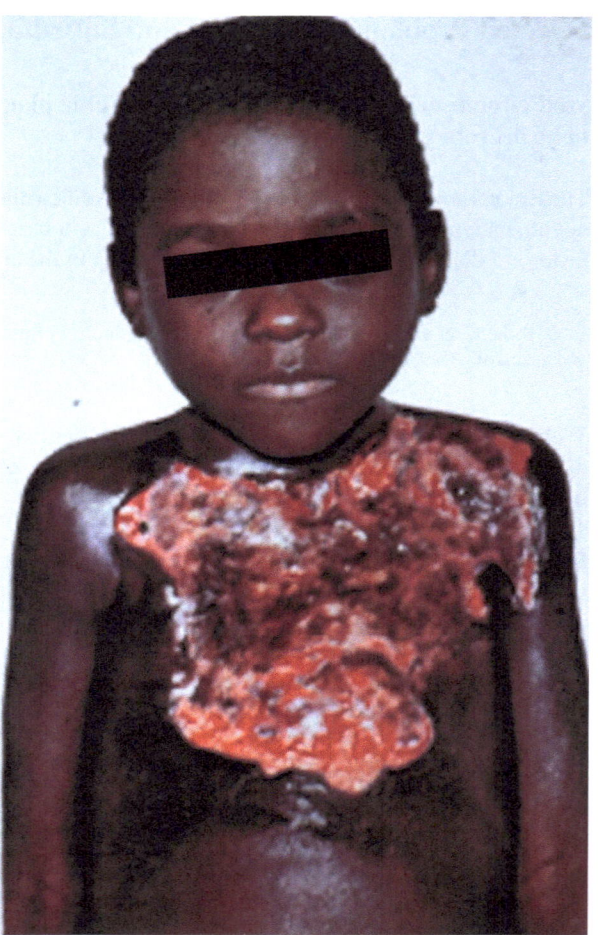

An indolent necrotizing disease of skin and subcutaneous tissue might be Buruli ulcer, caused by infection with *Mycobacterium ulcerans*.

Also known as ulcerans disease, Buruli ulcer is the world's third most common mycobacterial disease, after tuberculosis and leprosy. It occurs chiefly in Africa and also in South America and is associated with slow-moving or stagnant waters. A case of Buruli ulcer has been reported in a tourist who had been on a canoe trip in Brazil [1, 2] (see Fig. 12.12).

1. Portaels F, et al. Buruli ulcer. Clin Dermatol. 2009;27:291.
2. McGann H, et al. Buruli ulcer in United Kingdom tourist returning from Latin America. Emerg Infect Dis. 2009;15:1827.

Skin and nails can offer some unexpected insights.

Here are two of them:

> *Skin wrinkles*: There seems to be an inverse relationship between skin wrinkles and bone health, according to a paper presented in 2011 [1].
>
> *Thumbnail pattern*: Here is a way to assess handedness, a determination that might be pertinent in a comatose patient. According to Shearn: "The dominant thumbnail has a wider base and the angles formed by the base and the lateral aspects of the nail are more obtuse" [2].

1. Skin wrinkles may provide a glimpse into bone health. Presented at the Endocrine Society 93rd Annual Meeting. Abstract P3-126. Presented June 4, 2011.
2. Shearn MA. Nails and systemic disease. West J Med. 1978;129:358.

Chapter 13
The Endocrine and Metabolic Systems

*It would indeed be rash for a mere pathologist to venture forth
on the uncharted sea of the endocrines, strewn as it is with the
wrecks of shattered hypotheses, where even the most wary
marine may easily lose his way as he seeks to steer his bark
amid the glandular temptations whose siren voices have proved
the downfall of many who have gone before.*

Scottish-Canadian pathologist
William Boyd (1885–1979) [1]

Contents

R.B. Taylor, *Diagnostic Principles and Applications*,
DOI 10.1007/978-1-4614-1111-6_13, © Springer Science+Business Media, LLC 2013

As a medical student, long ago, my course textbook was "Boyd's Pathology," a heavy tome which I dutifully read—cover to cover—and underlined to be sure I had noted the important parts. My task was made easier because, as evidenced in the quotation presented, Boyd wrote with a flair rarely found in current medical writing. Extended metaphors and classical allusions, such as the one above to the sirens of ancient Greek mythology, are seldom encountered today. In 1955, Boyd metaphorically likened the endocrines to uncharted seas. Today these oceans are somewhat better "charted." Yet, in both the endocrine and metabolic systems, there are dozens of rare diseases we everyday practicing clinicians may encounter once in a professional lifetime, but, when we do, we want to recognize the pathologic entity before us.

1. Boyd W. Pathology for the surgeon. 7th ed. Philadelphia: Saunders;1955. chapter 32.

Hypoglycemia

In a patient with symptomatic hypoglycemia, think of three diseases: diabetes mellitus (DM), alcoholism, and sepsis.

In a study of 125 emergency department visits for symptomatic hypoglycemia, these three diseases, alone or in combination, accounted for 90 % of cases [1]. Low blood sugar causes two types of symptoms: Autonomic symptoms include hunger, sweating, tremor, and palpitations, and neuroglycemic manifestations may include confusion, impaired coordination, strange behavior, and drowsiness [2].

The most common cause of symptomatic low blood sugar is insulin-induced hypoglycemia, which occurs three or more times per patient per year in those who have been diabetic for more than 15 years [3]. Insulinoma is a rare cause of hypoglycemia but is the most commonly occurring hormone-secreting islet cell tumor [4]. In patients who have had gastric surgery, postprandial hypoglycemia related to excessive insulin effect may occur [4].

1. Malouf R, et al. Hypoglycemia: causes, neurologic manifestations, and outcome. Ann Neurol. 1985;17:421.
2. Adukauskiene D, et al. Causes, diagnosis, and treatment of hypoglycemia. Medicina (Kaunas). 2006;42:860.
3. Frier BM. The incidence and impact of hypoglycemia in type 1 and type 2 diabetes. Int. Diabetes Monit. 2009;21:210.
4. Pourmotabbed G, et al. Hypoglycemia. Obstet Gynecol Clin North Am. 2001;28:383.

Obesity

Obesity can complicate the physical examination by obscuring important physical findings.

For example, jugular venous pressure in the neck may be difficult to determine, layers of adipose tissue may muffle heart sounds, breath sounds may appear diminished, and the liver edge may elude palpation [1]. Obese women, who tend to have large and often pendulous breasts, have an increased risk of non-palpable breast tumors [2]. Here are some key facts regarding clinical examination of the obese person:

- More than one-third of American adults are obese [3].
- Many medical students and residents receive little or no formal training regarding how to perform a physical examination on an obese patient [1].
- Approximately 40 % of American physicians hold negative attitudes toward obese persons [4].

Aronne offers the following opinion: "Obesity meets all the criteria of a medical illness, including a known etiology, recognized signs and symptoms, and a range of structural and functional changes that culminate in pathologic consequences." He goes on to point out that excess adipose tissue acts as an endocrine organ producing bioactive molecules, such as tumor necrosis factor-alpha, that are associated with the development of diabetes, endothelial damage, and other conditions [5].

1. Silk AW, et al. Reexamining the physical examination for obese patients. JAMA. 2011;305:193.
2. Chagpar AB, et al. Body mass index influences palpability but not stage of breast cancer at diagnosis. Am Surg. 2007;73:555.
3. National Center for Health Statistics. Health, United States, 2009; With special feature on medical technology. Hyattsville: National Center for Health Statistics; 2010.
4. Fujioka K, et al. Office-based management of obesity. Mt Sinai J Med. 2010;77:466.
5. Aronne LJ, et al. Obesity as a disease state: a new paradigm for diagnosis and treatment. Clin Cornerstone. 2009;9:9.

Obesity is the best predictor of undiagnosed diabetes mellitus.

In a disease that will affect one in three Americans born since year 2000 and that has severe complications that can sometimes be lessened by early detection and treatment, sentinel clues are important [1]. According to the results of the Diabscreen study, "The yield of opportunistic targeted screening was fair; obesity alone was the best predictor of undiagnosed diabetes" [2].

1. Kirk JK, et al. Diabetes: rethinking risk and the Dx that fits. J Fam Pract. 2009;58:248.
2. Woolthuis EP, et al. Yield of opportunistic targeted screening for type 2 diabetes in primary care: the Diabscreen study. Ann Fam Med. 2009;7:422.

Diabetes Mellitus

Based on hemoglobin A1c (HbA1c) levels, about one-fifth of patients admitted to the hospital may have "unrecognized probable diabetes."

This conclusion follows a study of 696 adult non-obstetric patients admitted over 11 days to an acute care general hospital. Yet, the authors report that few of these individuals were diagnosed with diabetes in the year following their hospital stay [1]. The apparent paradox may be explained by another report pointing out that hyperglycemia in hospitalized patients can be due to stress, and the elevated blood sugar levels will normalize in nondiabetic patients when the acute disease is controlled [2].

1. Wexler DJ, et al. Prevalence of elevated hemoglobin A1c among patients admitted to the hospital without a diagnosis of diabetes. J Clin Endocrinol Metabol. 2008;93:4238.
2. Song SH, et al. Not all raised blood sugars are diabetes! QJM. 2011;104:711.

Be suspicious of diabetes in women who experienced abuse during childhood.

Based on findings from the Nurses' Health Study involving 67,853 women, those who experienced moderate or severe physical abuse during childhood had a 26–54 % increased risk of developing diabetes in adulthood. There was a 16 % higher risk of diabetes in those who reported unwanted sexual touching and a "dose-related" 34–69 % increased risk with forced sexual activity before adulthood [1].

1. Richard-Edwards JW, et al. Abuse in childhood and adolescence as a predictor of type 2 diabetes in adult women. Am J Prev Med. 2010;39:529.

The "prayer sign" can be a clue to the diagnosis of diabetes.

Limited joint mobility in diabetics may yield a positive prayer sign in which the patient, when attempting to hold the hands together in a praying position, cannot completely close the gap between opposing palms (see Fig. 13.1). This finding may improve with control of the patient's hyperglycemia. The prayer sign should not be confused with other hand abnormalities that are more common in diabetic patients: Dupuytren contracture, tenosynovitis with thickening of the flexor tendon sheaths of the fingers, and complex regional pain syndrome (aka reflex sympathetic dystrophy) [1].

1. Somai P, et al. Limited joint mobility in diabetes mellitus: the clinical implications. J Musculoskel Med. 2011;28:118.

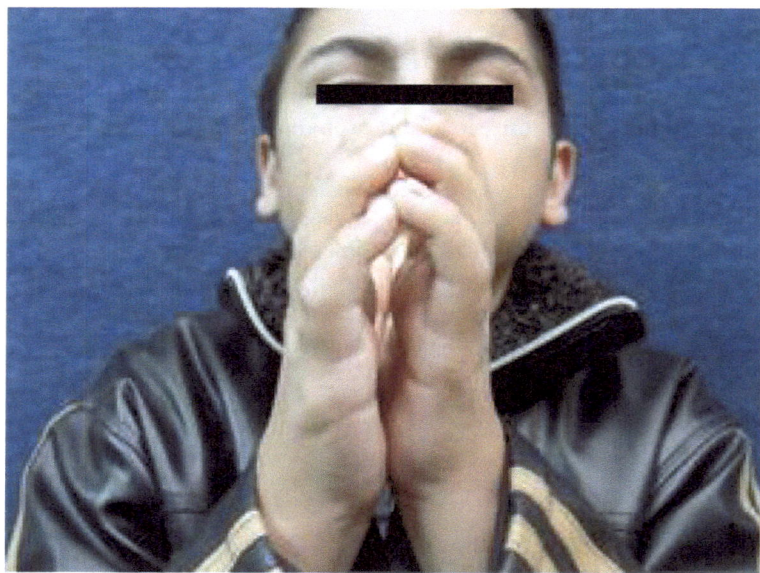

Fig. 13.1 A positive prayer sign in a 23-year-old man with type 1 diabetes since age one. This patient was unable to oppose the palms of his hands

Consider screening your diabetic patients for symptoms of anxiety and depression.

These two conditions have a much higher prevalence in diabetic patients than in the general population, according to a study of 2,049 persons with types 1 and 2 diabetes. Risk factors for anxiety and depression in diabetics were smoking, complications of diabetes, being an ex-drinker or a current heavy drinker, and uncertainty about blood sugar control [1].

1. Collins MM. Anxiety and depression symptoms in patients with diabetes. Diabetic Med. 2009;26:153.

Thyroid Disease

Difficulty swallowing or exertional dyspnea may be the tip-off to the diagnosis of substernal goiter.

In a large series (872) of thyroidectomies, 50 (5.7 %) were substernal goiters (see Fig. 13.2). In addition to the presence of a cervical mass in 69 %, dysphagia was described by 33 % of patients and dyspnea by 28 % [1].

In addition to the usual causes of goiter, I came across two "zebras": One is Pendred syndrome, an autosomal recessive disorder with congenital hearing loss associated with thyroid enlargement owing to reduced iodine organification [2]. The other is amyloid goiter as part of primary systemic amyloidosis [3].

1. Allo MD, et al. Rationale for the operative management of substernal goiter. Surgery. 1983;94:969.
2. Vázquez AG, et al. Pendred syndrome: a cause of goiter associated with deafness. Endocrinol Nutr. 2009;56:428.
3. Siddique MA, et al. Amyloid goiter as a manifestation of primary systemic amyloidosis. Thyroid. 2007;17:77.

Many of the symptoms of hypothyroidism—such as constipation, tiredness, poor memory, weight gain, and dry skin—are found in "normal" persons.

Other symptoms and signs that may, or may not, point to the presence of hypothyroidism are cold intolerance, cognitive dysfunction, hoarseness, muscle pains, joint

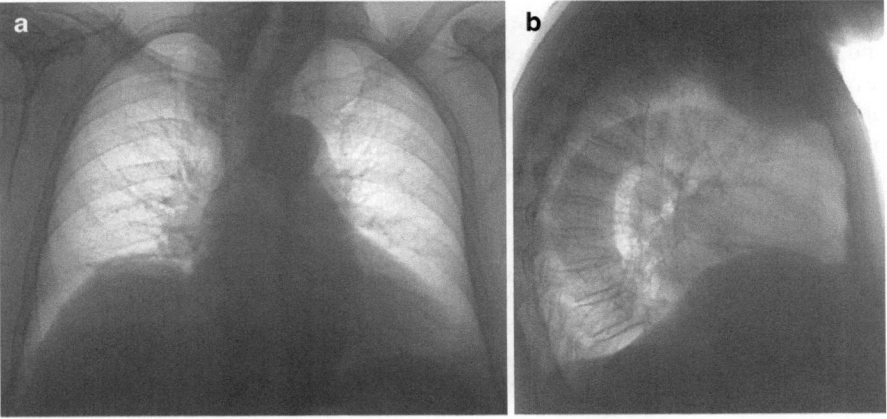

Fig. 13.2 Substernal goiter. Chest x-ray

pains, sluggish deep tendon reflexes, puffy face, and bradycardia [1]. For this reason, many clinicians have a low threshold for obtaining a thyroid-stimulating hormone (TSH) level in persons with multiple symptoms and signs suggesting that a thyroid hormone deficiency may be the cause.

1. McDermott MT, et al. Hypothyroidism. Ann Intern Med. 2009;151:ITC6-1.

Most patients with subclinical hypothyroidism are asymptomatic.

Because of the paucity of symptoms and signs, subclinical hypothyroidism, aka mild thyroid failure, is a laboratory diagnosis: the finding of an elevated TSH level in the face of normal thyroxine concentrations. The condition affects 3–8 % of the general population [1]. Although not all experts agree, there are well-designed studies linking subclinical hypothyroidism to an increased risk of coronary heart disease (CHD) and CHD mortality [2].

1. Fatourechi V. Subclinical hypothyroidism: an update for primary care physicians. Mayo Clin Proc. 2009;84:65.
2. Rondondi N, et al. Subclinical hypothyroidism and the risk of coronary heart disease and mortality. JAMA. 2010;304:1365.

Suspect hyperthyroidism in a patient who loses weight in the face of an increased appetite.

Although the same pair of seemingly paradoxical manifestations may be seen with uncontrolled diabetes, the patient with hyperthyroidism is also likely to have some combination of a fine tremor of the hands, heat intolerance, palpitations, weakness, and emotional lability [1]. However, a cross-sectional study of 3,049 older patients revealed that the seniors in your practice may not present with the classic symptoms of thyroid hormone excess [2]. Experienced clinicians evaluating patients with suspicious findings listen for a systolic bruit, best heard over a lateral lobe, present in about a third of patients with hyperthyroidism [3].

1. Trivalle C, et al. Differences in the signs and symptoms of hyperthyroidism in older and younger patients. J Am Geriatr Soc. 1996;44:50.
2. Boelaert K, et al. Older subjects with hyperthyroidism present with a paucity of symptoms and signs: a large cross-sectional study. J Clin Endocrinol Metabol. 2010;95:2715.
3. Orient JM, editor. Sapira's art & science of bedside diagnosis. 3rd ed. Philadelphia: Lippincott, Williams & Wilkins; 2005. p. 278.

Hyperthyroidism traced to hamburger consumption has been reported.

The cause of "hamburger thyrotoxicosis" is meat that contains bovine thyroid tissue that has been mixed into ground beef [1].

1. Malvinder S, et al. Recurrent hamburger thyrotoxicosis. CMAJ. 2003;169:415.

Not all exophthalmos is caused by Graves disease.

The hallmark of Graves disease is exophthalmos (proptosis), but other disorders can cause the abnormal physical finding. Among 82 patients with exophthalmos, there were 23 persons with Graves disease, 20 with inflammatory pseudotumor, 16 with angioma, five with carotid cavernous fistula, five with cranial neurogliocytoma, four with retinal glioblastoma, three with metastatic tumor, three with lymphangioma, and three with nasosinusitis. The authors highlight the value of computed tomography (CT) in the evaluation of exophthalmos [1].

1. Li X, et al. Value of CT in the diagnosis of exophthalmos. J China Clin Med Imag. 2008. Available at: http://en.cnki.com.cn/Article_en/CJFDTOTAL-LYYX200802012.htm.

Be alert for thyroid cancer in women with benign thyroid disease, benign breast disease, asthma, and/or obesity.

In a long-term study of 69,506 women and 21,207 men, investigators found 242 women and 40 men with thyroid cancer. They report "Elevated risks were observed for women with benign thyroid conditions (HR 2.35, 95 % CI 1.73–3.20), benign breast disease (HR 1.56, 95 % CI 1.08–2.26), asthma (HR 1.68, 95 % CI 1.00–2.83), and body mass index ≥35.0 versus 18.5–24.9 kg/m^2 (HR 1.74, 95 % CI 1.03–2.94; P-trend 0.04). Current smoking was inversely associated with thyroid cancer risk (HR 0.54)" [1].

1. Meinhold CL, et al. Non-radiation risk factors for thyroid cancer in US radiologic technologists study. Am J Epidem. 2010;171:242.

No single negative test can conclusively rule out the presence of follicular cancer of the thyroid gland.

The statement above is the authors' conclusion following a retrospective study comparing the reliability of physical examination (PE), ultrasonography (US), and fine-needle aspiration (FNA) cytology in the evaluation of 242 euthyroid patients with thyroid nodules. In the report, the sensitivity and specificity of the three modalities are as follows [1]:

Test	Sensitivity (%)	Specificity (%)
PE	63	98
US	78	90
FNA	80	98

1. Okamoto T, et al. Test performances of three diagnostic procedures in evaluating thyroid nodules: physical examination, ultrasonography and fine needle aspiration cytology. Endocrinol J. 1994;41:243.

Gout

During an acute attack of gout, the serum uric acid (SUA) level may be normal or even low.

Based on a selective literature review of gout diagnosis and management, Tausche et al. conclude that better information regarding the serum urate level is obtained when blood is drawn 2–3 weeks following an attack [1]. In a study of patients with acute gouty arthritis, Urano et al. found "SUA was significantly lower in the acute phase (7.5 ± 1.4 mg/dL) than in the intercritical phase (8.5 ± 0.9 mg/dL) ($p < 0.0001$)." Of the 41 patients in the study, a normal SUA level was found during the acute attack in 20 (49 %) patients [2]. Presumptive diagnosis of the acute gout attack rests on history and physical findings, while synovial fluid urate crystal identification remains the gold standard [3] (see Fig. 13.3).

1. Tausche AK, et al. Gout—current diagnosis and treatment. Dtsch Arztebl Int. 2009;106:549.
2. Urano W, et al. The inflammatory process in the mechanism of decreased serum uric acid concentrations during acute gouty arthritis. J Rheumatol. 2002;29:1950.
3. Malik A, et al. Clinical diagnostic criteria for gout: comparison with the gold standard of synovial fluid crystal analysis. J Clin Rheumatol. 2009;15:22.

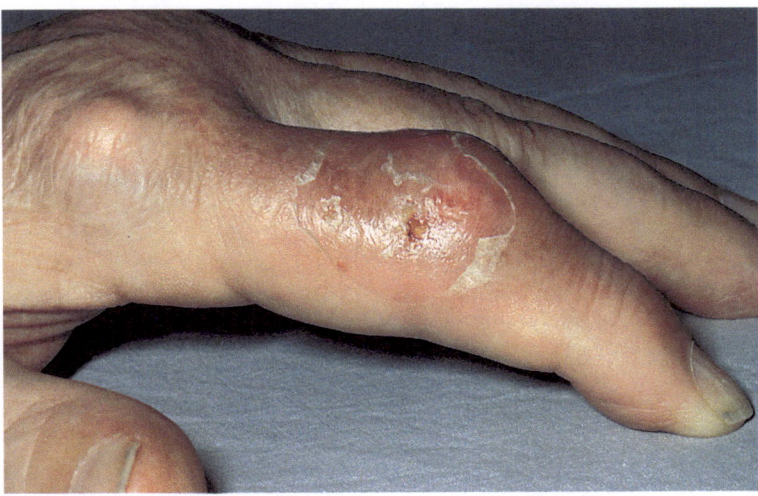

Fig. 13.3 Tophaceous gout produced chronic swelling and serous drainage in this finger. Examination of a drop of this fluid under the polarizing microscope confirmed the diagnosis

Pseudogout can be misdiagnosed as gout, but there are helpful clinical differences.

Much less common than gout, pseudogout tends to affect the knee or wrist versus the first metatarsophalangeal joint classically involved in acute gouty attacks. Gout is more likely than pseudogout to occur following surgery, trauma, or severe disease occurrence [1]. An acute inflammatory arthritis occurring following parathyroidectomy is especially suspicious for pseudogout [2]. In pseudogout, synovial fluid analysis reveals calcium pyrophosphate dihydrate crystals, rather than the monosodium urate crystals characteristic of gout.

1. Dieppe PA, et al. Pyrophosphate arthropathy: a clinical and radiologic study of 105 cases. Ann Rheum Dis. 1982;41:371.
2. Bilezikian JP, et al. Pseudogout after parathyroidectomy. Lancet. 1973;1(7801):445.

Gynecomastia

Up to 10 % of cases of male gynecomastia can be traced to drugs.

A distressing condition affecting males at any stage of life, gynecomastia can often be the result of medication use. Aiman et al. tell that both furosemide (Lasix) and digoxin (Lanoxin), both used in patients with heart failure, can cause gynecomastia, and they report such a finding in a patient using both drugs [1]. Young athletes attempting to increase muscle mass by using anabolic androgenic steroids may find that they have also increased the size of their mammary glands [2]. Among the other drugs that might cause gynecomastia are fenofibrate (Lipofen and other brands) [3], isoniazid [4], and spironolactone (Aldactone) [5]. In addition, there is a report of breast enlargement associated with soy product consumption [6].

1. Aiman U, et al. Gynecomastia: an ADR due to drug interaction. Indian J Pharmacol. 2009;41:286.
2. Orlandi MA, et al. Gynecomastia in two young men with histories of prolonged use of anabolic androgenic steroids. J Ultrasound. 2010;13:46.
3. Gardette V, et al. Gynecomastia associated with fenofibrate. Ann Pharmacother. 2007;41:508.
4. Garg R, et al. Isoniazid induced gynecomastia: a case report. Indian J Tuberc. 2009;56:51.
5. Haynes BA, et al. Male gynecomastia. Mayo Clin Proc. 2009;84:672.
6. Martinez J, et al. An unusual case of gynecomastia associated with soy product consumption. Endocrinol Pract. 2008;14:415.

Approximately 5 % of males with testicular germ cell tumors (GCTs) will have gynecomastia.

The abnormal stimulation of breast tissue may also be seen with the less common Leydig cell tumor of the testis [1, 2].

1. Tseng A Jr, et al. Gynecomastia in testicular cancer patients: prognostic and therapeutic implications. Cancer. 1985;56:2534.
2. Bertola G, et al. An uncommon cause of gynecomastia: testicular Leydig cell tumor. Hormonal profile before and after orchiectomy. Recent Prog Med. 2006;97:85.

Males with gynecomastia have an increased risk of breast cancer.

In a study of 642 men with primary breast cancer, "significant risks were seen for Klinefelter syndrome (16.83, 6.81–41.62), gynecomastia (5.08, 3.21–8.03), obesity (1.91, 1.50–2.44), and orchitis/epididymitis (1.80, 1.08–3.01)" [1]. Johnson et al. recommend a stepwise diagnostic approach to gynecomastia to include laboratory studies and imaging to rule out the presence of tumors or endocrinopathy [2].

1. Brinton LA et al. Etiologic factors for male breast cancer in the US Veterans Affairs medical care system database. Breast Cancer Res Treat. 2010;119:185.
2. Johnson RE, et al. Gynecomastia: pathophysiology, evaluation, and management. Mayo Clin Proc. 2009;84:1010.

Disorders of Pubertal Development

Approximately 3 % of children will experience some variation of normal pubertal development [1].

Here are some of the possible variations and causes:

Delayed puberty in children with idiopathic short stature (ISS): Children with ISS will often exhibit late puberty [2].

Girls with precocious puberty (PP): In girls with secondary sexual characteristics before age eight, pelvic ultrasound may help differentiate PP from a functioning ovarian cyst [3].

Swyer syndrome: Also known as gonadal dysgenesis, Swyer syndrome describes women with delayed puberty associated with primary amenorrhea, normal vagina, and normal to tall stature. In the study of 29 women with Swyer syndrome by Michala et al., all patients had a confirmed karyotype showing 46XY, and one had an abnormal Y chromosome. The patient with Swyer syndrome has an increased risk of developing dysgerminoma [4].

Kallmann syndrome: The combination of hypogonadotropic hypogonadism and anosmia/hyposmia should be suspected in a male with microphallus and/or cryptorchidism, especially if hearing loss is present. Many persons with impaired sense of smell are unaware of their defect. A renal ultrasound may reveal renal agenesis [5].

1. Bramswig J, et al. Disorders of pubertal development. Dtsch Arztebl. 2009;1067:295.
2. Mariani A, et al. Puberty and pubertal growth dynamics in children with idiopathic short stature. J Pediatr Endo Metabol. 2011;24:319.
3. de Vries L, et al. Role of pelvic ultrasound in girls with precocious puberty. Horm Res Pediatr. 2011;75:148.
4. Michala L, et al. Swyer syndrome. Br J Obstet Gyn. 2008;115:734.
5. Kaplan JD, et al. Clues to an early diagnosis of Kallmann syndrome. Am J Med Genet A. 2010;152A:2769.

Selected Problems of the Endocrine and Metabolic Systems

Acute intermittent porphyria can have protean manifestations, but the most common acute presentation is abdominal pain.

This autosomal dominant disorder with incomplete penetrance is well known by medical historians as the probable cause of the "Madness of King George 3rd," also the title of a 1994 motion picture. Neurologic and psychiatric manifestations, such as an agitated psychosis, evoking the image of the "insane" King, are common [1, 2]. Some patients exhibit peripheral neuropathy, and there may be muscle weakness beginning in the proximal muscles of the legs. The urine may develop a port-wine color following exposure to sunlight. Acute attacks may be precipitated by alcohol, acute illness, surgery, inadequate nutrition, or drugs such as sulfonamides and barbiturates [3].

1. Grandchamp B. Acute intermittent porphyria. Semin Liver Dis. 1998;18:17.
2. Macalpine I, et al. The "insanity" of King George 3rd: a classic case of porphyria. Br Med J. 1966;1(5479):65.
3. Burgovne K, et al. Porphyria: reexamination of psychiatric implications. Psychother Psychosom. 1995;64:121.

The combination of liver function abnormalities, splenomegaly, movement disorders, and/or psychiatric manifestations such as depression may indicate the presence of Wilson disease (WD).

Many of these patients will have Kayser–Fleischer brown-green rings in the cornea and/or sunflower cataracts caused by copper deposition in the lens. Other possible manifestations include headaches, cardiomyopathy, pancreatitis, asymptomatic hepatomegaly, and acute liver failure. There may be degenerative joint change in various joints, including the metacarpophalangeal joints [1] (see Fig. 13.4). Laboratory investigation of suspected WD will classically reveal reduced levels of serum ceruloplasmin, an increased urinary copper excretion, and high concentrations of copper on liver biopsy [2]. Acute liver failure of WD is fatal if the patient does not receive liver transplantation [3].

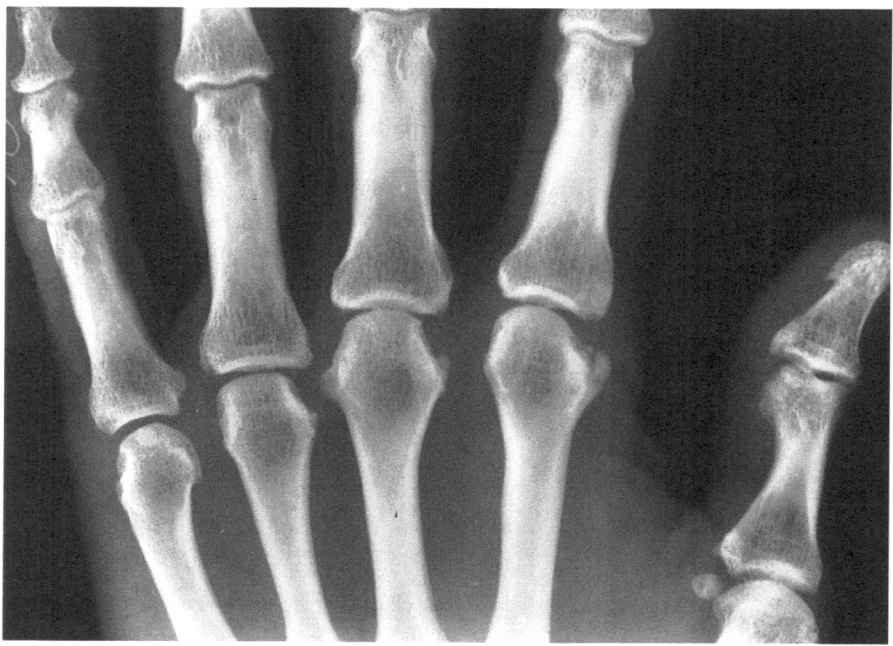

Fig. 13.4 Wilson disease. The radiograph is from a 39 year old man with ataxia, tremor, and dysarthria. Kayser–Fleischer rings were present on ophthalmologic examination. Degenerative changes were present in multiple joints. Several joints, including the metacarpophalangeal joints, were surrounded by small ossicles, characteristic of Wilson disease

1. Roberts EA, et al. Diagnosis and treatment of Wilson disease: an update. Hepatology. 2008;47:2089.
2. Medici V, et al. Wilson disease—a practical approach to diagnosis, treatment and follow-up. Digest Liver Dis. 2007;7:601.
3. Korman JD, et al. Screening for Wilson disease in acute liver failure: a comparison of currently available diagnostic tests. Hepatology. 2008;48:1167.

The presentation of a triad of dark skin, cirrhosis, and diabetes probably represents late stage hereditary hemochromatosis (HH) that should have been diagnosed years before.

The classic triad of late stage hemochromatosis is seldom seen today, even though a study of 2,851 patients revealed an average time lag from symptom onset to definitive diagnosis of 10–12 years [1]. A common inherited disease of persons of Northern European ancestry, HH is a disorder of iron metabolism resulting in iron overloading in the liver and other organs such as the pancreas [2]. The key to early diagnosis is recognition of subtle and non-localizing manifestations: weakness and lethargy, joint pains, and impotence in males [3] (see Fig. 13.5).

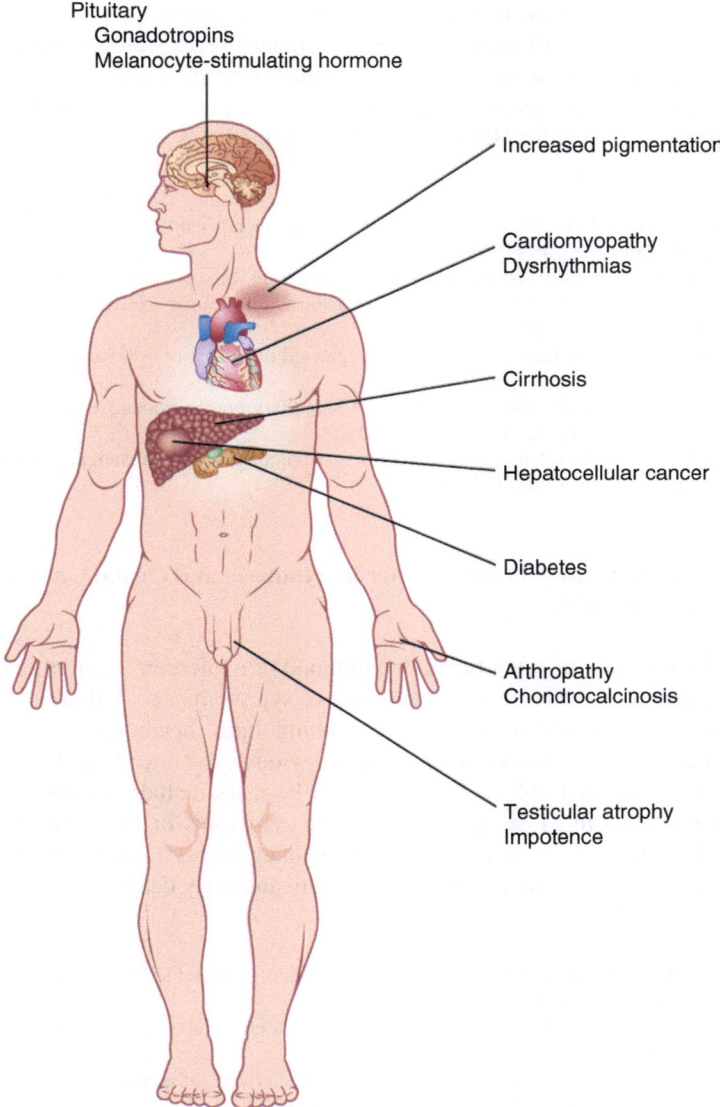

Fig. 13.5 Clinical manifestations of hereditary hemochromatosis. The clinical manifestations of HH are protean. The most common abnormalities are found in the liver, and the development of hepatocellular carcinoma is 100 times more common in patients with untreated hemochromatosis than in the general population

Many HH patients are referred to orthopedic surgeons for joint replacement because of secondary osteoarthritis [4]. And there is a 20-fold increased risk of hepatocellular cancer in patients with hemochromatosis [5]. Because of the nonspecificity of early symptoms and the serious implications of the disease, the possibility of screening for HH has been discussed [6].

1. McDonnell SM, et al. A survey of 2851 patients with hemochromatosis: symptoms and response to treatment. Am J Med. 1999;106:619.
2. Bacon BR. Hemochromatosis: diagnosis and management. Gastroenterology. 2001;120:718.
3. Niederau C, et al. Epidemiology, clinical spectrum and prognosis of hemochromatosis. Adv Exp Med Biol. 1994;356:293.
4. Carlsson A. Hereditary hemochromatosis: a neglected diagnosis in orthopedics. Acta Orthop. 2009;80:351.
5. Elmberg M, et al. Cancer risk in patients with hereditary hemochromatosis and in their first-degree relatives. Gastroenterology. 2003;125:1733.
6. Edwards CQ, et al. Prevalence of hemochromatosis among 11,065 presumably healthy blood donors. N Engl J Med. 1988;318:1355.

Fabry disease (FD) may begin with acroparesthesia and chronic, burning pain in the lower extremities.

The first manifestations often begin in childhood or adolescence, and there is typically a decade-long delay between the onset of symptoms and definitive diagnosis [1, 2]. An X-linked inborn error of glycosphingolipid metabolism, FD has been described as occurring more commonly than previously assumed [2]. Manifestations reported in a series of 1,765 patients in a Fabry Registry include: neurologic pain in 62 %, skin lesions in 31 %, gastroenterologic symptoms in 19 %, renal signs in 17 %, and eye signs in 11 % of patients [3]. Kidney biopsy findings are diagnostic of this disease that can cause major organ failure and early death [4].

1. Samiy N. Ocular features of Fabry disease: diagnosis of a treatable life-threatening disorder. Survey Ophthal. 2008;53:416.
2. Hoffman B, et al. Fabry disease: often seen, rarely diagnosed. Dtsch Arztebl Int. 2009;106:440.
3. Eng CM, et al. Fabry disease: baseline medical characteristics of a cohort of 1765 males and females in a Fabry Registry. J Inherit Metab Dis. 2007;30:184.
4. Houge G, et al. Fabry disease defined: baseline clinical manifestations of 366 patients in the Fabry Outcome Survey. Eur J Clin Invest. 2004;34:236.

Chapter 14
Blood and the Hematologic System

Blood is a very special juice.
German author Johann Wolfgang von Goethe (1749–1832) [1]

Contents

R.B. Taylor, *Diagnostic Principles and Applications*,
DOI 10.1007/978-1-4614-1111-6_14, © Springer Science+Business Media, LLC 2013

Today's medical student is no longer dispatched to the patient's bedside to perform the time-consuming Lee–White clotting time test and community-based physicians are unlikely to be found peering through microscopes at stained blood smears. Nevertheless, findings related to circulating blood cells and the hematopoietic and lymphatic systems can have profound diagnostic and prognostic implications. Just some examples would be the unexpected finding of anemia in a long-distance runner or the detection of leukopenia in a person taking a psychotropic drug, as discussed below.

1. Goethe JW. Faust, Part I, Act I, Sc iv.

Anemia

Anemia, which is fundamentally a manifestation of some underlying disorder, may cause no symptoms at all.

Anemia is a common clinical problem. When symptoms occur, they are likely to be fatigue, diminished physical endurance, and impaired cognition [1, 2]. The most common cause of anemia worldwide is iron deficiency, described by Brunner et al. as "the most prevalent single nutrient deficiency [2]."

1. Clark SF. Iron deficiency anemia: diagnosis and management. Curr Opin Gastroenterol. 2009;25:122.
2. Brunner C, et al. Iron deficiency and iron deficiency anemia: symptoms and therapy. Ther Umsch. 2010;67:219.

Clinical pallor of the conjunctiva and palm is useful in detecting anemia, at least severe anemia; nail pallor, maybe; pallor of the palmar creases, probably not.

Three US physicians made individual assessments at various sites on 103 patients. They found that pallor of the conjunctiva, face, and palms together help confirm the presence of anemia, but the nail beds and palmar creases were not helpful in determining the presence or absence of anemia [1]. In another study conducted in Nepal and Zanzibar, where anemia is more prevalent than in the USA, 5,760 persons were examined. Of these, 3,072 were anemic and 192 had severe anemia (hemoglobin <7.0 g/L). Three sites were examined for pallor: conjunctiva, palm, and nail beds. These investigators concluded, "Pallor at any of these three sites detected severe anemia with >84 % specificity" [2].

Both reports suggest that the absence of pallor at various sites is not useful in excluding the presence of anemia. The Nepal/Zanzibar study found that the overall sensitivity of clinical pallor of the various sites was about 50 %, which, in the population studied, seems to me to be a *coin toss* [2].

1. Nardone DA, et al. Usefulness of physical examination in detecting the presence or absence of anemia. Arch Intern Med. 1990;150:201.
2. Stoltfus RJ. Clinical pallor is useful to detect severe anemia in populations where anemia is prevalent and severe. J Nutr. 1999;129:1675.

Iron-deficiency anemia (IDA) can be the tip-off to the presence of serious disease.

In a study of 148 patients, mean age 66.2 years, with IDA, 12.2 % were found to have cancer, 6.8 % had benign tumors, and 64.9 % had other nonmalignant disorders.

No underlying cause was detected in 16.2 % of patients [1]. Here are just some of the possible causes you may encounter:

> *Colorectal cancer*: Of 101 patients with colorectal cancer admitted to a hospital in Taiwan, 51 % were found to be anemic. Women were more likely to be anemic than men [2].
> *Celiac disease*: IDA may be the sole initial symptom of celiac disease and, in one study, was found in half of 30 patients with confirmed celiac disease [3, 4].
> *Malaria*: About a third of deaths associated with *P. falciparum* malaria are caused by severe malarial anemia [5].

Whether or not the anemia is caused by iron deficiency is noteworthy, because bleeding gastrointestinal lesions "are infrequently found in anemic patients without evidence of iron deficiency and alternative causes should be sought," although the authors hedge a little in this dictum in the case of elderly patients [6].

1. Ho CH, et al. Predictive risk factors and prevalence of malignancy in patients with iron deficiency anemia in Taiwan. Am J Hematol. 2005;78:108.
2. Ho CH, et al. The prevalence of iron deficiency anemia and its clinical implications in patients with colorectal carcinoma. J Chin Med Assoc. 2008;71:119.
3. Jones S, et al. Patterns of clinical presentation of adult coeliac disease in a rural setting. Nutr J. 2006;14:24.
4. Hin H, et al. Coeliac disease in primary care: case-finding study. BMJ. 1999;318(7177):164.
5. Haldar K, et al. Malaria, erythrocytic infection, and anemia. Hematology. 2009;1:87.
6. Powell N, et al. Gastrointestinal evaluation of anemic patients without evidence of iron deficiency. Eur J Gastroenterol Hepatol. 2008;20:1094.

The anemia of chronic disease is generally normochromic and normocytic, with a mild to moderate decrement in the level of hemoglobin (Hb).

The second most prevalent anemia, following IDA, anemia of chronic disease is an immune response to some ongoing disorder. Weiss et al. call it the *anemia of inflammation* [1]. Possible causes include: infection; cancer; chronic kidney disease; rejection of a transplanted solid organ; or an autoimmune disease such as connective tissue disease, inflammatory bowel disease, vasculitis, or sarcoidosis [1, 2]. Determining the serum concentration of iron and transferrin saturation is unlikely to be helpful, because the values are generally reduced in both IDA and anemia of chronic disease [1].

1. Weiss G, et al. Anemia of chronic disease. N Engl J Med. 2005;352:1011.
2. Masson C. Rheumatoid arthritis. Joint Bone Spine. 2011;78:131.

When the patient with anemia is a long-distance runner, consider the diagnosis of *runner's anemia*.

In runner's anemia, there is hemolysis of older, more mature red blood cells resulting from the pounding of feet on pavement. The result is a relative macrocytosis. Gastrointestinal blood loss and plasma volume expansion may contribute to the anemia [1]. Eichner suggests that footstrike hemolysis, ridding the system of aging erythrocytes, may actually be a theoretical benefit to the runner [2].

1. Dang CV. Runner's anemia. JAMA. 2001;286:714.
2. Eichner ER. Runner's macrocytosis: a clue to footstrike hemolysis. Am J Med. 1985;78:321.

In the case of young children in developed countries, finding an *anemic* hemoglobin concentration does not necessarily mean that the toddler has an iron deficiency.

White reports on children 12–35 months of age involved in the US National Health and Nutrition Examination Survey III (NHANES III). He found that those with an Hb concentration of <110 g/L had a positive predictive value for iron deficiency of only 29 % (95 % CI 20–38 %). The author concludes that although iron deficiency remains common in the USA, "anemia in toddlers in developed countries is more likely to be due to causes other than iron deficiency." And the report goes on to tell that most children with iron deficiency are not anemic [1].

1. White KC. Anemia is a poor predictor of iron deficiency among toddlers in the United States: for heme the bell tolls. Pediatrics. 2005;115:315.

In an elderly person found to be anemic, consider nutrient deficiency as a cause.

In the case of elderly persons in the NHANES III study, 34 % of anemia found was caused by deficiencies of iron, folate, and vitamin B12, alone or in combination [1].

1. Andrés E, et al. Role of B12 in anemia in old age. Arch Intern Med. 2009;169:1167.

Polycythemia

Although polycythemia vera (PV) may be discovered incidentally on a blood count, many patients first present with a venous or arterial thrombosis.

In a study of 1,213 patients with PV, arterial or venous thromboses were recorded in 485 patients, with 64 % of these occurring either at presentation or before diagnosis [1]. Other symptoms that may be reported include lightheadedness, headache, cough, and easy fatigability. This treatable disease is characterized by recurrent thrombotic events, and if untreated, the survival time of patients with PV is approximately 2 years, making PV a *must-not-miss diagnosis* [2].

1. Gruppo Italiano Studio Policitemia. Polycythemia vera: the natural history of 1213 patients followed for 20 years. Ann Intern Med. 1995;123:656.
2. Pleyer L, et al. Polycythemia vera. In: Greil R, et al., editors. Chronic myeloid neoplasias and clonal overlap syndromes. New York: Springer; 2010. p. 52.

Pruritus aggravated by hot shower or bath water is a *defining feature* of PV [1].

This so-called aquagenic pruritus occurs in 30–40 % of patients with PV and may be pathognomonic of the disease [1, 2]. Although pruritus is often highly distressing to the patient, the occurrence of pruritus is curiously associated with a lower rate of arterial thrombosis [3].

1. Saini KS, et al. Polycythemia vera-associated pruritus and its management. Eur J Clin Invest. 2010;40:828.
2. Broudy VC. The polycythemias. Sci Am Med. 1996;5 Hema V:1.
3. Gangat N, et al. Pruritus in polycythemia vera is associated with a lower risk of arterial thrombosis. Am J Hematol. 2008;6:451.

Coagulation Disorders

Think expansively regarding possible causes when you encounter a patient with petechiae.

In addition to thrombocytopenia (discussed below), other possible diagnoses include:

> *Child abuse*: Look for other evidence, including the possibility of fractures in differing stages of healing [1].
>
> *Coining*: Often seen in young children of immigrants from Southeast Asia, coining or coin rubbing (*cao gio*) is a Vietnamese method of treating febrile illness. Coining characteristically causes linear petechiae, erythema, and even abrasions [1]. See Fig. 14.1.
>
> *Dermatitis herpetiformis*: This disease, discussed in Chap. 12, can cause palmar petechiae and purpura [2].
>
> *Rocky Mountain spotted fever*: Look for petechiae on the dorsum of the hand, found in 85–90 % of infected patients [3]. See Fig. 14.2.
>
> *Impending death in cancer patients*: Petechiae on the fingers and palms have been described occurring on cancer patients not long before death, speculated to be a result of "systemic deterioration in terminally ill patients" [4].

Also, van Onna et al. report that in a young person with both coma and petechiae, the most likely diagnoses are meningococcal septicemia and intracerebral bleeding resulting from head trauma [5].

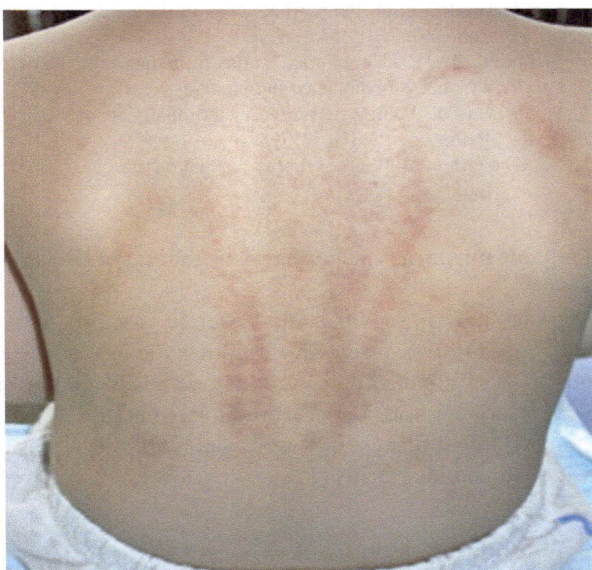

Fig. 14.1 Coining. Note linear lesions on the back of this young person

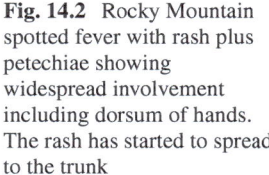

Fig. 14.2 Rocky Mountain
spotted fever with rash plus
petechiae showing
widespread involvement
including dorsum of hands.
The rash has started to spread
to the trunk

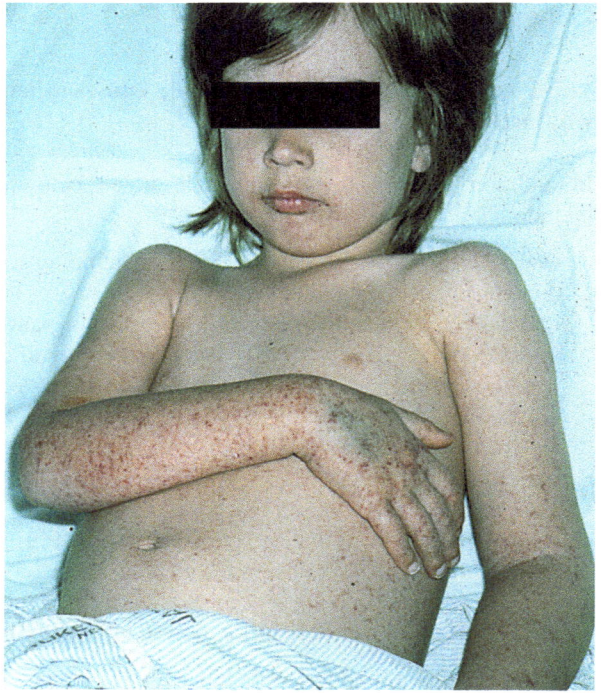

1. Ermertcan AT, et al. Skin manifestations of child abuse. Indian J Dermatol Venereol Leprol. 2010;76:317.
2. McCleskey PE, et al. Palmar petechiae in dermatitis herpetiformis: a case report and clinical review. Cutis. 2002;70:217.
3. Lichtman MA, et al. Lichtman's atlas of hematology. New York: McGraw Hill. Available at: http://www.accessmedicine.com/content.aspx?aID=2783420.
4. Shinjo T, et al. Palmar petechiae in terminally ill patients with cancer: a sign of impending death. J Palliat Med. 2010;13:615.
5. van Onna M, et al. Black and blue . . . and unconscious. BMJ. 2009;339:b2864.

Palpable purpura is a characteristic finding in Henoch–Schönlein purpura (HSP).

The classic triad of this acute systemic vasculitis is palpable purpura (seen in all patients), arthritis (seen in 75 % of patients), and abdominal pain (occurring in 60–75 % of affected persons). Platelet levels are normal. Most patients with HSP will describe a prior upper respiratory infection. HSP can cause diagnostic confusion and might be misdiagnosed as polyarteritis nodosa, Kawasaki disease, or juvenile rheumatoid arthritis [1].

1. Reamy BV, et al. Henoch-Schönlein purpura. Am Fam Physician. 2009;80:697.

A young patient with severe gastrointestinal bleeding or intracranial hemorrhage probably has something other than immune thrombocytopenic purpura (ITP).

Also called idiopathic thrombocytopenic purpura, ITP is much more likely to cause petechiae and purpura, or perhaps gingival bleeding, nosebleed, or menorrhagia, although the more serious bleeding manifestations may occur in older patients. The fundamental pathology of ITP is immune-mediated platelet damage resulting in platelet phagocytosis by the reticuloendothelial system [1–3]. The diagnosis, essentially one of exclusion, is based on finding thrombocytopenia in the setting of an otherwise normal hemogram and in the absence of an apparent other cause such as a disease (hepatitis C infection is one possibility) or use of a suspect medication, as described in the next section [3, 4].

1. Yang R, et al. Pathogenesis and management of chronic idiopathic thrombocytopenic purpura; an update. Int J Hematol. 2000;71:18.
2. Provan D, et al. International consensus report on the investigation and management of primary immune thrombocytopenia. Blood. 2010;115:168.
3. Pilleaux CL, et al. Immune thrombocytopenic purpura associated with hepatitis C virus infection: report of one case. Rev Med Chil. 2010;138:1140.
4. Rodeghiero F, et al. Standardization of terminology, definitions and outcome criteria in immune thrombocytopenic purpura of adults and children. Blood. 2009;113:2386.

Thrombocytopenia can be caused by any of a number of drugs.

Heparin-induced thrombocytopenia is the most common immune-mediated platelet deficiency state caused by drugs [1]. Quinine and quinidine are classical offenders, and one intriguing example is so-called *cocktail purpura*, thrombocytopenic bruising that follows ingestion of the quinine *tonic water* used in cocktail mixes [2]. Even widely used atorvastatin has been reported to cause reduced platelet levels [3]. Thrombocytopenia may also be associated with the use of sulfonamides, beta-lactam antibiotics, rifampin (Rifadin), vancomycin, alemtuzumab (Campath), valproic acid (Depakote), phenytoin (Dilantin), carbamazepine (Tegretol), and even the measles–mumps–rubella vaccine [4].

1. McCrae KR, et al. Platelets: an update on diagnosis and management of thrombocytopenic disorders. Hematology Am Soc Hematol Educ Program. 2001:282.
2. Korbitz BC, et al. Cocktail purpura: quinine-dependent thrombocytopenia. Rocky Mt Med J. 1973;70:38.
3. Narayanan D, et al. Atorvastatin-related thrombocytopenic purpura. BMJ Case Reports. 2010;1136:2614.
4. Aster RH, et al. Drug-induced immune thrombocytopenia: pathogenesis, diagnosis, and management. J Thromb Hemost. 2009;7:911.

Low platelet counts—gestational thrombocytopenia—may be noted during pregnancy.

A low platelet count is also the *LP* in the HELLP (hemolysis, elevated liver enzymes, low platelet count) syndrome of pregnancy and in preeclampsia/eclampsia [1, 2].

1. Brass E. Thrombocytopenia in pregnancy. Postgrad Obstet Gynecol. 2010;30:1.
2. McCrae KR, et al. Platelets: an update on diagnosis and management of thrombocytopenic disorders. Hematology Am Soc Hematol Educ Program. 2001:282.

Bleeding that seems disproportionate to a situation—such as a minor wound—is characteristic of von Willebrand disease.

von Willebrand disease is the most common of the inherited bleeding disorders [1]. Patients may present with trivial wounds that bleed more than 15 min, epistaxis lasting longer than 10 min, easy bruising, oral cavity bleeding, or menorrhagia [2]. The cause is a defect in von Willebrand factor resulting in abnormalities of both platelets and Factor VIII [3]. There may be profound bleeding with orthopedic procedures or following childbirth, making timely recognition of this disease clinically important [1, 4].

1. Kroonen LT, et al. Orthopedic manifestations of patients with von Willebrand disease. Orthopedics. 2008;31:263.
2. Crownover B, et al. Diagnosing von Willebrand disease. Am Fam Physician. 2010;81:1415.
3. Nichols WL, et al. von Willebrand disease: evidence-based diagnosis and management guidelines, the National Heart, Lung, and Blood Institute Expert Panel Report (USA). Hemophilia. 2008; 14:171.
4. Pacheco LD, et al. von Willebrand disease and pregnancy: a practical approach for the diagnosis and treatment. Am J Obstet Gynecol. 2010;203:194.

Leukocytosis

There seems to be an *obesity-related leukocytosis*.

Of 327 persons evaluated for persistent leukocytosis, 15.3 % were found to be obese and, in these patients, no other cause for the elevated white blood cell count could be found. The authors attribute the association of leukocytosis and obesity to the production of inflammatory cytokines by fatty tissue [1]. Recognition of this association might help some patients avoid needless diagnostic tests.

1. Herishanu Y, et al. Leukocytosis in obese individuals: possible link in patients with unexplained persistent neutrophilia. Eur J Hematol. 2006;76:516.

In some settings, leukocytosis can have unfavorable prognostic implications.

Leukocytosis can be a predictor for noninfective morbidity and mortality [1]. Here are some examples:

Sickle cell disease (SCD): In children with SCD, leukocytosis and hemolysis have been found to be independent risk factors for early lung volume decline [2].
Polycythemia vera: In patients with polycythemia vera, white blood counts above 15×10^9/L have a significantly increased risk of thrombosis, with an increased risk of myocardial infarction [3].
Hospital admission: Based on a study of 1,650 patients, leukocytosis in the early stages of general hospital admission is described by one team of investigators as "an alarming sign for mortality" [4].

1. Asadollahi K, et al. Leukocytosis as a predictor of non-infective mortality and morbidity. QJM. 2010;103:285.
2. Tassel C, et al. Leukocytosis is a risk factor for lung function deterioration in children with sickle cell disease. Respir Med. 2011;105:788.
3. Landolfi R, et al. Leukocytosis as a major thrombotic risk factor in patients with polycythemia vera. Blood. 2007;109:2446.
4. Asadollahi K, et al. Leukocytosis as an alarming sign for mortality in patients hospitalized in general wards. Iran J Med Sci. 2011;36:45.

Not all extreme leukocytosis is leukemia.

Halkes et al. report on three patients with leukocytosis greater than 50×10^9/L. One had a hepatic sarcoma; the second, a *Salmonella* infection; and the third, a necrotic leg abscess [1].

1. Halkes CJM, et al. Extreme leukocytosis: not always leukemia. Netherlands J Med. 2007;65:248.

Leukopenia

Leukopenia can follow the use of iodinated contrast material (ICM), and may be due to other causes, as well.

Kovoor et al. report on this phenomenon following the use of ICM for hysterosalpingography [1]. Leukopenia can also be associated with the use of other compounds such as clozapine (Clozaril), carbamazepine (Tegretol), risperidone (Risperdal), sulfasalazine (Azulfidine), and even the widely used cephalosporins [2–4].

A patient with systemic lupus erythematosus (SLE) may have a low white blood cell count [5], as also may a person with human immunodeficiency virus (HIV) infection [6] or anorexia nervosa [7].

1. Kovoor E, et al. Severe transient leukocytopenia following hysterosalpingography. Gynecol Obstet Invest. 2009;69:190.
2. Sedky K, et al. Psychotropic medications and leukopenia. Curr Drug Targets. 2006;7:1191.
3. Uzun S, et al. Leukopenia during therapy with risperidone long-acting injectable: two case reports. J Clin Psychopharmacol.2008;28:713.
4. Whitman CB. Cephalosporin-induced leukopenia following rechallenge with cefoxitin. Ann Pharmacother. 2008;42:1327.
5. Dias AMB, et al. White blood cell count abnormalities and infections in one-year follow-up of 124 patients with SLE. Ann NY Acad Sci. 2009;1173:103.
6. Costantini A, et al. HIV-induced abnormalities in myelopoiesis and their recovery following antiretroviral therapy. Curr HIV Research. 2010;8:336.
7. Polli N, et al. Low insulin-like growth factor I and leukopenia in anorexia nervosa. Int J Eat Disord. 2008;41:355.

Many recipients of solid organ transplants have leukopenia.

In a study of 102 adult kidney and/or pancreas transplant recipients, 59 (58 %) had leukopenia or neutropenia, with the initial occurrence noted at a mean of 91 days following the organ transplantation [1].

1. Hartmann EL, et al. Management of leukopenia in kidney and pancreas transplant recipients. Clin Transplant. 2008;22:822.

Some patients have an inherited paucity of neutrophils.

Keep in mind that most leukocytes are neutrophils, and thus a deficiency of neutrophils results in a leukopenia. The disorder, called *congenital neutropenia*, results in both a tendency to develop serious bacterial infections and an increased risk of leukemia [1].

1. Boztug K, et al. A syndrome with congenital neutropenia and mutations in G6PC3. N Engl J Med. 2009;360:32.

Eosinophilia

Three disease categories account for most cases of eosinophilia: infestations, drugs, and hypersensitivity disorders.

The classic infection/infestation is parasitic, which may be *Giardia*, hookworm, roundworm, *Schistosoma*, or filaria [1]. Bryant et al. describe helminthic parasites as the most common cause of eosinophilia in children who are either travelers returning from an exotic locale or immigrants from a developing country [2]. See Fig. 14.3, showing the life cycle of hookworm, and why we should be very careful about going barefoot in locations where sanitation is uncertain. Among the drugs that can cause eosinophilia are sulfonamides, penicillin, phenytoin (Dilantin), aspirin, and carbamazepine. Asthma, atopic dermatitis, and acute urticaria are among the hypersensitivity disorders that can be associated with eosinophilia [1].

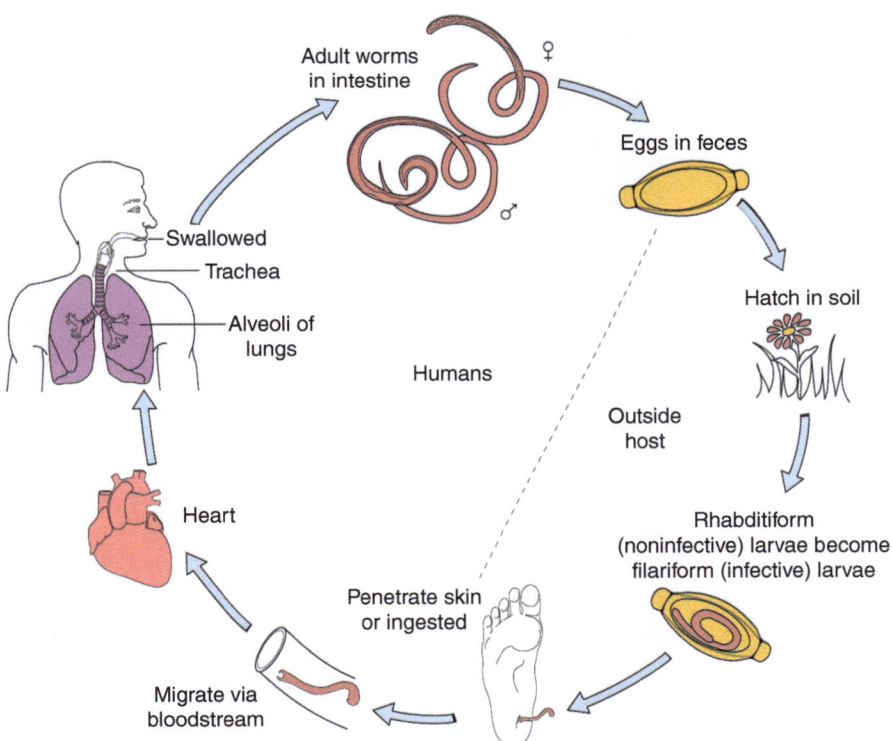

Fig. 14.3 Hookworm life cycle. Hookworm larvae enter the human body via the skin. They are transported to the small intestine via the heart and lungs in a fashion similar to Ascaris larvae. Adults mature in the intestine and pass unembryonated eggs in feces into the soil where filariform larvae develop

1. Sims H, et al. Investigation of an incidental finding of eosinophilia. BMJ. 2011;342:d2670.
2. Bryant P, et al. A practical approach to eosinophilia in a child arriving or returning from the tropics. Adv Expt Med Biology. 2011;697:289.

The patient with a very high eosinophil count may have the hypereosinophilic syndrome.

The rare disorder is diagnosed upon finding otherwise unexplained eosinophilia of $\geq 1.5 \times 10^9$/L associated with evidence of tissue damage [1, 2]. For example, Sethi et al. describe three patients with cerebral infarcts occurring as part of the hypereosinophilic syndrome [3].

1. Gleich GJ, et al. The hypereosinophilic syndromes: current concepts and treatments. Br J Hematol. 2009;145:271.
2. Roufosse F, et al. Practical approach to the patient with hypereosinophilia. J Allergy Clin Immunol. 2010;126:39.
3. Sethi HS, et al. Cerebral infarcts in the setting of eosinophilia: three cases and a discussion. Arch Neurol. 2010;67:1275.

Lymphadenopathy

Lymphadenopathy is an important manifestation of a number of diseases.

Here are a few disorders in which lymphadenopathy can be important in early diagnosis:

HIV disease: Enlargement of lymph nodes is a common HIV presentation, which may begin early in the seroconversion phase [1].

Epstein–Barr virus (EBV) infection: In a study of 160 children presenting with cervical lymphadenopathy, 24 (15 %) had serologic evidence of EBV infection [2].

Cat-scratch disease: Regional lymph node enlargement, developing 1–2 weeks following initial infection, is characteristically ipsilateral [3].

Systemic lupus erythematosus: Extensive lymphadenopathy can be part of the early presentation of SLE [4].

1. Jacobs W. The problem of HIV-related lymphadenopathy. CME. 2010:8:364. Available at: http://www.ajol.info/index.php/cme/article/viewFile/71847/60805.
2. Abdel-Aziz M, et al. Epstein-Barr virus infection as a cause of cervical lymphadenopathy in children. Int J Pediatr Otorhinolaryngol. 2011;75:564.
3. Klotz SA, et al. Cat-scratch disease. Am Fam Physician. 2011;83:152.
4. Tuinman PR, et al. A young woman with generalized lymphadenopathy. Netherlands J Med. 2011;69:284.

When a young woman presents with severe cervical lymphadenopathy and fever, consider the diagnosis of Kikuchi disease.

Also known as histiocytic necrotizing lymphadenitis, Kikuchi disease is a rare, self-limited entity typically found in young women. Biopsy findings confirm the diagnosis. The disease is unresponsive to antibiotic therapy, and a correct diagnosis spares the patient unnecessary antimicrobial exposure [1, 2]. It has been speculated that Kikuchi may be a manifestation of SLE [3].

1. Quari F, et al. Kikuchi disease: an important cause of cervical lymphadenopathy. Clin Med. 2007;7:82.
2. Lien CH, et al. Kikuchi disease (histiocytic necrotizing lymphadenitis): report of one case. Acta Pediatr Taiwan. 1999;40:344.
3. Chen YH, et al. Kikuchi disease in systemic lupus erythematosus: clinical features and literature review. J Microbiol Immunol Infect. 1998;31:187.

Of all sites of possible lymphadenopathy, the supraclavicular nodes are the most worrisome for malignancy [1].

In a study of 457 patients, ages less than 19 years, with peripheral lymphadenopathy, 346 had benign causes and 111 had malignant disease. Among these subjects, the supraclavicular area was involved only in the malignant group [2]. The left supraclavicular lymph node, known as Virchow's node, may be the site of cancer metastatic from tumors in the lung, abdomen, or pelvis [3]. See Fig. 14.4.

1. Ferrer R. Lymphadenopathy: differential diagnosis and evaluation. Am Fam Physician. 1998;58:1313.
2. Oguz A, et al. Evaluation of peripheral lymphadenopathy in children. Pediatr Hematol Oncol. 2006;23:549.
3. Cervin JR, et al. Virchow's node revisited: analysis with clinicopathologic correlation of 152 fine-needle aspiration biopsies of supraclavicular lymph nodes. Arch Path Lab Med. 1995;119:727.

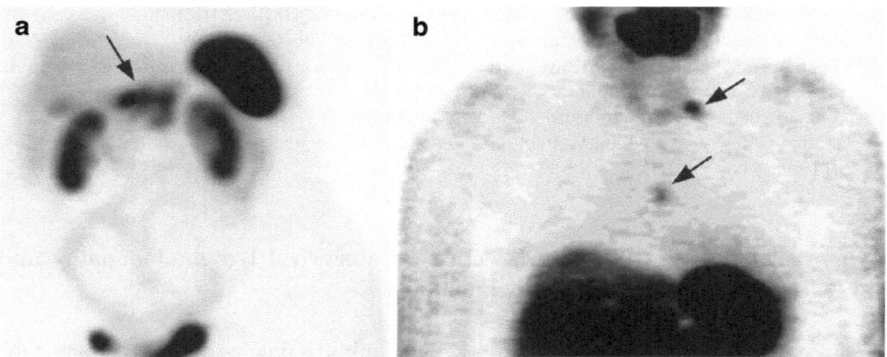

Fig. 14.4 A 76-year-old woman with duodenal carcinoid (*arrow*) detected accidentally at gastroscopy, carried out because of mild, nonspecific abdominal symptoms. (**a**) Virchow and mediastinal lymph node metastases (*arrows*) are detected (**b**)

Splenomegaly

In the patient with splenomegaly, think of hematologic disease, especially lymphoma, or chronic liver disease.

In two studies involving a total of 619 patients with splenomegaly, the top causes were hematologic and hepatic diseases, accounting for more than half of all patients. Other disorders causing enlargement of the spleen included infectious diseases, notably the acquired immunodeficiency syndrome (AIDS), heart failure, and splenic vein thrombosis [1, 2].

In some other areas of the world, the differential diagnosis of splenomegaly is different. A report from India of 100 patients with splenomegaly describes malaria as the most common cause, found in 22 (22 %) of patients [3].

1. O'Reilly RA. Splenomegaly in 2505 patients at a large university medical center from 1913 to 1995, 1963 to 1995: 449 patients. West J Med. 1988;169:88.
2. O'Reilly RA. Splenomegaly at a United States hospital: diagnostic evaluation of 170 patients. Am J Med Sci. 1996;312:160.
3. Sundaresan JB, et al. A hospital-based study of splenomegaly with special reference to the group of indeterminate origin. J Indian Med Assn. 2008;106:150.

"Massive splenomegaly always indicates underlying pathology" [1].

Described as a spleen weighing at least 500–1,000 g, massive splenomegaly results in a readily palpable organ. Luo et al. describe the chronic leukemias as the most common causes [1]. On the other hand, O'Reilly found myelofibrosis the disease most frequently encountered [2]. Other, less common, diseases to be considered with massive splenomegaly include lymphoma, thalassemia major, visceral leishmaniasis (kala-azar), Gaucher disease, and, of course, malaria [1]. See Fig. 14.5.

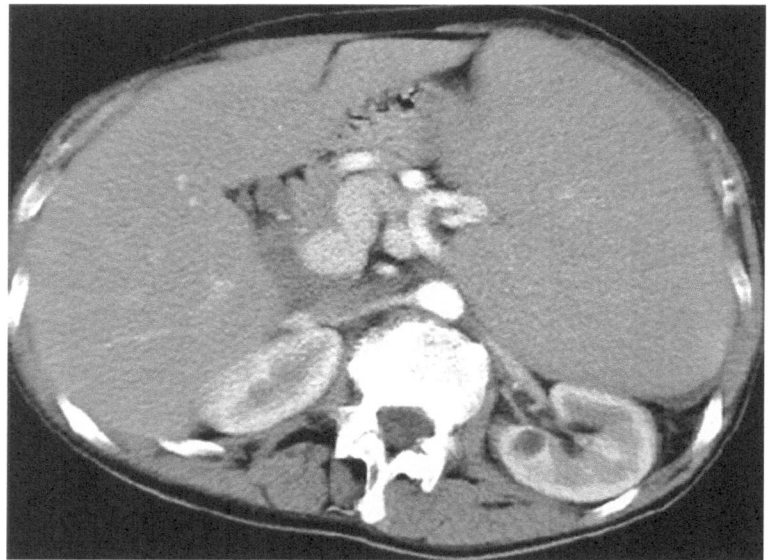

Fig. 14.5 A computerized tomography scan of the abdomen showing massive splenomegaly and enlarged lymph nodes in retroperitoneum

1. Luo EJ, et al. Massive splenomegaly. Hosp Physician. 2008;5:31.
2. O'Reilly RA. Splenomegaly at a United States hospital: diagnostic evaluation of 170 patients. Am J Med Sci. 1996;312:160.

Selected Problems Related to the Hematologic and Lymphatic Systems

Cyanosis unresponsive to oxygen therapy is the classical clinical picture of methemoglobinemia.

Methemoglobinemia, an example of cyanosis and dyspnea unrelated to heart or lung disease, can be caused by drugs such as nitrites, aniline dyes, metoclopramide (Reglan), and phenacetin, and also by inhalation of automobile exhaust fumes [1]. One report describes five patients with severe methemoglobinemia caused by the use of 20 % benzocaine spray [2]. In another article, the hemoglobin abnormality is traced to sniffing mephedrone [3].

1. Suyama H, et al. Methemoglobinemia induced by automobile exhaust fumes. J Anesth. 2005;19:333.
2. Ash-Bernal R, et al. Acquired methemoglobinemia: a retrospective series of 138 cases at 2 teaching hospitals. Medicine (Baltimore). 2004;83:265.
3. Ahmed N, et al. Methemoglobinemia due to mephedrone ("snow"). BMJ Case Reports. 2010; doi.10.1136/bcr.04.2010.2879.

The picture of episodes of severe crisis-like pain lasting several days is the defining feature of sickle cell disease.

The painful crisis commonly affects the abdomen, although almost any region of the body can be affected. These episodes are the sentinel symptom in one quarter of patients, are the most common symptoms after age 2 years, and are the leading cause of hospital admissions for SCD [1, 2]. The hemogram and reticulocyte count have not proved helpful in evaluating the acute pain crisis and not been demonstrated to affect clinical decision-making [3]. Kirkham points out that these blood tests have—inappropriately—been used to "prove" that a patient is a drug seeker, rather than in acute pain [4].

1. Bainbridge R, et al. Clinical presentation of homozygous sickle cell disease. J Pediatr. 1985;106:881.
2. Brozovic M, et al. Sickle cell disease in Britain. J Clin Pathol. 1984;37:1321.
3. Bernard AW, et al. Best evidence topic report: full blood count and reticulocyte count in painful sickle crisis. Emerg Med J. 2006;23:302.
4. Kirkham K. Adult sickle cell anemia. Primary Care Rep. 2011;17:121.

The finding of microcytic, hypochromic anemia with basophilic stippling of the red blood cells suggests the presence of lead poisoning.

Lead can be found in paint, food, water, and utensils used every day. In adults, most exposure occurs in the workplace [1]. Clinical manifestations of chronic lead poisoning include hyperactivity, cognitive impairment, anorexia, abdominal pain, and renal disease [1, 2].

1. Papanikolaou NC, et al. Lead toxicity update. Med Sci Monitor. 2005;11:RA329.
2. Janus J, et al. Evaluation of anemia in children. Am Fam Physician. 2010;81:1462.

Chapter 15
Infections and Infestations

"You and I may not live to see the day," Snow explained to the
young curate, *"and my name may be forgotten when it comes;
but the time will arrive when great outbreaks of cholera will be
things of the past; and it is the knowledge of the way in which
the disease is propagated which will cause them to disappear."*
English physician John Snow (1813–1858) [1]

Contents

R.B. Taylor, *Diagnostic Principles and Applications*,
DOI 10.1007/978-1-4614-1111-6_15, © Springer Science+Business Media, LLC 2013

John Snow is remembered for his meticulous study of the 1854 cholera epidemic in Soho, England, culminating in his dramatic removal of the pump handle from the community well that he had deduced to be the source of the disease. Although we no longer see major cholera outbreaks—at least in the developed world—communicable diseases of various types are still with us. As we consider the stories of the various infectious diseases, we should remind ourselves that many more lives have been saved by the introduction of proper hygienic measures, such as hand washing and the development of pure drinking water, than by all the antibiotics ever administered to humankind.

1. Snow J. Quoted in: Johnson S. The ghost map: the story of London's most terrifying epidemic—and how it changed science, cities, and the modern world. New York: Riverhead Books; 2006. p. 181.

Viral Infections

Pharyngitis/tonsillitis is part of the typical clinical spectrum of infectious mononucleosis (IM), which may lead to the inappropriate prescription of antibiotics.

Infectious mononucleosis, the most widely recognized type of Epstein–Barr virus (EBV) infection, is characterized by malaise, sore throat, headache, fever, and cervical lymphadenopathy [1]. Unwarranted use of antibiotics can be unfortunate because up to 80 % of patients with IM who receive ampicillin develop a maculopapular rash; a similar dermatitis also occurs in some IM patients given amoxicillin and other beta-lactam antibiotics [2]. See Fig. 15.1.

1. Luzuriaga K, et al. Infectious mononucleosis. N Engl J Med. 2010;362:1993.
2. Jenson HB. Epstein-Barr virus. Pediatr Rev. 2011;32:375.

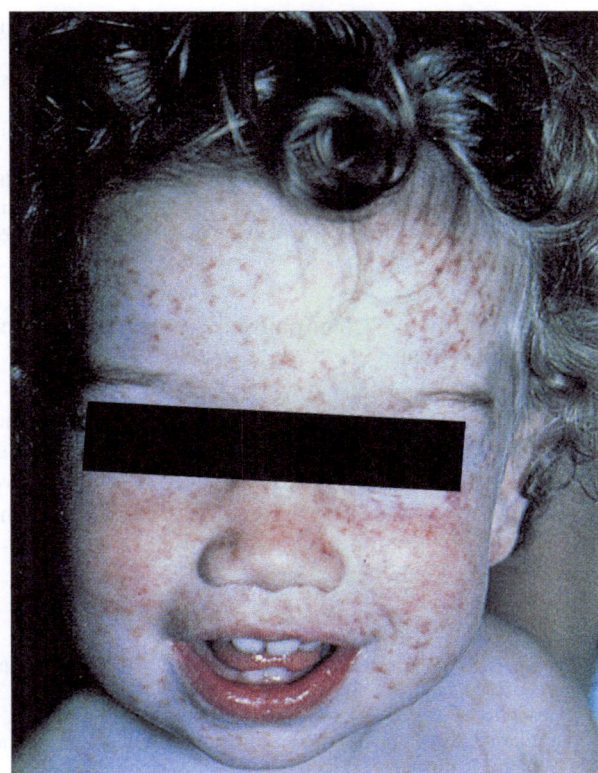

Fig. 15.1 Ampicillin rash in Epstein–Barr virus (EBV) infection. Patients with EBV infection often respond to an ampicillin challenge with a diffuse, nonpruritic, maculopapular rash, which may superficially resemble measles

In addition to its usual more-or-less benign manifestations, IM can have some serious sequelae.

Here are some of the risks that attend a diagnosis of IM:

Chronic fatigue syndrome (CFS): In a study of 301 adolescents with IM, 13 % met criteria for a diagnosis of CFS 6 months later, and 7 % carried the CFS diagnosis at 1 year [1].

Splenic infarction or rupture: Both have been reported [2, 3], and all patients with suspected IM should have a careful abdominal examination to check for splenic enlargement.

Multiple sclerosis: A study of 104 patients with multiple sclerosis occurring following IM led the investigators to conclude, "The risk of multiple sclerosis was persistently increased for more than 30 years after infectious mononucleosis and uniformly distributed across all investigated strata of sex and age" [4].

Systemic lupus erythematosus (SLE): Exposure to EBV has been linked to mild SLE [5].

1. Katz BZ. Chronic fatigue syndrome after infectious mononucleosis in adolescents. Pediatrics. 2009;124:189.
2. van Hal S, et al. Splenic infarction due to transient antiphospholipid antibodies induced by Epstein-Barr virus infection. J Clin Virol. 2005;32:245.
3. Aldrete JS. Spontaneous rupture of the spleen in patients with infectious mononucleosis. Mayo Clin Proc. 1992;67:910.
4. Nielsen TR, et al. Multiple sclerosis after infectious mononucleosis. Arch Neurol. 2007;64:72.
5. Zandman-Goddard G, et al. Exposure to Epstein-Barr virus infection is associated with mild systemic lupus erythematosus disease. Ann NY Acad Sci. 2009;1173:658.

Think of norovirus when pain is a prominent accompaniment of acute vomiting and diarrhea.

Feared as the scourge of cruise ships and restaurants, norovirus causes up to 90 % of nonbacterial epidemic acute foodborne illness. In a study of one norovirus outbreak with 40 cases in which 32 subjects were interviewed, the key symptoms were abdominal pain, 90.6 %; vomiting, 71.9 %; and diarrhea, 71.9 % [1]. In another study of a gastroenteritis outbreak caused by norovirus involving 709 individuals, 78.6 % reported abdominal pain [2].

1. Sala MR, et al. An outbreak of food poisoning due to a genogroup I norovirus. Epidemiol Infect. 2004;133:187.
2. Papadoupoulos VP, et al. A gastroenteritis outbreak due to norovirus infection in Xanthi, Northern Greece: management and public health consequences. J Gastrointest Liver Dis. 2006;15:27.

The most common neurologic sequela of a varicella infection is acute cerebellar ataxia (ACA).

Occurring in about one in 4,000 cases of varicella, ACA causes impaired gait, slurred speech, and, sometimes, nystagmus. These manifestations generally last days to weeks before subsiding [1]. My initial encounter with this varicella complication came in my first year in private practice, when a 10-year-old boy was brought to my office with waning chicken pox lesions and a rather sudden inability to stand or walk. The findings terrified the parents (and also me, the young physician who had not learned in medical school of this uncommon complication of what was then a common disease). A telephone consultation with a senior pediatrician was reassuring to us all.

1. Salas AA, et al. Acute cerebellar ataxia in childhood: initial approach in the emergency department. Emerg Med J. 2010;27:956.

Flu-like manifestations in a biphasic pattern with the second phase including headache, nuchal rigidity, and myalgia may represent poliomyelitis in the unvaccinated person, such as an immigrant from a developing country.

The description above characterizes nonparalytic poliomyelitis. Less than 1 % of infected persons will develop paralysis, as the virus invades the anterior horns of the spinal cord [1]. A classic finding in paralytic polio is the *tripod sign*: As the patient sits in bed, the head tends to fall backward and the body, with weakened muscles of the back, must be supported with the arms spread out behind [2].

1. Solomon T, et al. Infectious causes of acute flaccid paralysis. Curr Opin Infect Dis. 2003;16:375.
2. Anderson T. Is it polio? BMJ. 1955;2:485.

Measles can be followed by subacute sclerosing panencephalitis (SSP), as the measles virus is reactivated 1–35 years following the original disease.

Symptoms of SSP include aberrant behavior, visual disturbances, myoclonus, and ataxia. Most patients with this disorder have a poor prognosis [1]. It seems to me, as a veteran clinician, that the differential diagnosis of these findings, occurring perhaps years after having measles, would be perplexing; presented with these manifestations today, a pertinent question will be: Had the patient received the measles vaccine or not?

1. Sever JL. Persistent measles infection of the central nervous system: subacute sclerosing panencephalitis. Rev Infect Dis. 1983;5:467.

Bacterial Infections

Some specific clinical signs can help differentiate between group A beta-hemolytic strep (GABHS) infection and viral pharyngitis.

Sore throat with cervical adenopathy, tonsillar exudate, and temperature above 100.4 °F suggest GABHS infection, while coryza and cough are more likely to be seen with a viral infection [1]. The frequency with which clinicians see patients complaining of sore throat and the specter of complications such as rheumatic fever make identification of GABHS infection important. For the record, 1.3 % of visits to healthcare providers are for sore throat, accounting for some 15 million visits annually in the USA [2].

Some useful statistics in the diagnosis of GABHS pharyngitis are as follows [3]:

Anterior cervical adenopathy: Swollen or enlarged anterior cervical nodes have a 55–82 % sensitivity and a 34–73 % specificity.

Absence of cough: In the diagnosis of GABHS pharyngitis, absence of cough has a 51–79 % sensitivity and a 36–68 % specificity.

Palatine petechiae: Petechiae located on the palate have only a 7 % sensitivity but an 88 % specificity for GABHS.

1. Choby BA. Diagnosis and treatment of streptococcal pharyngitis. Am Fam Physician. 2009;79:383.
2. Wessels MF. Streptococcal pharyngitis. N Engl J Med. 2011;364:648.
3. Regoli M, et al. Update on the management of acute pharyngitis in children. Ital J Pediatr. 2011;37:10.

In the evaluation of the complaint of sore throat, what the patient tells us can bias what we perceive on physical examination.

In a study involving 32 physicians on two separate visits, Kiderman et al. presented each physician with healthy simulated patients who recited one of two scripts suggesting either a bacterial or viral infection. No actor had pharyngitis or cervical adenopathy; the presence of normal throats was documented photographically before each visit. The investigators found, "Physicians generally perceived some abnormal finding, and more often so with the 'bacterial' script." Most physicians reported abnormal physical findings in healthy simulated patients, findings suggesting the diagnosis of GABHS infection and justifying antibiotic therapy [1].

1. Kiderman A, et al. Bias in the evaluation of pharyngitis and antibiotic overuse. Arch Intern Med. 2009;169:524.

When a community-acquired *Staphylococcus aureus* infection is encountered, there are some epidemiologic risk factors that might be clues to methicillin-resistant *S. aureus* (MRSA) infection versus methicillin-susceptible *S. aureus* (MSSA) infection.

In a study of 108 patients with MRSA infection and 78 with MSSA infection, MRSA infection was more likely in patients of younger age ($p < 0.0001$); snorting/smoking illegal drugs ($p = 0.1$); skin or soft tissue infection ($p = 0.015$); recent incarceration ($p = 0.03$); and more recent visits to bars, raves, or clubs ($p = 0.3$). The investigators go on to point out, however, that clinical and epidemiologic factors such as those listed above cannot reliably distinguish between methicillin-sensitive and methicillin–resistant infection [1]. See Fig. 15.2.

1. Miller LG, et al. Clinical and epidemiologic characteristics cannot distinguish community-associated methicillin-resistant Staphylococcus aureus infection from methicillin-susceptible S. aureus infection: a prospective investigation. Clin Infect Dis. 2007;44:471.

In children, the cause of most abscesses is community-acquired (CA) MRSA infection.

The above is the conclusion of Hasty et al., following review of the records of 920 children presenting to two geographically distant pediatric emergency departments in the USA with skin and soft tissue infections. Of these children, bacterial cultures were obtained in 270 instances, with MRSA found in 60 (22 %). The findings were different when the skin/soft tissue infection was an actual abscess, and 53 % of these lesions were found on culture to be caused by MRSA [1].

1. Hasty MB, et al. Cutaneous community-associated methicillin-resistant Staphylococcus aureus among all skin and soft-tissue infections in two geographically distant pediatric emergency departments. Acad Emerg Med. 2007;14:35.

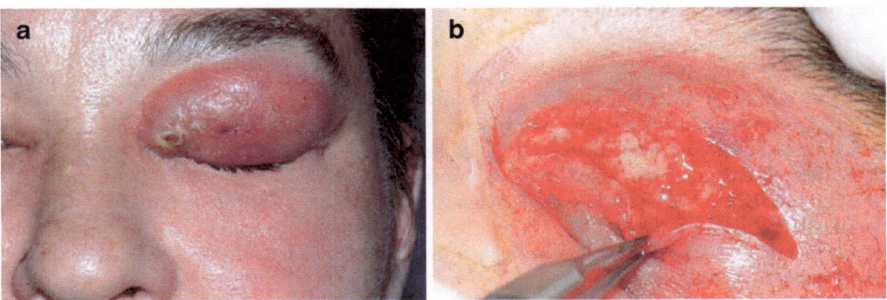

Fig. 15.2 Patient who had been plucking her brows and lashes developed severe onset of cellulitis. On opening the lid for drainage, there was diffuse infection of the soft tissue with multiple microabscesses consistent with MRSA: before surgery (**a**) and upon opening the lid for drainage (**b**)

In addition to the classic clues to the diagnosis of meningitis—high fever, rash, headache, confusion, and neck stiffness—be suspicious of the febrile child who has leg pain and/or cold hands and feet.

In fact, the classic manifestations of meningococcal disease may occur late, and most children have only nonspecific symptoms in the early hours [1]. For this reason, early clues suggesting sepsis may be helpful in recognition of meningitis. In a study of 345 children with meningococcal disease compared with 924 children with acute self-limited infection, cold hands and feet were found in 40.3 % of those with meningococcal disease compared with 18.2 % of those with minor febrile infections. Leg pain was reported by 37.6 % of children with meningococcal disease but by only 5.7 % of those with minor febrile infection [2].

1. Thompson MJ, et al. Clinical recognition of meningococcal disease in children and adolescents. Lancet. 2006;367:397.
2. Haj-Hassan TA, et al. Which early "red flag" symptoms identify children with meningococcal disease in primary care? Br J Gen Pract. 2011;61:e97.

Most cases of gas gangrene are related to penetrating injury, but the disease can be related to a diverse group of other causes.

Clostridial myonecrosis, aka gas gangrene, characteristically follows penetrating trauma that creates an anaerobic environment. This is the scenario in approximately 70 % of cases, with *Clostridium perfringens* the culprit in most of these [1]. See Fig. 15.3. Other, less common, causes of clostridial myonecrosis include obstetrical complications such as intrauterine fetal demise, prolonged rupture of the membranes, retained placenta, and induced abortion. The disease should be suspected in infections in persons who inject heroin [2].

The first evidence of gas gangrene is typically severe pain at the site of injury (or surgery). Misdiagnosis can occur, and one report described patients with gas gangrene with initial diagnoses of compartment syndrome and appendicitis [3]. One case has been reported of simultaneous involvement of both lower extremities arising in the absence of trauma or surgery [4].

1. Awad MM, et al. Virulence studies on chromosomal alpha-toxin and theta-toxin mutants constructed by allelic exchange provide genetic evidence for the essential role of alpha-toxin in Clostridium perfringens-mediated gas gangrene. Mol Microbiol. 1955;15:191.
2. Christie B. Gangrene bug killed 35 heroin users. West J Med. 2000;173:82.
3. Schropfer E, et al. Diagnosis and misdiagnosis of necrotizing soft tissue infections. Cases J. 2008;1:252.
4. Lu J, et al. Gas gangrene without wound: both lower extremities affected simultaneously. Am J Emerg Med. 2008;26:970.

Fig. 15.3 X-ray reveals soft-tissue gas (*arrows*) consistent with gangrene. This patient also had osteomyelitis, but the soft-tissue gas is much more prominent

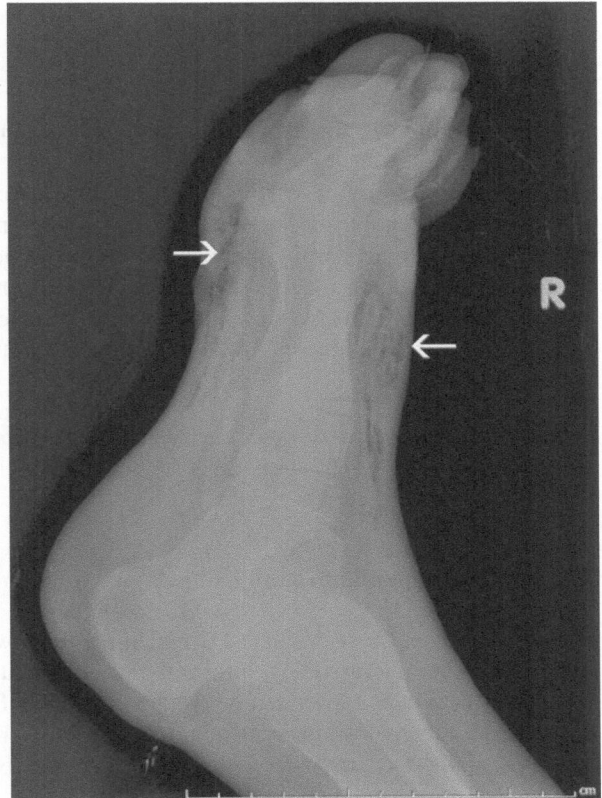

Although watery diarrhea is the classic manifestation of *Clostridium difficile* infection, most infected persons do not have symptoms or signs of disease.

In one series, 83 (21 %) of 399 patients who entered the hospital with negative cultures acquired *C. difficile* during their stay, although 52 of these persons had no symptoms, 31 reported diarrhea, and none had the textbook picture of colitis [1]. Suspect the infection when unexplained leukocytosis is found.

In the long-term care setting, approximately half of all patients may carry *C. difficile* [2]. In both settings, asymptomatic carriers represent a source for potential spread of disease. The increasingly widespread use of acid-suppressive therapy may contribute to the high levels of *C. difficile* presence reported, and patients using these drugs may be considered to be at higher risk [3].

1. McFarland LV, et al. Nosocomial acquisition of Clostridium difficile infection. N Engl J Med. 1989;320:204.
2. Riggs MM, et al. Asymptomatic carriers are a potential source for transmission of epidemic and non-epidemic Clostridium difficile strains among long-term care facility residents. Clin Infect Dis. 2007;45:992.

3. Howell MD, et al. Iatrogenic gastric acid suppression and the risk of nosocomial Clostridium difficile infection. Arch Intern Med. 2010;170:784.

Consider pertussis in the differential diagnosis of chronic cough.

Classic manifestations of whooping cough are: paroxysmal cough, inspiratory whoop, and post-tussive emesis. The latter two symptoms are especially helpful in diagnosis, but chronic, paroxysmal cough is less specific for the disease [1]. When the chief manifestation of disease is chronic cough, other diagnoses to consider include laryngotracheitis (croup), bacterial tracheitis, reactive airway disease, cardiogenic cough, cystic fibrosis, and foreign body aspiration [2].

1. Cornia PB, et al. Does this coughing adolescent or adult have pertussis? JAMA. 2010;204:890.
2. Teng MS, et al. Whooping cough: management and diagnosis of pertussis. Prim Care Rep. 2011;17:40.

The most common manifestation of primary tuberculosis (TB) is fever.

Even in the twenty-first century, TB remains a worldwide problem, with human immunodeficiency virus (HIV) infection and poverty as key factors in its persistence [1]. Unexplained fever can be an important clue. Present in 70 % of subjects with primary tuberculosis described in one study, the temperature elevation is typically low grade. Occurring less commonly, in about one quarter of primary TB patients, are chest pain, including pleuritic chest pain, cough, fatigue, and joint pain [2]. Occasionally, an early manifestation of primary TB will be erythema nodosum, described in Chap. 12 [3].

1. Campbell IA, et al. Pulmonary tuberculosis: diagnosis and treatment. BMJ. 2006;332:1194.
2. Poulsen A. Some clinical features of tuberculosis. Acta Tuberculosis Scand. 1951;33:37.
3. Mert A, et al. Primary tuberculosis cases presenting with erythema nodosum. J Dermatol. 2004;31:66.

The chief manifestations of reactivation TB are weight loss, fatigue, and cough.

Night sweats have long been described as a key tip-off to the presence of pulmonary tuberculosis. They occur, with or without fever, in about half of patients with reactivation TB [1, 2].

1. MacGregor RR. A year's experience with tuberculosis in a private urban teaching hospital in the post-sanitarium era. Am J Med. 1975;58:221.
2. Arango L, et al. The spectrum of tuberculosis as currently seen in a metropolitan hospital. Am Rev Respir Dis. 1973;108:805.

Sexually Transmitted Diseases

Syphilis should be considered in the differential diagnosis of puzzling cutaneous, ocular, and neurologic findings.

A sexually transmitted disease (STD) that has a colorful history and that has afflicted humankind for centuries, syphilis is making a comeback after previous decades of some success in prevention and management. The "sexual revolution" and the rise of HIV infections have played key roles, and today's newly minted clinicians lack the familiarity of their older colleagues with the protean manifestations of syphilis.

The stage most likely to be encountered in the office is secondary syphilis, which can cause a polymorphic skin eruption, mucous membrane lesions (that are highly infectious), ocular manifestations, and systemic findings [1]. Skin lesions can take various forms, and one report describes a papulo-erythemato-squamous eruption that could be misdiagnosed as psoriasis [2].

Ocular manifestations of secondary syphilis include retinitis, chorioretinitis, uveitis, episcleritis, and optic neuritis [3, 4].

In one study of 80 cases of secondary syphilis, 21 (26.3 %) were associated with neurologic symptoms. Of these patients, 50 were HIV positive [5]. Clinicians must keep in mind that patients co-infected with syphilis and HIV can have atypical clinical findings [6].

1. Ramoni S, et al. An atlas of syphilis in a single case. Arch Dermatol. 2011;147:869.
2. Lanjouw E, et al. Unusual late nodular presentation of secondary syphilis. Int J STD AIDS. 2009;20:271.
3. Peuch C, et al. Ocular manifestations of syphilis: recent cases over a 2.5 year period. Graesfes Arch Clin Exp Ophthal. 2010;248:1623.
4. Muldoon EG, et al. Syphilis consequences and the implications in delayed diagnosis: five cases of secondary syphilis presenting with ocular symptoms. Sex Transm Infect. 2010;86:512.
5. Dumortier C, et al. Non-cutaneous manifestations of secondary syphilis. Ann Dermatol Venereal. 2008;135:451.
6. Lautenschlager S. Cutaneous manifestations of syphilis: recognition and management. Am J Clin Dermatol. 2006;7:291.

Every seventh patient with syphilis may have contracted the disease through oral sex, an activity that the patient may neglect to report to the clinician.

A Centers for Disease Control and Prevention (CDC) report describing 1,582 cases of primary and secondary syphilis in Chicago offers some interesting facts and conclusions [1]. In the most recent data described, men who have sex with men (MSM) accounted for 60 % of cases described. Many of these MSM engaged in only oral sex and were astonished to learn that they could contract syphilis in this manner. Overall, 13.7 % of patients with primary or secondary syphilis described in the report contracted their disease through oral sex [1].

1. Centers for Disease Control and Prevention. Transmission of primary and secondary syphilis by oral sex –Chicago, Illinois, 1998–2002. MMWR Morb Mortal. Wkly Rep. 2004;53:966.

Oral gonorrhea, described as "rare" in some studies, may be missed because of a failure to look and test.

In my search of the literature, I came across two studies describing oral gonorrhea as *rare* [1, 2]. When it occurs, the pharynx may have varying degrees of painful erythema or perhaps ulceration with a pseudomembranous coating. Or there may be no pharyngeal symptoms at all [1, 2]. In a study of gonorrhea in women involving 525 adolescents (age 14–21) and adults (age >21), investigators found a pharyngeal gonorrhea prevalence of 2.5–6.8 % in women tested in the various study sites. They conclude, "Culturing only the cervix missed 20–40 % of adult STD, 14–26 % of adolescent STD, and 11 % of adolescent hospital infected cases" [3].

1. Bruce AJ, et al. Oral manifestations of sexually transmitted diseases. Clin Dermatol. 2004; 22:520.
2. Little JW. Gonorrhea: update. Oral Surg Oral Med Oral Pathol Oral Radiol Endod. 2006; 101:137.
3. Giannini CM, et al. Culture of non-genital sites increases the detection of gonorrhea in women. J Pediatr Adol Gynecol. 2010;23:246.

Be suspicious of HIV infection in men who have sex with men (MSM) with a history of childhood sexual abuse (CSA).

Although HIV infection is not strictly an STD and can be acquired perinatally or via contaminated blood, I deal with it in this section because, after all, sexual congress is the classical mode of transmission. In a study of 4,295 men who have sex with men, 39.7 % had a history of childhood sexual abuse, and those with a history of CSA were found to be at increased risk for HIV infection (adjusted HR 1.30, 95 % CI 1.02–1.69) [1].

1. Mimiaga J, et al. Childhood sexual abuse is highly associated with HIV risk-taking behavior and infection among MSM in the EXPLORE Study. J Acq Imm Def Syndr. 2009;51:340.

Oral candidiasis can be an early clue to the presence of HIV disease.

The most common of the opportunistic infections found in HIV patients, oral candidiasis occurs in up to half of all persons with HIV infection during the course of their disease. Manifestations range from angular cheilitis to the pseudomembranous candidiasis found in patients with more advanced disease [1]. See Fig. 15.4.

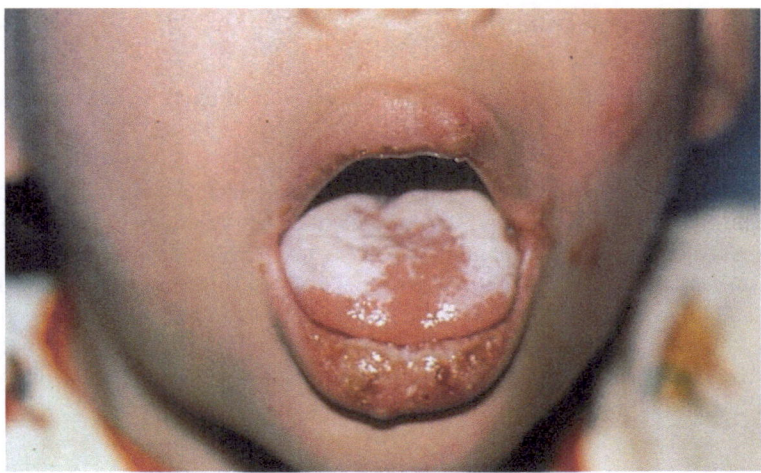

Fig. 15.4 Oral candidiasis in an HIV-infected patient

1. Nokta M. Oral manifestations associated with HIV infection. Current HIV/AIDS Reports. 2008;5:5.

Be alert for the development of dementia in the patient with HIV infection.

With the advent of highly active antiretroviral therapy (HAART), the incidence of dementia in HIV-infected patients has dropped. But, and this is a big consideration, the number of patients with HIV dementia has actually risen owing to two factors: the increased numbers of HIV-infected patients and the longer life expectancy afforded by the newer drugs [1].

1. Anthony IC, et al. The neuropathology of HIV/AIDS. Int Rev Psychiat. 2008;20:15.

Arthropod-Borne Infections

Erythema migrans (EM), the signature skin lesion of early Lyme disease, may not present in a *bull's-eye* pattern.

Lyme disease, the most common tick-borne disease in the United States, begins with a flu-like syndrome and, in 80 % of patients, an erythematous skin lesion that develops a clear center. The diagnostic pearl is this: EM begins as a homogeneous eruption, and the bull's-eye pattern with central clearing develops as the lesion enlarges. In one series of 118 cases, the EM first observed had a homogeneous pattern in 59 % of instances, central erythema in 32 %, and central clearing in only 9 % [1]. In a series of 165 cases of Lyme disease reported in Maryland, 13 % of patients lacked EM at the time of presentation [2].

1. Smith RP, et al. Clinical characteristics and treatment outcome of early Lyme disease in patients with microbiologically confirmed erythema migrans. Ann Intern Med. 2002;136:421.
2. Aucott J, et al. Diagnostic challenges of early Lyme disease: Lessons from a community case series. BMC Infect Dis. 2009;9:79.

Disseminated Lyme disease can cause a variety of neurologic manifestations, which can occasionally be the initial sign of infection.

Neurologic features of Lyme disease may include: peripheral neuropathy, cranial nerve palsies, lymphocytic meningitis, and radiculopathy. The facial or abducens nerves may be involved [1–3]. See Fig. 15.5.

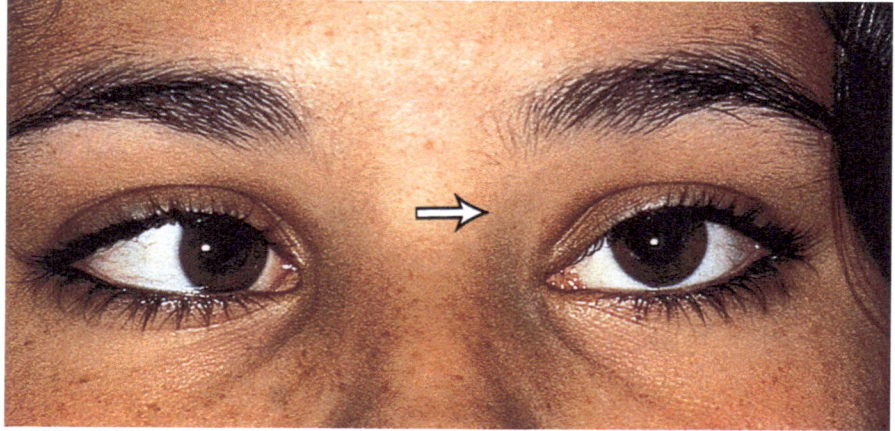

Fig. 15.5 Abducens palsy occasionally seen with Lyme disease

1 McKay G, et al. Lyme disease: an unusual case of peripheral nerve palsy. J Bone Joint Surg Br. 2010;92:713.
2. Zajkowska JM, et al. Peripheral neuropathies in Lyme borreliosis. Pol Merkur Lekaarski. 2010;29:115.
3. Sauer A, et al. Five cases of paralytic strabismus as a rare feature of Lyme disease. Clin Infect Dis. 2009;48:756.

Headache is generally the earliest manifestation of Rocky Mountain spotted fever (RMSF) and is also the symptom most likely to be described.

More than 80 % of patients with RMSF report headache [1]. Cephalgia, fever, and rash make up the classic troika of RMSF, although Jaffe et al. report that this full combination of manifestations is absent in most patients who develop RMSF [2]. Malaise and myalgia occur commonly. The especially helpful finding is detection of a maculopapular eruption that begins peripherally, spreads proximally, and evolves to exhibit petechiae. Lacz describes, "The cutaneous centripetal pattern is a result of cell to cell migration by the causative organism Rickettsia rickettsii" [3].

1. Glaser C, et al. Rickettsial and Ehrlichial infections. Handb Clin Neurol. 2010;96C:143.
2. Jaffe J, et al. Rocky Mountain spotted fever. In: Current diagnosis and treatment: emergency medicine. New York: McGraw Hill; 2011, chapter 42.
3. Lacz NL, et al. Rocky Mountain spotted fever. J Eur Acad Dermatol Venereol. 2006;20:411.

Although most patients with West Nile virus infection are asymptomatic or exhibit nonspecific flu-like symptoms, a few will experience neuroinvasive disease.

So named because the organism was first isolated in 1937 from the blood of a patient in the West Nile province of Uganda, the West Nile virus causes no symptoms in most infected persons. When present, the manifestations mimic viral influenza: fever, fatigue, and headache. The presence of muscle weakness or difficulty concentrating may be a slightly helpful clue that one is dealing with something more than simple flu. When neuropathology is seen, the picture may be one of meningitis, encephalitis, or flaccid paralysis [1, 2].

1. Kramer LD, et al. West Nile virus. Lancet. 2007;6:171.
2. Sejvar JJ, et al. Neurologic manifestations and outcome of West Nile virus infection. JAMA. 2012;307:223.

Cat-scratch disease can be an arthropod-borne disease.

A common disease, especially of children, cat-scratch disease does not necessarily arise from an animal scratch or bite. The organism, *Bartonella henselae*, can also be

Fig.15.6 Cat-scratch disease with postauricular adenopathy and purulent drainage

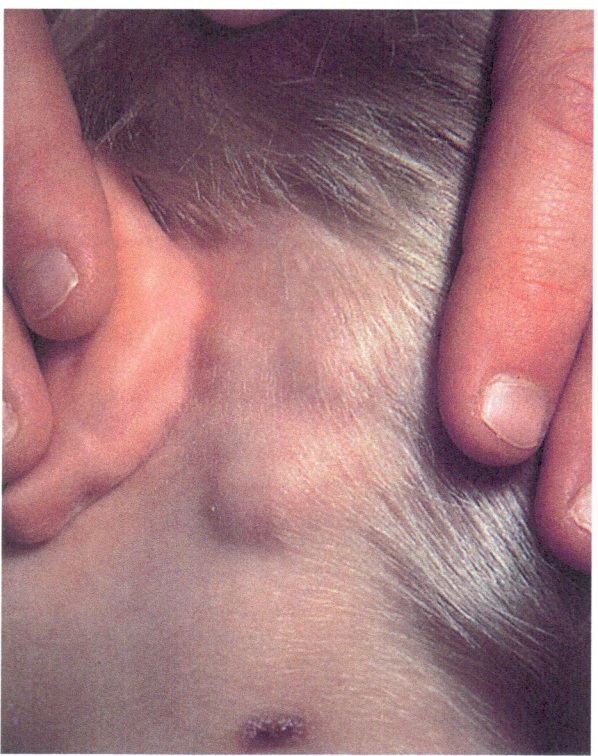

transmitted by fleas or ticks [1]. Consider that fleas feed on animals but *reside* independently, typically where the animals sleep. Thus one could enter a home where there are animals, but the animals are gone, perhaps boarded during a vacation, and the visitor could be bitten by the very hungry fleas left behind.

In recognizing the presence of cat-scratch disease, look for the most common manifestation—regional lymphadenopathy [2]. See Fig. 15.6.

1. Mosbacher M, et al. Cat scratch disease and arthropod vectors: more to it than a scratch? J Am Board Fam Med. 2010;23:685.
2. English R. Cat scratch disease. Pediatr Rev. 2006;27:123.

Travel-Related Infections and Infestations

The returned international traveler who develops fever may have a serious illness.

Wilson et al. describe 24,920 returned travelers evaluated at a GeoSentinel clinic, one of a network of facilities specializing in travel-related or tropical medicine, over a 9-year period. Of those with fever, 35 % had a systemic febrile illness, 15 % had a diarrheal disease, and 14 % had a disease of the respiratory tract. The authors report, "More than 17 % of travelers with fever had a vaccine-preventable infection or falciparum malaria, which is preventable with chemoprophylaxis" [1].

1. Wilson ME, et al. Fever in returned travelers; results from the GeoSentinel Surveillance Network. Clin Infect Dis. 2007;44:1560.

Among returned ill travelers with fever, malaria must be high on the differential diagnosis list.

Here are some pertinent facts about malaria in travelers, a *must-not-miss diagnosis*:

A common cause of fever: Malaria is one of the most common causes of systemic febrile illnesses in travelers from every region, according to a study of 17,353 ill returned travelers [1].

The risk of chemoprophylaxis avoidance: The risk of malaria associated with staying in an endemic region of sub-Saharan Africa for 1 month without taking chemoprophylaxis is 1:5 [2].

Poor adherence with chemoprophylaxis: In a report of 57 US travelers who returned with confirmed malaria, only 13 (23 %) had adhered to a recommended prophylactic regimen [3].

Efficacy of chemoprophylaxis: In the same study of 57 US returned travelers with malaria, 12 developed *Plasmodium vivax* or *Plasmodium ovale* infection in spite of taking appropriate chemoprophylaxis, but none who followed the recommended mefloquine regimen contracted falciparum malaria [3].

Suggestive findings: Think of malaria in the febrile returned traveler who is found to have an enlarged spleen, thrombocytopenia, and hyperbilirubinemia [4].

1. Freedman DO, et al. Spectrum of disease and relation of place to exposure among ill returned travelers. N Engl J Med. 2006;354:119.
2. Kain KC, et al. Malaria in travelers: epidemiology, disease, and prevention. Infect Dis North Am. 1998;12:267.
3. Dorsey G, et al. Difficulties in the prevention, diagnosis and treatment of imported malaria. Arch Intern Med. 2000;160:2505.
4. Bottieau E, et al. Fever after a stay in the tropics: diagnostic predictors of the leading tropical conditions. Medicine. 2007;86:18.

The febrile traveler returning from the tropics with headache and extremely painful myalgia may have dengue fever.

Sometimes called *breakbone fever* because of the severe myalgia, dengue is found in both Southeast Asia and Latin America. It is carried by the day-stinging *Aedes* mosquito and has an incubation period of 3–8 days, often just enough time to fly home from the vacation in the tropics. There may be low platelet and leukocyte counts and elevated serum transaminase levels [1, 2].

1. Choudhary IA, et al. Update on fever in the returning traveler. Patient Care. 2006;6:14.
2. Allwin R. Significant increase in travel-associated dengue fever in Germany. Med Microbiol Immun. 2011;200:155.

In returning international travelers with continuing diarrhea, consider the strong possibility of parasitic disease.

In a study of patients at 30 GeoSentinel sites on six continents, travelers from all regions except Southeast Asia who described diarrhea were more likely to have parasite-induced diarrhea than bacterial diarrhea [1].

1. Freedman DO, et al. Spectrum of disease and relation of place to exposure among ill returned travelers. N Engl J Med. 2006;354:119.

The clue to the recognition of a bedbug bite is finding itchy lesions in clusters or a linear pattern.

There may be maculopapular lesions, wheals, or hemorrhagic blisters. The bites of these flat, brown hematophagous insects can, at times, cause urticaria and even anaphylaxis [1, 2]. One author has reported a case of severe anemia, with a hemoglobin level of 8 g/dL in a 60-year-old man who suffered multiple bedbug bites [3].

You might tell your frequently traveling patients that there is a commercial web site—bedbugregistry.com—that can provide readers reports of bedbug findings in many hotels, sometimes even with identification of specific rooms with infestations reported by travelers.

1. Davis RF, et al. Recognition and management of common ectoparasitic diseases in travelers. Am J Clin Dermatol. 2009;10:1.
2. Delauray P, et al. Bedbugs and infectious diseases. Clin Infect Dis. 2011;52:200.
3. Hwang SW. Severe anemia from bedbugs. CMAJ. 2009;181:287.

Selected Problems Related to Infectious Diseases

There are red flags that every clinician should know suggesting serious infection in children.

Van den Bruel et al. analyzed 30 studies, concluding that there are four findings that suggest serious infections in a child: petechial rash (LR 6.18–83.70); cyanosis (LR 2.66–52.20); poor peripheral perfusion (LR 2.39–38.80); and rapid breathing (LR 1.26–9.78). The authors also cited the risk of severe infection being present in the face of parental concern (LR 14.40, 95 % CI 9.30–22.10) and clinician instinct (LR 23.50, 95 % CI 16.80–32.70) [1].

1. Van den Bruel A, et al. Diagnostic value of clinical features at presentation to identify serious infection in children in developed countries: a systematic review. Lancet. 2010;375:834.

Anemia and evidence of renal impairment following 5–10 days of diarrhea is the classic picture of hemolytic–uremic syndrome (HUS).

Hemolytic–uremic syndrome follows infection with enterohemorrhagic *E. coli* bacteria. In one epidemic, 9 % of 501 cases of *E. coli* 0157:H7-associated diarrhea were followed by HUS [1]. Bloody diarrhea is an important clue, noted in approximately half of patients with HUS. The full picture of HUS includes: hemolytic anemia with erythrocyte fragmentation, thrombocytopenia, and evidence of acute renal damage [1, 2].

1. Bell BP, et al. A multistate outbreak of Escherichia coli O157:H7-associated bloody diarrhea and hemolytic uremic syndrome from hamburgers. The Washington experience. JAMA. 1994;272:1349.
2. Gerber A, et al. Clinical course and the role of shiga toxin-producing Escherichia coli infection in the hemolytic-uremic syndrome in pediatric patients, 1997–2000, in Germany and Austria: a prospective study. J Infect Dis. 2002;186:493.

Recurrent infections associated with high serum levels of IgE describes Job syndrome, a rare disorder of infancy and childhood.

Job syndrome is also known as the hyperimmunoglobulin E syndrome. The infections, typically involving the skin and respiratory tract, are characteristically caused by *Staphylococcus aureus* and *Haemophilus influenzae*. Coarse facial features are part of the syndrome. See Fig. 15.7. The disease, which has both autosomal dominant and recessive variants, is named for Job, described in the Bible as being smitten with boils by Satan [1, 2].

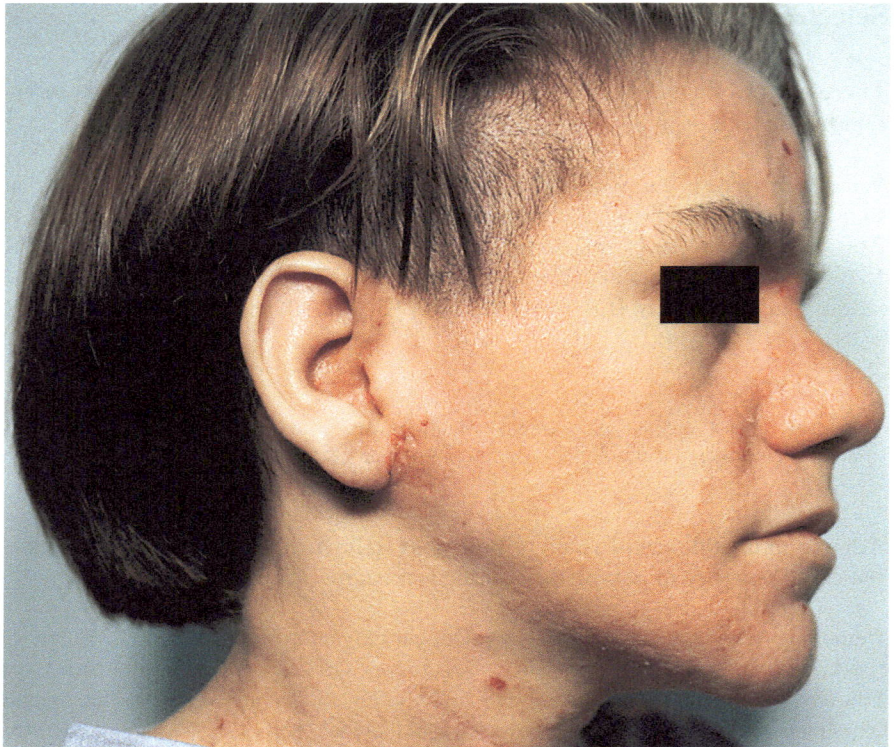

Fig.15.7 *Staphylococcus aureus* pyoderma in a child with hyper-IgE syndrome (Job syndrome). Note the coarse facial features that tend to become more prominent with age

1. Donabedian H. The hyperimmunoglobulin E recurrent infection (Job's) syndrome: a review of the NIH experience and the literature. Medicine. 1983;62:195.
2. Brandao M, et al. Hyper-IgE syndrome: report of three cases and review of the literature. J Med Cases. 2011;2:213.

A cutaneous infection that follows tattooing may be caused by mycobacteria.

In my research, I came across several reports of mycobacteria of various species that followed tattooing, including the inoculation of tubercle bacilli [1–3].

1. Kluger N, et al. Atypical mycobacteria infection following tattooing: review of an outbreak in eight patients in a French tattoo parlor. Arch Dermatol. 2008;144:941.
2. Drage LA, et al. An outbreak of Mycobacterium chelonae infections in tattoos. J Am Acad Dermatol. 2009;62:501.
3. Wong HW, et al. Papular eruption on a tattoo: a case of primary inoculation tuberculosis. Australasian J Dermatol. 2005;46:87.

Chapter 16
Mental Health Problems

The separation of psychology from the premises of biology is purely artificial, because the human psyche lives in indissoluble union with the body.

Swiss psychiatrist Carl Jung (1875–1961) [1]

Contents

R.B. Taylor, *Diagnostic Principles and Applications*,
DOI 10.1007/978-1-4614-1111-6_16, © Springer Science+Business Media, LLC 2013

Mental health problems are distressingly prevalent in the general population. Primary care clinicians have learned the full impact of this fact as US federal and state agencies have cut funding for mental health services, sending patients with both complex and severe psychiatric problems to seek care in generalist practices. Just to give you an idea of the prevalence of DSM-IV mental disorders in the general population, a study of 9,282 adult individuals revealed a 12-month prevalence of the following disorders: anxiety, 18.1 %; mood, 9.5 %; impulse control, 8.9 %; substance abuse, 3.8 %; and any mental health disorder, 26.2 %. Of the cases described, 22.3 % were considered serious; and 23 % of patients had three or more DSM-IV diagnoses [2].

1. Jung CG. Psychological factors determining human behavior. Boston: Harvard Univ. Press; 1937.
2. Kessler RC, et al. Prevalence, severity, and comorbidity of 12-month DSM-IV mental disorders. Arch Gen Psychiatry. 2005;62:617.

Anxiety Disorders

In the patient with general anxiety disorder (GAD), look for other psychiatric diseases, present in the majority of patients with anxiety.

In a study of 109 patients with GAD, 25 (23 %) had social phobia, 23 (21 %) had simple phobia, and 46 (42 %) had suffered one or more major depressive episodes [1]. Another survey of US persons age 15–45 years revealed that GAD is highly comorbid and that those with the diagnosis of GAD have a 90.4 % lifetime comorbidity with other psychiatric diagnoses [2]. The authors of this latter study go on to report that GAD is not a benign annoyance and that those with the disease experience "substantial interference with their lives, a high degree of professional help-seeking, and a high use of medication because of their GAD symptoms" [2].

Yet another study looked at 217 patients with one or more anxiety disorders and concurrent comorbidity with depression. The investigators found that those with a single anxiety disorder ($n=119$) had a 20.1 % comorbidity with major depressive disorder (MDD). Patients with two anxiety diagnoses ($n=75$) had a 45.3 % comorbidity MDD, and patients with three or more anxiety disorders ($n=23$) had an 87.0 % comorbidity with MDD [3].

1. Brawman-Mintzer O, et al. Psychiatric comorbidity in patients with generalized anxiety disorder. Am J Psychiatry. 1993;150:1216.
2. Wittchen HU, et al. DSM-III-R generalized anxiety disorder in the National Comorbidity Survey. Arch Gen Psychiatry. 1994;51:355.
3. Miyhazaki M, et al. Diagnosis of multiple anxiety disorders predicts the concurrent comorbidity of major depressive disorder. Compr Psychiatry. 2010;51:15.

Patients with anxiety symptoms are at increased risk of suicide.

A study of 2,778 patients found that those with self-reported anxiety symptoms were at double risk of reporting suicidality, after controlling for the usual variables [1].

1. Diefenbach GJ, et al. The association between self-reported anxiety symptoms and suicidality. J Nerv Ment Dis. 2009;197:92.

Be alert for the possibility of alcohol or cannabis dependence in the patient with social anxiety disorder.

A 14-year longitudinal study in Florida found social anxiety disorder to be associated with 4.5 greater odds of alcohol dependence (but not abuse) and a 6.5 greater risk of cannabis dependence (but not abuse) [1].

1. Buckner JD, et al. Specificity of social anxiety disorder as a risk factor for alcohol and cannabis dependence. J Psychiatr Res. 2008;42:230.

When a patient who complains of chest pain is found to have little or no coronary artery disease (CAD), the answer may be panic disorder.

A review of 38 articles led Fleet et al. to conclude, "Panic disorder is present in 30 % or more of chest pain patients with no or minimal CAD and may coexist with CAD." They go on to suggest that physicians often fail to recognize the presence of panic disorder in this setting [1].

1. Fleet RP, et al. Panic disorder, chest pain and coronary artery disease: literature review. Can J Cardiol. 1994;10:827.

Eating Disorders

Patients with bulimia nervosa (BN) are more likely to come to the clinician requesting assistance with weight control or for management of a physical problem related to their psychiatric disease than they are for care of the BN itself [1].

Extreme weight control measures and excessive concern regarding body image coupled with binge eating characterize BN. A curious case is described by Myers, who tells of a woman who swallowed her toothbrush while she was using it as a bulimic tool [2]. Here are some instructive facts about BN:

> *Normal weight*: Most patients coming to your office with BN will be of normal weight, not obese or emaciated [3].
>
> *Erosion of anterior teeth*: Gastric acid, coupled with the head posture and velocity of regurgitation, can result in severe erosion of the maxillary front teeth and the lingual surfaces of the maxillary first molars [4]. This finding may be first noted by the dentist.
>
> *Cigarette smoking*: There are higher rates of cigarette smoking among bulimic persons [5].
>
> *Childhood sexual abuse (CSA)*: A study of 1,936 persons with eating disorders revealed that the incidence of BN in adolescence was 2.5 times higher (95 % CI 0.80–8.0) with a past history of one episode of CSA and 4.9 times higher (95 % CI 1.9–12.7) with two or more episodes, compared with those reporting no incidence of CSA [6].

1. Hay PJ. Understanding bulimia. Aust Fam Physician. 2007;36:708.
2. Myers R. The woman who swallowed a toothbrush. New York: MFJ Books; 2003. p. 166.
3. Ghomas JG, et al. A prospective test of the relation between weight change and risk for bulimia nervosa. Int J Eating Disorders. 2011;44:295.
4. Spear F. A patient with severe wear on the anterior teeth and minimal wear on the posterior teeth. J Am Dent Assoc. 2008;139:1399.
5. Kendzor DE, et al. Cigarette smoking is associated with body shape concerns and bulimia symptoms among young adult females. Eating Behav. 2009;10:56.
6. Sanci L, et al. Childhood sexual abuse and eating disorders in females. Arch Pediatr Adolesc Med. 2008;162:261.

Russell sign—calluses on the knuckles—is a telltale sign of bulimia nervosa.

The calluses arise as the patient places the hand in the mouth to induce vomiting, thus abrading the dorsal skin of the fingers and hand with the superior incisors [1]. See Fig. 16.1. However, not all patients use this method, and some will take ipecac to induce vomiting [2].

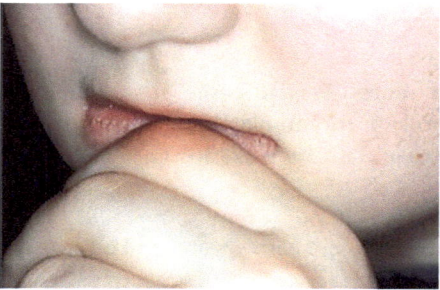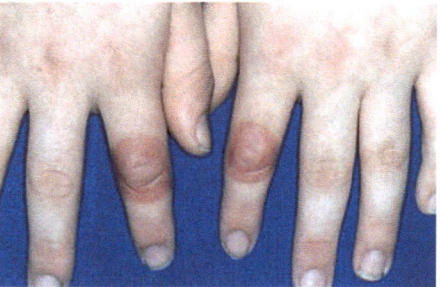

Fig. 16.1   Russell sign: calluses of the knuckles seen in some patients with bulimia

1. Glorio R, et al. Prevalence of cutaneous manifestations in 200 patients with eating disorders. Int J Dermatol. 2000;39:348.
2. Mehler PS. Medical complications of bulimia nervosa and their treatments. Int J Eating Disorders. 2011;44:95.

Skin manifestations of anorexia nervosa (AN) include melasma, hyperpigmentation, factitial dermatitis, abdominal striae, and poor wound healing.

Also reported in patients with AN are cheilitis, carotenoderma, and diffuse hypertrichosis [1, 2].

1. Sturmia R, et al. Skin signs in anorexia nervosa. Dermatology. 2001;203:314.
2. Sturmia R, et al. Dermatologic signs in patients with eating disorders. Am J Clin Dermatol. 2005;6:165.

The patient with a puzzling electrolyte abnormality may have an eating disorder.

Among the medical complications of eating disorders are sodium depletion and hypovolemia, hypomagnesemia, and hypophosphatemia. Other medical complications that may be seen are liver dysfunction, gastric dilation, cardiac arrhythmia, and osteopenia/osteoporosis [1, 2].

1. Mitchell JE, et al. Medical complications of anorexia nervosa and bulimia nervosa. Curr Opin Psychiatry. 2006;19:438.
2. Buchanan R, et al. Prolonged QT interval in bulimia nervosa. BMJ Case Reports. 2001: doi:10.1136/bcr.01.2011.3780.

A patient may be misdiagnosed as having AN when another disease is the cause of symptoms.

In the literature are several reports of instances in which achalasia was misdiagnosed as AN [1, 2].

Also, AN is not solely found in women and, according to one report, the disease affects more than a million men each year [3].

1. Rosenzweig S, et al. The diagnosis and misdiagnosis of achalasia: a study of 25 consecutive cases. Clin Gastroenterol. 1989;11:147.
2. Desseilles M, et al. Achalasia may mimic anorexia nervosa, compulsive eating disorder, and obesity problems. Psychosomatics. 2006;47:270.
3. Crosscope-Happel C, et al. Male anorexia nervosa: a new focus. J Ment Health Counseling. 2000;22:365.

Personality Disorders

The patient with wildly fluctuating mood changes throughout the day may have borderline personality disorder (BPD).

Of the DSM-IV-TR diagnostic criteria for BPD, affective instability leads the list, present in 95 % of patients in one study [1]. With a prevalence of up to 4 % in the community, BPD is described by Kernberg et al. as a serious psychiatric disorder that is difficult to treat [2]. From moment to moment, the mood of these patients may swing from euphoria to depression to anger. The following are some other facts pertinent to BPD:

> *Link to ADHD*: In one study of 118 women with BPD, there was a history of childhood attention-deficit hyperactivity disorder (ADHD) in 41.5 % of patients, and adult ADHD in 16.1 % [3].
> *Link to childhood events*: Several studies have linked BPD to childhood neglect and physical and sexual abuse [4, 5].
> *Persistent manifestations*: Of all the various features of BPD, affective symptoms and interpersonal difficulties reflecting dependency and abandonment issues tend to be the ones to be most stable over the years [1, 6].

1. McGlashan TH, et al. Two year prevalence and stability of individual DSM-IV criteria for schizotypal, borderline, avoidant, and obsessive-compulsive personality disorders: toward a hybrid model of axis II disorders. Am J Psychiatry. 2005;162:883.
2. Kernberg OF, et al. Borderline personality disorder. Am J Psychiatry. 2009;166:505.
3. Philipsen A, et al. Attention-deficit hyperactivity disorder as a potentially aggravating factor in borderline personality disorder. Br J Psychiatry. 2008;192:118.
4. Widom CS, et al. A prospective investigation of borderline personality disorder in abused and neglected children followed up into adulthood. J Pers Disord. 2009;23:433.
5. Lieb K, et al. Borderline personality disorder. Lancet. 2004;364:453.
6. Zanarini MC, et al. The subsyndromal phenomenology of borderline personality disorder: a 10-year follow-up study. Am J Psychiatry. 2007;164:929.

Problems delegating tasks can be an important clue to the recognition of obsessive–compulsive disorder (OCD).

A common disorder of both children and adults, OCD can be severe, even disabling. The course tends to be chronic, and the disease causes serious social and occupational problems in those afflicted [1, 2]. McGlashan reports that problems delegating tasks represent the most prevalent and least changeable criteria for the diagnosis of obsessive–compulsive personality disorder [3].

1. Markarian Y, et al. Multiple pathways to functional impairment in obsessive-compulsive disorder. Clin Psychol Rev. 2010;30:78.
2. Abramowitz JS, et al. Obsessive-compulsive disorder. Lancet. 2009;374:491.
3. McGlashan TH, et al. Two year prevalence and stability of individual DSM-IV criteria for schizotypal, borderline, avoidant, and obsessive-compulsive personality disorders: toward a hybrid model of axis II disorders. Am J Psychiatry. 2005;162:883.

Depression

The diagnosis of depression is sometimes missed because the patient may not disclose depressive symptoms to the primary care clinician.

A survey of 1,054 adults revealed that 43 % of respondents described one or more reasons for not reporting depressive symptoms to their primary care physician. The leading reason described was concern that they would be prescribed antidepressants (22.9 %; 95 % CI 18.8–27.5 %). Patients with no prior history of depression attributed nondisclosure to two reasons: a belief that primary care clinicians do not manage depression and concern that disclosure of depressive symptoms may prompt a psychiatric referral [1]. Another report tells that men are consistently less likely than women to seek help for depressive symptoms [2].

1. Bell RA, et al. Suffering in silence; reasons for not disclosing depression in primary care. Ann Fam Med. 2011;9:439.
2. Möller-Leimkühler AM. Barriers to help-seeking by men: a review of sociocultural and clinical literature with particular reference to depression. J Affect Disord. 2002;71:1.

A handy two-question screening tool can be an efficient way to identify the depressed patient.

The two questions address mood and anhedonia:

1. During the past month, have you felt down, depressed, or hopeless?
2. During the past month, have you felt little interest or pleasure in doing things?

This two-question screening tool was evaluated in two studies. The first involved 421 patients and, with a positive response to both questions, demonstrated a sensitivity of 97 % (95 % CI 83–99 %) and a specificity of 67 % (95 % CI 62–72 %) [1]. In the second study, which compared the two-question tool to six commonly used, longer instruments, demonstrated a sensitivity of 96 % (95 % CI 90–99 %) and a specificity of 57 % (95 % CI 53–62 %) for the two-question screening tool [2].

1. Arroll B, et al. Screening for depression in primary care with two verbally asked questions: cross-sectional study. BMJ. 2003;327:1144.
2. Whooley MA, et al. Case-finding instruments for depression: two questions are as good as many. J Gen Intern Med. 1997;12:439.

Low blood pressure is often seen in depressed persons and might just be one more clue to the diagnosis.

In Norwegian study involving 60,799 adults, investigators found that subjects with blood pressure in the lowest ranges were more likely to have depression (OR 1.22; 95 % CI 1.03–1.46) or anxiety (OR 1.31; 95 % CI 1.16–1.49) [1]. A second study reported from the Netherlands had similar findings, with authors reporting that current and remitted depressed patients had lower mean systolic blood pressure and were significantly less likely to have isolated systolic hypertension than controls [2].

1. Hildrum B, et al. Association of low blood pressure with anxiety and depression: the Nord-Trøndelag Health Study. J Epidemiol Community Health. 2007;61:53.
2. Licht CM, et al. Depression is associated with decreased blood pressure, but antidepressant use increases the risk for hypertension. Hypertension. 2009;53:681.

When making a diagnosis of depression, look for the presence of comorbidities.

There is an increased incidence of numerous diseases in patients with depression. Some of these are chronic obstructive pulmonary disease (COPD), neurologic disease, impaired vision, and diabetes mellitus [1, 2]. Depression confers a relative risk between 1.5 and 2.0 for the onset of coronary artery disease (CAD) in otherwise healthy individuals, according to Lett et al. [3]. Many Alzheimer patients have depression, which is often unrecognized, with symptoms attributed to the dementia [4].

Depression is also a risk factor for death, comparable in strength to smoking, a conclusion based on a 3–6-year study involving 61,349 subjects [5].

1. Schneider C, et al. COPD and the risk of depression. Chest. 2010;137:341.
2. Lyness JM, et al. The relationship of medical comorbidity and depression in older, primary care patients. Psychosomatics. 2006;47:435.
3. Lett HS, et al. Depression as a risk factor for coronary artery disease: evidence, mechanisms, and treatment. Psychosomatic Med. 2004;66:305.
4. Porta-Etessam J, et al. Depression in patients with moderate Alzheimer disease: a prospective observational cohort study. Alzheimer Dis Assoc Disord. 2011;25:317.
5. Mykletun A, et al. Levels of anxiety and depression as predictors of mortality: the HUNT Study. Br J Psychiatry. 2009;195:118.

Delusions, Hallucinations, and Psychoses

The hallmark of a psychosis is a disturbed sense of reality, which can involve delusions, hallucinations, or a disorder of logical thought.

There are a variety of psychotic disorders, with schizophrenia occurring most commonly and substance-induced psychotic disorders in second place. Among the general population, the lifetime prevalence of all psychotic disorders is about 3 %, suggesting that one of about every 33 patients will have a psychotic episode during his or her lifetime [1]. Men are affected more often than women, and those in urban settings experience more psychoses than those who live in rural areas [2]. Psychotic symptoms may occur in association with somatic disorders, including central nervous system tumors, infections, and vascular events; Alzheimer disease; hypoglycemia, hypoxia, or electrolyte disorders; endocrine dysfunction including thyroid disease; hepatic and renal disease; and systemic lupus erythematosus [3, 4].

1. Peräläj SJ, et al. Lifetime prevalence of psychotic and bipolar I disorders in a general population. Arch Gen Psychiatry. 2007;64:19.
2. van Os J, et al. Prevalence of psychotic disorders and community levels of psychotic symptoms: an urban-rural comparison. Arch Gen Psychiatry. 2001;58:663.
3. Patkar AA, et al. Psychotic symptoms in patients with medical disorders. Curr Psychiatry Rep. 2004;6:216.
4. Appenzeller S, et al. Acute psychosis in systemic lupus erythematosus. Rheumatol Int. 2008;28:237.

A good example of a delusion is the Ekbom syndrome of delusionary parasitosis.

A delusion is a firmly held, but factually incorrect, belief. Some delusions can be bizarre, indeed. Persons with the Ekbom syndrome report an infestation with insects, lice, or mites that no one else can see—the *invisible bugs*. The delusional belief is firmly rooted and does not respond to logical persuasion or evidence [1, 2]. See Fig. 16.2.

1. Hinkle NC. Ekbom syndrome: the challenge of the "invisible bug" infestation. Ann Rev Entomology. 2010;55:77.
2. Nicolato R, et al. Delusional parasitosis or Ekbom syndrome: a case series. Gen Hosp Psychiatry. 2006;28:85.

A delusional belief regarding spousal infidelity describes the Othello syndrome.

Named for the Shakespearean character Othello who, believing his wife Desdemona to be an adulteress (she wasn't), kills her. Although both men and women can suffer

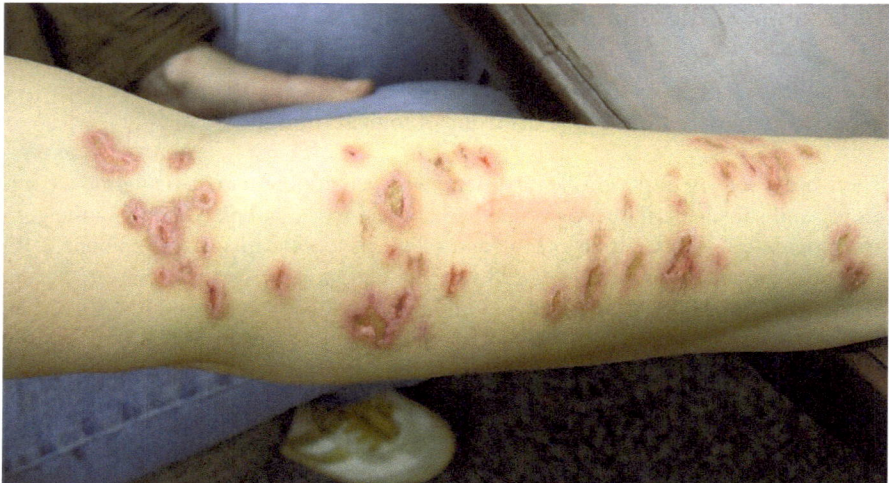

Fig. 16.2 Results of a patient with Ekbom syndrome having spent hours every evening removing scabs with tweezers. She explained that she had to help the *bugs* emerge from her skin

the Othello syndrome, the pathologic jealousy characteristic of the disorder is more common and more volatile in the male [1]. The syndrome has been described in association with Parkinson disease and in a single case in which symptoms began following a stroke in a 25-year-old woman [2, 3].

1. Todd J, et al. The Othello syndrome: a study in the psychopathology of sexual jealousy. J Nerv Ment Dis. 1955;122:367.
2. Georgiev D, et al. Othello syndrome in patients with Parkinson's disease. Psychiatria Danubina. 2010;22:94.
3. Westlake RJ, et al. Pathological jealousy appearing after cerebrovascular infarction in a 25-year old woman. Aust New Zeal J Psychiatry. 1999;33:105.

False sensory perceptions characterize hallucinations, which may affect any of the five senses.

Auditory hallucinations are most common and one of Meador's *doctors' rules* holds that, in general, auditory hallucinations are psychotic in origin, while visual hallucinations are more likely to be caused by chemicals [1]. The chemicals may include drugs of various kinds, or alcohol withdrawal, in the case of delirium tremens. As with many clinical "rules", there are noteworthy exceptions, and yet the adage may be helpful at times.

The auditory hallucination—*hearing voices* in the absence of acoustical input— is a leading manifestation of schizophrenia, occurring in 60–80 % of cases [2, 3].

With many entities, experienced clinicians have a single, memorable *personal index case* that serves as a reminder of the disease. In the case of psychotic hallucinations, my most vividly recalled case was a young man, brought to my office by his concerned parents for an initial visit because of what they considered "odd behavior". The patient seemed quite normal to me until, late in the visit, he confided that he had masturbated and that the voices in his head were compelling him to cut the muscles out of his right arm in atonement for his actions.

Up to 40 % of patients with Parkinson disease experience visual hallucinations, typically described as complex visual images that occur when the subject is alert with the eyes open [4].

Sapira suggests that a tactful way to inquire about the possibility of hallucinations is use of the question: Have you ever heard or seen something that others couldn't hear or see? [5]

1. Meador CK. A little book of doctor's rules II. Philadelphia: Hanley & Belfus; 1999, Rule 157.
2. Hugdahl K. "Hearing voices:" auditory hallucinations as failure of top-down control of bottom-up processes. Scand J Psychol. 2009;50:553.
3. Hoffman RE, et al. Time course of regional brain activation associated with onset of auditory/verbal hallucinations. Br J Psychiatry. 2008;193:424.
4. Barnes J, et al. Visual hallucination in Parkinson's disease: a review and phenomenological survey. J Neurol Neurosurg Psychiatry. 2001;70:727.
5. Orient JM, editor. Sapira's art and science of diagnosis. 3rd ed. Philadelphia: Lippincott, Williams & Wilkins; 2005. p. 641.

The sense that one's thoughts and actions are controlled externally is an important clue to the diagnosis of schizophrenia.

Sometimes termed a *disturbance of self*, the battle with—and sometimes, surrender to—external forces can lead to periodic turmoil in the patient's social, occupational, and personal domains [1]. The disease ranks among the top ten leading causes of disability worldwide and often has a lifelong course with periodic exacerbations [2]. Here are some important facts about schizophrenia:

Hereditary influence: Heredity plays a role in many instances of schizophrenia, estimated at 80 % in one report [2].

Socioeconomic considerations: There is a higher prevalence of schizophrenia in lower socioeconomic groups [2].

Cannabis use: A systematic review of the literature suggests that cannabis use is an independent risk factor for the development of psychosis [3].

Other environmental factors: There is a small increased risk of schizophrenia with older parental age, perinatal infection, obstetrical complications, and winter/spring birth [2].

Relationship to epilepsy: Episodic schizophrenia-like psychosis has been reported as the first manifestation of epilepsy [4].

1. Waters FAV, et al. First-rank symptoms in schizophrenia: reexamining mechanisms of self-recognition. Schizophr Bull. 2010;36:510.
2. Tandon R, et al. Schizophrenia: "just the facts:" what we know in 2008. Schizophr Res. 2008;100:4.
3. Le Bec PY, et al. Cannabis and psychosis: search for a causal link through a critical and systematic review. Encephale. 2009;35:377.
4. Verhoeven WMA, et al. Recurrent schizophrenia-like psychosis as first manifestation of epilepsy: a diagnostic challenge in neuropsychiatry. Neuropsychiatr Dis Treat. 2010;6:227.

Suicide

There are diverse risk factors that might help identify the potentially suicidal patient, a _must-not-miss diagnosis_.

Here are some of the risk factors for suicide:

Sadness: In a nationally representative study of high school students in 2007, 6.9 % of adolescents attempted suicide. The leading risk factor was sadness, with an adjusted OR of 5.74 for girls and 10.96 for boys [1].

Huffing glue: In the study of adolescents cited above, huffing glue was another important risk factor for suicide: girls, adjusted OR 1.63; and boys, adjusted OR 2.04. Other risk factors cited in this study were weapon carrying, forced sex, dating violence (girls), hard drug use (boys), and sports involvement (boys) [1].

Moving residence: A study of children in Denmark revealed an increased risk of suicide with a move in residence [2].

High-altitude living: In a study of suicide rates in US counties, there was a "strong positive correlation" between county altitude and suicide rates ($p < 0.001$). Altitude- induced hypoxia is suggested as a possible mechanism [3].

Body weight: A Swedish study of 1,133,019 men revealed an increased risk of attempted suicide in lower weight men [4].

Presence of cancer: In older adults, the risk of suicide is higher if there is a cancer diagnosis [5].

1. West BA, et al. Children at risk for suicide attempt and attempt-related injuries: findings from the 2007 Youth Risk Behavior Study. West J Emerg Med. 2010;11:257.
2. Qin P, et al. Frequent change of residence and risk of attempted and completed suicide among children and adolescents. Arch Gen Psychiatry. 2009;66:628.
3. Brenner BE, et al. Positive association between altitude and suicide in 2584 US counties. High Alt Med Biol. 2012;12:31.
4. Batty GD, et al. Body mass index and attempted suicide: cohort study of 1,133,019 Swedish men. Am J Epidemiol. 2010;172:890.
5. Miller M, et al. Cancer and the risk of suicide in older Americans. J Clin Oncol. 2008;26:4720.

Selected Problems Related to Mental Health

The patient with bipolar disease is most likely to seek professional help during an episode of depression.

Bipolar disease affects 3–5 % of all Americans, a not insignificant prevalence for this troublesome disorder [1]. Manic episodes may be readily identified, but the person in the depressed phase of bipolar disorder will be misdiagnosed unless the clinician inquires about the possibility of agitation, restlessness, or disease-related disruption of personal or family life [2].

Manic episodes and depression represent the two poles of bipolar disease. In between is hypomania, often missed by clinicians, and sometimes actually embraced by patients reveling in the elevated sense of well-being, the increased energy that permits enhanced productivity on the job and at home, and perhaps even the reduced need for sleep.

1. Goodwin FK, et al. Manic-depressive illness: bipolar disorders and recurrent depression. 2nd ed. New York: Oxford; 2007.
2. Loganathan M, et al. When to suspect bipolar disorder. J Fam Pract. 2010;59:682.

The unexpected onset of agitation and confusion in a person taking several prescription medications and, perhaps, also herbal drugs may signal the onset of serotonin syndrome.

The serotonin syndrome, aka serotonin toxicity, occurs when there is a drug-induced increase in the serotonin levels causing stimulation of postsynaptic serotonin$_{2A}$ receptors in the central nervous system [1]. A classic scenario is the addition of a selective serotonin reuptake inhibitor (SSRI) to a drug regimen that already includes a medication from the following list: opioids such as meperidine; triptans such as sumatriptan (Imitrex); tricyclic antidepressants; monoamine oxidase inhibitors; valproate (Depakote); ergot alkaloids; amphetamine derivatives such as methylphenidate (Ritalin); serotonin–norepinephrine reuptake inhibitors; cocaine; and/or herbal remedies such as nutmeg, Panax ginseng, and St. John's wort [2, 3]. Other manifestations of serotonin toxicity may include shivering, fever, tachycardia, hyperreflexia, myoclonus, and tremor [2]. Arora et al. present a simplified approach to the diagnosis, which they report to be 84 % sensitive and 97 % specific for the diagnosis of serotonin syndrome. See Fig. 16.3 [4].

1. Sun-Edelstein C, et al. Drug-induced serotonin syndrome: a review. Expert Opin Drug Safety. 2008;7:587.
2. Rehman HU. Recent onset of confusion, limited mobility, and disturbed sleep-wake cycle. J Fam Pract. 2011;60:261.
3. Taylor RB. Essential medical facts every clinician should know. New York: Springer; 2011. p. 215.
4. Arora B, et al. The serotonin syndrome—the need for physician's awareness. Int Emerg Med. 2010;3:373.

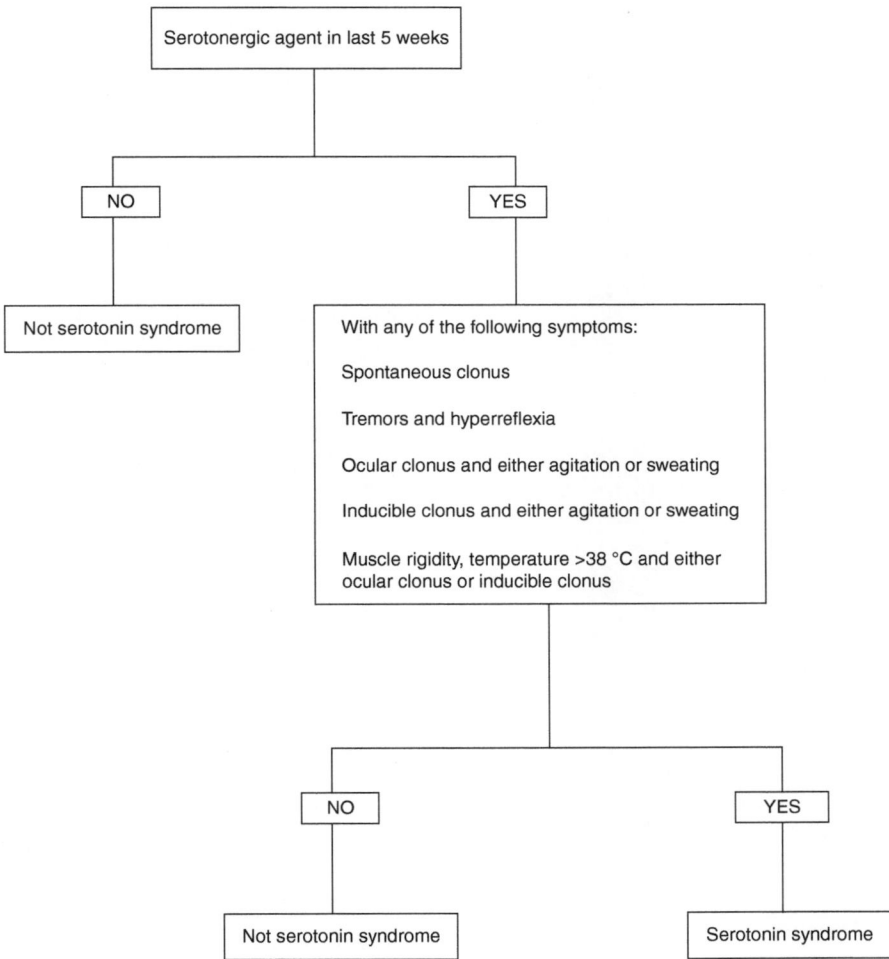

Fig. 16.3 Diagnostic criteria for serotonin syndrome

A single question may help identify the patient who misuses drugs.

The single question is this: "How many times in the past year have you used an illegal drug or used a prescription medication for nonmedical reasons?" In a study of 394 adults surveyed in a waiting room setting, the question was found to be 100 % sensitive (95 % CI 90.6–100 %) and 73.5 % specific (95 % CI 67.7–78.6 %) in identifying the patient with a drug use problem [1].

1. Smith PC, et al. A single-question screening test for drug use in primary care. Arch Intern Med. 2010;170:1155.

Chapter 17
Laboratory and Imaging Diagnosis

I have been surprised to note the readiness with which
high-grade young men, graduates from medical institutions
which are models for our time, yield to the temptation of
machine-made diagnosis.

America surgeon William J. Mayo (1861–1939) [1]

Contents

R.B. Taylor, *Diagnostic Principles and Applications*,
DOI 10.1007/978-1-4614-1111-6_17, © Springer Science+Business Media, LLC 2013

It may seem odd to begin the chapter on laboratory and imaging diagnosis by quoting Dr. Mayo's words disparaging *machine-made* diagnosis. Certainly we all value the tremendous advances that have been made in both the clinical laboratory and the various types of diagnostic imaging. However, the ready availability of just this sort of testing has fostered an attitude that the medical history and physical examination are just not as important as they were a generation ago. Based on a three-plus-decade-long career as a medical school professor, I can attest that this belief system has resulted in half-hearted instruction in history-taking and physical examination skills in teaching the current generation of medical students and residents, a skill deficit which, I believe, would sadden the brothers Mayo and the other medical giants of their day. This book has, in contrast to current trends, focused on the diagnostic clues to be found in the medical history and on physical examination. The laboratory and imaging options we have today must supplement, not replace, basic clinical acumen. With that preface, let us look at some of the benefits that the use of machines can provide.

1. Mayo WJ. Aphorisms. In: Willius FA, editor. Aphorisms of Dr. Charles Horace Mayo and Dr. William James Mayo. Rochester: Mayo Foundation for Medical Education and Research; 1988. p. 55.

Hematology Testing

Hemoglobin (HBG), hematocrit (HCT), and erythrocyte counts obtained from skin puncture capillary blood are slightly higher than those found in venous blood [1, 2].

This makes intuitive sense to me: The capillary blood lies between arterial blood leaving the lungs and venous blood on its way back to the heart. Although the difference is small, about 2 % in one study, considering the specimen source may be important when borderline results are evaluated [1].

1. Daae LN, et al. A comparison between hematological parameters in "capillary" and venous blood samples from hospitalized children aged 3 months to 14 years. Scand J Clin Lab Invest. 1991;51:651.
2. Bellamy GJ, et al. Venous and skin puncture blood counts compared. Clin Lab Hematol. 1998;10:329.

Low hemoglobin levels may be found in three groups: highly trained athletes, African-Americans, and the elderly.

Here are some reported findings:

Highly trained athletes: Low levels of hemoglobin and haptoglobin may be found in highly trained athletes, especially runners, attributed to plasma volume expansion or to running-induced hemolysis [1–3].

African-Americans: In a study of 1,491 African-American (AA) and 31,005 white subjects, when iron-deficient and thalassemic persons were eliminated from consideration, 6.1 % of AA women would be considered anemic, compared to 2.77 % of whites; for men, the figures were 4.29 % versus 3.6 % [4].

Elderly individuals: Anemia is present in up to 10 % of persons age 65 or older. The percentage of persons with anemia increases with age, with anemia present in one quarter of community-dwelling octogenarians [5].

1. Merkel D, et al. Incidence of anemia and iron deficiency in strenuously trained adolescents: results of a longitudinal follow-up study. J Adol Health. 2009;45:286.
2. Shaskey DJ, et al. Sports hematology. Sports Med. 2000;29:27.
3. Defaux B, et al. Serum ferritin, transferrin, haptoglobin in middle- and long-distance runners, elite rowers, and professional racing cyclists. Int J Sports Med. 1981;2:43.
4. Buetler E, et al. Hematologic differences between African-Americans and whites; the roles of iron deficiency and alpha-thalassemia on hemoglobin levels and mean corpuscular volume. Blood. 2005;106:740.
5. Eisenstaedt R, et al. Anemia in the elderly: current understanding and emerging concepts. Blood Rev. 2006;20:213.

Smokers have higher levels of hemoglobin than nonsmokers.

Findings from the Second National Health and Nutrition Examination Survey revealed that both men and women had hemoglobin levels approximately 0.4 g/dL higher than never-smokers. No such difference was noted when hemoglobin levels of ex-smokers were compared with those of never-smokers. The authors suggest that the differences noted may result in a masking effect in the detection of anemia [1].

1. Nordenberg D, et al. The effect of cigarette smoking on hemoglobin levels and anemia screening. JAMA. 1990;264:1556.

Neurotic bloodletting can result in factitious anemia: the Lasthénie de Ferjol syndrome.

The namesake of this rare disease is a fictitious 16-year-old girl in a French novel, *The Story without a Name*, by Barbey d'Aurevilly (1808–1889). Impregnated by a priest, the tragic heroine gives birth to a stillborn infant. She subsequently stabs 18 needles into her heart (inducing anemia) and dies [1]. The literature contains several case reports of Lasthénie de Ferjol syndrome, an entity that occurs chiefly in women [1, 2].

1. Karamanou M, et al. Lasthénie de Ferjol syndrome: a rare disease with a fascinating history. Int Med J. 2010;40:381.
2. Piccillo GA, et al. Eighteen needles to forget. . . an unnamed past. J Forensic Legal Med. 2007;14:304.

Do not count on white blood cell (WBC) indicators to identify or rule out serious infection.

A systematic review of 14 studies of the diagnostic value of laboratory tests in identifying serious infections in febrile children led to the conclusion that white blood cell markers (WBC count, absolute neutrophil count, band count, and left shift) "are less valuable than inflammatory markers in ruling in serious infection (positive LR, 0.87–2.43) and have no value in ruling out serious infection (negative LR, 0.61–1.14) [1]".

1. Van den Bruel A, et al. Diagnostic value of laboratory tests in identifying serious infections in febrile children: systematic review. BMJ. 2011;342:d3082.

The erythrocyte sedimentation rate (ESR) is most helpful when extreme elevations (>100 mm/h) are found.

Haque et al. studied 100 consecutive patients found to have an ESR >100 mm/h. The causes identified included: hematologic disorders, 41 %; infectious diseases, 36 %; and connective tissue disorders, 17 %. Among these patients, 30 % were found to have hematologic malignancies, including leukemia, lymphoma, and multiple myeloma. In only 4 % of cases could no cause be identified for the elevated ESR [1].

One report describes an extremely elevated ESR in association with Legionnaires disease [2].

A study of C-reactive protein and ESR in patients with suspected acute epididymitis revealed that both of these levels were much more elevated in patients with epididymitis when compared with patients with spermatic cord torsion or other noninflammatory causes of an acute scrotum [3].

1. Haque Z, et al. Clinical study on patients with grossly elevated erythrocyte sedimentation rate. J Med. 2007;8:64.
2. Cunha BA, et al. Extremely elevated erythrocyte sedimentation rates in Legionnaires disease. Eur J Clin Microbiol Inf Dis. 2010;29:1567.
3. Asgari SA, et al. Diagnostic accuracy of C-reactive protein and erythrocyte sedimentation rate in patients with acute scrotum. Urol J. 2006;3:108.

ESR and platelet counts can be useful in identification of Kawasaki disease (KD).

A study compared 33 KD patients with 34 patients with somewhat similar symptoms but who did not have KD. Both ESR and platelet counts were significantly higher in the KD patients ($p < 0.05$). With a cutoff of 15 mm/h, ESR had a sensitivity of 93.9 % and a specificity of 83.3 %. At a cutoff of 336.5×10^9/L, platelet elevations had a sensitivity of 70.6 % and a specificity of 75 % for the diagnosis of KD [1].

1. Xiu-Yu S, et al. Platelet count and erythrocyte sedimentation rate are good predictors of Kawasaki disease: ROC analysis. J Clin Lab Anal. 2010;24:385.

Serum and Plasma Chemistry Tests

Fasting glucose and glycosylated hemoglobin (HbA1c) together may have a role in the prediction of diabetes.

A population based analysis of 13,176 subjects in whom fasting glucose and HbA1c levels were studied in regard to the prediction of diabetes led investigators to two conclusions. First, HbA1c "performs well as a diagnostic tool when diabetes definitions that most closely resemble those used in clinical practice are used as the 'gold standard'." Also, they found that subjects with a fasting glucose ≥126 mg/dL and HbA1c ≥6.6 % at baseline had an 88 % 10-year risk of developing diabetes, compared with a 55 % risk among subjects with fasting glucose ≥126 mg/dL and HbA1c of 5.7 to <6.5 %. Thus the second conclusion, that there is a dual role for the two tests in prediction of diabetes [1].

As an aside, an exhaled breath analyzer to detect acetone in inhaled breath has been developed and may prove a helpful noninvasive tool to detect diabetes in the future [2].

1. Selvin E, et al. Performance of A1C for the classification and prediction of diabetes. Diabetes Care. 2011;34:84.
2. Wang L, et al. An acetone nanosensor for non-invasive diabetes detection. AIP Conf Proc. 2009;1137:206.

Hyponatremia can be the clue to a psychiatric disorder—polydipsia.

Hyponatremia is the most common electrolyte disorder in general hospital patients [1]. Other causes of low serum sodium levels include syndrome of inappropriate antidiuretic hormone release (SIADH), hypoalbuminemia, excessive use of diuretics, congestive heart failure, advanced liver disease, and exuberant intravenous fluid replacement with hypotonic solutions. Less common causes are adrenal insufficiency and hypothyroidism [2, 3].

1. Callahan MA, et al. Economic impact of hyponatremia in hospitalized patients: a retrospective cohort study. Postgrad Med. 2009;121:186.
2. Hoorn EJ, et al. Unexplained hyponatremia: seek and you will find. Nephron Physiol. 2011;118:66.
3. Liamis G, et al. Endocrine disorders: causes of hyponatremia not to neglect. Ann Med. 2011;43:179.

Think beyond the "usual suspects"—overuse of diuretics or possible aldosteronism— when you encounter a patient with hypokalemia.

Consider also severe glycosuria or rapidly falling blood glucose with insulin replacement in diabetes. Think also about the possibility of anorexia/bulimia, overuse of laxatives or enemas, mineralocorticoid administration, or heart failure. Other considerations include:

Severe emesis: Prolonged vomiting can result in dehydration and electrolyte abnormalities, including hypokalemia [1].

Magnesium deficiency: Although magnesium deficiency does not necessarily cause hypokalemia, it exacerbates the disorder and makes the condition refractory to treatment with potassium replacement [2].

Drugs: Low potassium levels have been associated with a number of drugs, including chloroquine (Aralen), beta-adrenergic drugs, ondansetron (Zofran), and nafcillin [3, 4].

Licorice consumption: There are more than 40 reported cases of hypokalemia caused by licorice in candy, chewing tobacco, medication, and herbal remedies [5]. In fact, licorice has been suggested to prevent hyperkalemia in dialysis patients [6].

Gitelman syndrome: This is rare inherited disorder manifested as hypokalemia associated with hypomagnesemia, hypocalciuria, and metabolic acidosis [7].

1. Garcia E, et al. Profound hypokalemia: unusual presentation and management in a 12-year-old boy. Pediatr Emerg Care. 2008;24:157.
2. Huang CL, et al. Mechanism of hypokalemia in magnesium deficiency. J Am Col Nephrol. 2007;18:2649.
3. Turner SR, et al. Ondansetron-associated hypokalemia in a 2-year-old with Pre-B-cell ALL. J Pediatr Hematol Oncol. 2008;30:58.
4. Qua DA, et al. Hypokalemia associated with nafcillin treatment. Inf Dis Clin Pract. 2009;17:130.
5. Elinav E. et al. Licorice consumption causing severe hypokalemic paralysis. Mayo Clin Proc. 2003;78:767.
6. Ferrari P. Licorice: a sweet alternative to prevent hyperkalemia in dialysis patients? Kidney Int. 2009;76:811.
7. Eren MA, et al. A rare cause of hypokalemia: Gitelman syndrome. Eur J Gen Med. 2011; 8:154.

In the patient with hyperkalemia, think of drugs, acute renal failure, and sepsis.

In a study of 45 patients with high levels of serum potassium, among the 34 with true hyperkalemia, the causes were found to be: medications (53 %), acute renal failure (32 %), sepsis (12 %), and rhabdomyolysis (3 %). What about the other 11 patients? They turned out to have pseudohyperkalemia owing to hemolysis of laboratory specimens [1].

Among the medications that can cause hyperkalemia are potassium-sparing diuretics such as spironolactone (Aldactone), beta-blockers, angiotensin receptor blockers (ARBs), angiotensin-converting enzyme (ACE) inhibitors, heparin, non-steroidal anti-inflammatory drugs (NSAIDs), trimethoprim (Proloprim), digitalis in toxic levels, and, of course, excessive consumption of potassium supplements [2, 3]. There is a reported case of elevated potassium levels attributed to orange juice ingestion in a diabetic patient with chronic renal failure [4, 5]. And Uthman reports

the possibility of *spurious hyperkalemia* if the patient vigorously exercises the arm
just prior to the blood draw [6].

1. Rajeev SP, et al. Hyperkalemia in a district general hospital. Endo Abstr. 2007;13:29.
2. Hollander-Rodriguez JC, et al. Hyperkalemia. Am Fam Physician. 2006;73:283.
3. Marinella MA. Trimethoprim-induced hyperkalemia: an analysis of reported cases. Gerontology. 1999;45:209.
4. Palmer BF. A physiologic-based approach to the evaluation of a patient with hyperkalemia. Am J Kid Dis. 2010;56:387.
5. Fan K, et al. Orange juice-induced hyperkalemia in a diabetic patient with chronic renal failure. Diab Care. 1996;19:1457.
6. Uthman E. Interpretation of lab test profiles. Available at: http://web2.airmail.net/uthman/lab_ test.html.

Vitamin D deficiency can reveal itself as unexplained hypocalcemia.

Hypocalcemia can have many other causes in addition to vitamin D deficiency:
nutritional deficiency, thyroid disease, growth hormone deficiency, and Cushing
disease [1, 2]. Critically ill patients may have hypocalcemia caused by hypoalbuminemia, hypomagnesemia, hyperphosphatemia, acute pancreatitis, malabsorption,
renal insufficiency, and sepsis [3]. The astute clinician will not forget to think about
parathyroid hormone (PTH) deficiency, either primary or surgically induced.

Bosworth et al. suggest a useful approach based on readily available testing: A
high level of parathyroid hormone with elevated serum phosphorus and creatinine
levels together suggests a diagnosis of renal failure. When the PTH is high but the
serum phosphorus is low or normal and the creatinine is normal, think of pancreatitis or vitamin D deficiency. If the PTH is low, the phosphorus level high, and the
creatinine level normal, the top diagnostic possibilities are hypoparathyroidism or
hypomagnesemia [4].

1. Noto H, et al. Vitamin D deficiency as an ignored cause of hypocalcemia in acute illness: report of 2 cases and review of the literature. Open Endocrinol J. 2009;3:1.
2. Mansoor R, et al. Frequency of occurrence of hypocalcemia in various disorders. Ann Pak Inst Med Sci. 2010;6:44.
3. Culleiton AL, et al. Keeping electrolytes and fluids in balance. Nurs Crit Care. 2011;6:27.
4. Bosworth M, et al. What is the best workup for hypoglycemia? J Fam Pract. 2008;57:677.

**Nine of every ten patients with hypercalcemia have hyperparathyroidism or
cancer.**

During the course of their disease, 5–30 % of cancer patients will have elevated
serum calcium levels, especially those with lung cancer and renal cell carcinoma
[1]. Other causes include renal failure, sarcoidosis, hyperthyroidism, and drug use,
notably thiazide diuretics [2].

Other causes to consider are:

Hypervitaminosis D: This is a not-unlikely scenario, given the current enthusiasm with which large doses of vitamin D are recommended [3].

Milk–alkali syndrome: Once a common outcome with the Sippy diet regimen of milk products and alkaline powders used to treat peptic ulcer, the syndrome has made a comeback as some individuals use nonprescription calcium-containing products to treat epigastric distress symptoms [4].

Familial benign hypercalcemia (*FBH*): Also called familial hypocalciuric hypercalcemia, this rare disease occurs in family clusters and symptoms are uncommon. It is important, however, that the clinician not mistakenly diagnose these patients as having hyperparathyroidism (and possibly subjecting them to needless surgery) [5, 6].

Blue diaper syndrome: This is another familial disease in which there is a defect in intestinal transport of tryptophan. The manifestations are hypercalcemia, nephrocalcinosis, and a telltale blue discoloration of the diaper owing to indicanuria which oxidizes to indigo blue [7].

1. Lumachi F, et al. Cancer-induced hypercalcemia. Anticancer Res. 2009;29:1551.
2. Desai HV, et al. Thiazide-induced severe hypercalcemia: a case report and review of the literature. Am J Therapeut. 2010;17:e234.
3. Joshi R. Hypercalcemia due to hypervitaminosis D: report of seven patients. J Trop Pediatr. 2011;55:396.
4. Ulett K, et al. Hypercalcemia and acute renal failure in milk-alkali syndrome: a case report. J Hosp Med. 2010;5:e18.
5. Auwerx J, et al. Familial hypocalciuric hypercalcemia–familial benign hypercalcemia: a review. Postgrad Med J. 1987;63:835.
6. Lietman SA, et al. Hypercalcemia in children and adolescents. Curr Opin in Pediatr. 2010;22:508.
7. Drummond KN, et al. The blue diaper syndrome: familial hypercalcemia with nephrocalcinosis and indicanuria. Am J Med. 1964;37:928.

Hyperphosphatemia could be caused by the ongoing use of phosphate-containing antacids or enemas.

Other possible causes of an elevated serum phosphate level are: chronic renal disease, hemolysis, rhabdomyolysis, and the tumor lysis syndrome [1, 2].

1. Shiber JR, et al. Serum phosphate abnormalities in the emergency department. J Emerg Med. 2002;23:395.
2. Sadarcan A, et al. Hyperphosphatemia in tumor lysis syndrome: the role of hemodialysis and continuous veno-venous hemofiltration. Pediatr Nephrol. 1994;8:351.

When an elevated serum alkaline phosphatase (SAP) is reported, consider the possibility of a spurious result caused by use of an anticoagulant tube for specimen collection or leaving the serum sample at room temperature for a prolonged period.

Once it has been determined that the result is valid, the search for a cause begins. Serum alkaline phosphatase comes chiefly from bones and liver. Bone-related causes of elevated SAP include: hyperparathyroidism, Paget disease, and cancer such as metastatic tumors of the breast, lung, kidney, ovary, or prostate. Hepatic causes of elevated SAP include: cirrhosis, fatty liver, hepatitis, primary biliary cirrhosis, sclerosing cholangitis, gallstones, and hepatic involvement in infections such as cytomegalovirus, toxoplasmosis, and infectious mononucleosis. Elevated plasma alkaline phosphatase levels have also been reported in patients with Alzheimer disease [1, 2].

1. Fisher JA, et al. Alkaline phosphatase, elevated. In: Taylor RB, editor. Manual of 10-minute diagnosis. Philadelphia: Lippincott, Williams & Wilkins; 2000. p. 339.
2. Vardy ERLC, et al. Alkaline phosphatase is increased in both brain and plasma in Alzheimer's disease. Neurodegen Dis. 2012;9:31.

When a mildly elevated aminotransferase level is found, think first of nonalcoholic liver disease (NALD).

Our tendency to order "comprehensive metabolic panels" as part of health maintenance examinations necessarily yields some unanticipated elevated values, often in aminotransferase levels. In fact, one study found the presence of high alanine aminotransferase (ALT) levels in 8.9 % of the US population and even in 7.3 % of persons who do not consume alcohol excessively or have viral hepatitis C [1]. The leading cause of elevated liver enzymes is nonalcoholic liver disease, present in up to 30 % of the population [2]. NALD is associated with higher body mass index, metabolic syndrome, and, according to a recent study, perhaps even obstructive sleep apnea (OSA) [3]. See Fig. 17.1. Among the other leading causes of elevated aminotransferase levels is hemochromatosis, discussed in Chap. 13.

1. Ioannou GN, et al. The prevalence and predictors of elevated serum aminotransferase activity in the United States in 1999–2002. Am J Gastroent. 2006;101:76.
2. OH RC, et al. Causes and evaluation of mildly elevated liver transaminase levels. Am Fam Physician. 2011;84:1003.
3. Norman D, et al. Serum aminotransferase levels are associated with markers of hypoxia in patients with obstructive sleep apnea. Sleep. 2008;31:121.

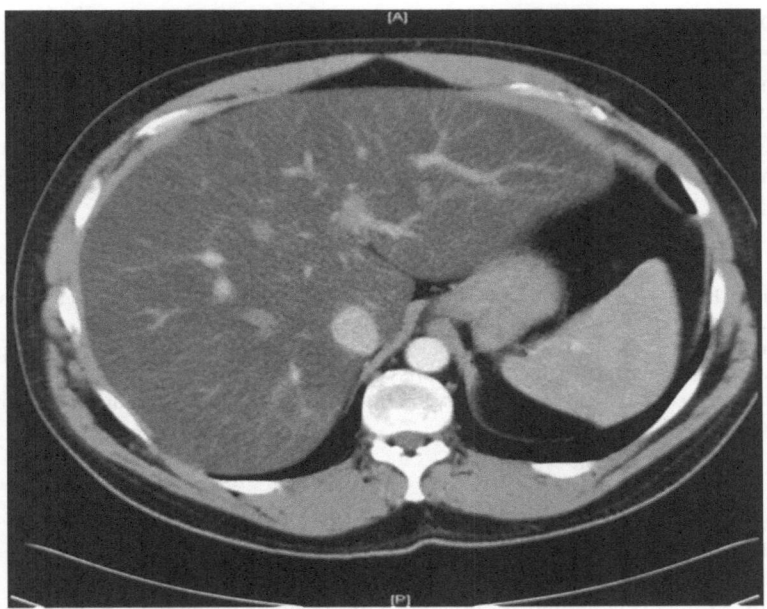

Fig. 17.1 Radiologic imaging in nonalcoholic fatty liver disease. Fatty infiltration lowers the CT attenuation of the liver parenchyma, causing hepatic vessels to stand out

An elevated uric acid level may be a clue to the presence of iron overload.

In a study of adults in the National Health and Nutrition Examination Survey 1999–2002, subjects with high uric acid levels (20.7 %) had high ferritin levels compared to those (8.8 %) with low uric acid levels ($p < 0.001$). Also, subjects with elevations of both uric acid and ferritin levels had higher liver enzyme levels than those with either elevated uric acid or ferritin. The significance of all this is stated by the authors in the conclusion: "Elevated levels of uric acid are associated with elevated ferritin levels and may serve as a risk stratification variable for presence of iron overload and hemochromatosis" [1].

1. Mainous AG, et al. Uric acid as a potential cue to screen for iron overload. J Am Board Fam Med. 2011;24:415.

Serum troponin levels can be elevated in patients with pulmonary embolism as well as in those with a myocardial infarction.

Although elevated serum troponin levels are well recognized as useful markers of acute myocardial infarction, high troponin levels may also be noted in patients with acute pulmonary embolism, offering the opportunity for misdiagnosis. In the first

24 h of a myocardial infarction, cardiac troponin-T has a high sensitivity (99 %) for acute myocardial infarction and a specificity of 86 % [1]. However, a study of 56 patients with confirmed acute pulmonary embolism showed an elevated troponin-T in 32 % of subjects [2].

There are other causes of elevated troponin levels, which include: unstable tachycardia, myocarditis, heart failure, severe aortic stenosis, gastrointestinal bleeding, pericarditis, and more than a dozen other, less common, entities [3].

1. Johnson PA. Cardiac troponin as a marker for myocardial ischemia in patients seen at the emergency department for acute chest pain. Am Heart J. 1999;137:1137.
2. Giannitis E, et al. Independent prognostic value of troponin T in patients with confirmed pulmonary embolism. Circulation. 2000;102:211.
3. Mahajan N, et al. Elevated troponin level is not synonymous with myocardial infarction. Int J Cardiol. 2006;111:442.

Elevated cysteine levels can help identify the patient with obstructive sleep apnea.

In study of 75 OSA patients compared with 75 control subjects, higher levels of plasma cysteine were found in OSA patients compared with controls ($p < 0.01$). The differences were found in both lean and obese groups of subjects. The elevated cysteine levels were reduced following effective OSA therapy [1].

1. Cintra F, et al. Cysteine: a potential biomarker for obstructive sleep apnea. Chest. 2011;139:246.

The best way to assess vitamin B_{12} activity is by determination of methylmalonate, not serum B_{12} levels.

In a study of 121 subjects age 65 or older followed for 4.6 years, elevated levels of B_{12} markers—notably methylmalonate—were associated with reduced cognitive function and brain volume [1]. When serum B_{12} levels decline, methylmalonate rises, and the methylmalonate level is more sensitive and specific for vitamin B_{12}-associated cognitive decline than serum B_{12} levels [1].

1. Tagney CC, et al. Vitamin B_{12}, cognition, and brain MRI measures. Neurology. 2011;77:1276.

Diagnostic Imaging

The discovery of a solitary pulmonary nodule (SPN) presents a diagnostic challenge, one that sometimes can be approached using commonsense clinical recommendations.

Since the introduction of computed tomography in the 1990s, more and more pulmonary nodules are being found, some as small as 1–2 mm in diameter [1]. See Fig. 17.2. The question, of course, arises: Is this nodule malignant? Soubani offers a reasonable approach that will be useful in some instances: "SPNs that are stable in size for >2 years and those with benign pattern of calcification do not need further studies. Lesions with clear change in size are malignant until proven otherwise and require tissue diagnosis" [2].

1. Beigelman-Aubry C, et al. Management of an incidentally discovered pulmonary nodule. Eur Radiol. 2007;17:449.
2. Soubani AO. The evaluation and management of the solitary pulmonary nodule. Postgrad Med J. 2008;84:459.

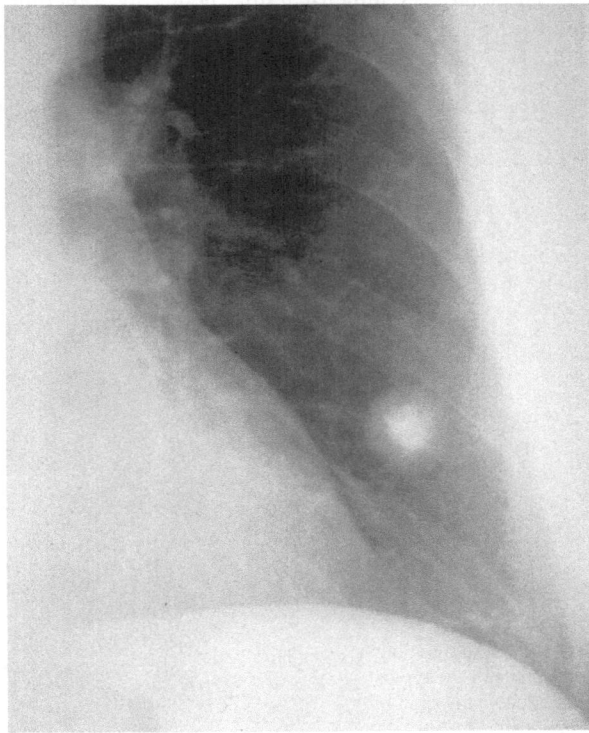

Fig. 17.2 Chest radiograph of a solitary pulmonary nodule (SPN). SPN is defined as a single spherical lesion ≤3 cm in diameter, surrounded by aerated lung and not associated with mediastinal adenopathy, atelectasis, pneumonitis, or satellite lesions. Lesions >3 cm in diameter are referred to as masses; 80–90 % of these masses are malignant

The most common tumor of the anterior mediastinum is a thymoma [1].

A thymoma may be asymptomatic and reveal itself only as an incidental finding on an imaging study. On the other hand, a mediastinal mass may cause cough, dyspnea, or chest pain. Hoarseness suggests recurrent laryngeal nerve involvement, and the presence of any symptom increases the chances that the tumor is malignant [1–3].

In addition to thymoma and thymic carcinoma, other diagnostic considerations when confronted with a mediastinal mass include: retrosternal goiter, lymphoma, germ cell tumors such as seminoma, mediastinal cysts, and even a normal thymus [3–6].

1. Alpet JB, et al. Increasing dyspnea due to an anterior mediastinal mass. Chest. 2011;139:217.
2. Siemienowicz M, et al. Massive anterior mediastinal mass causing cardiac compression. J Am Coll Cardiol. 2010;56:47.
3. Haas CS, et al. A mediastinal mass. J Fam Pract. 2010;59:347.
4. Matwiyoff GN, et al. A 28-year-old man with a mediastinal mass. Chest. 2008;134:648.
5. Gandara F, et al. Mediastinal seminoma: a case report. Internet J Int Med. 2011;9:1.
6. Gupta AK. Normal thymus mimicking "mediastinal mass." Pediatr Radiol. 2009;76:1067.

The asymptomatic patient with bilateral hilar adenopathy probably has sarcoidosis.

The most common chest manifestation of sarcoidosis is bilateral hilar adenopathy [1]. These large, symmetrical hilar nodes are sometimes described as *potato nodes*. See Fig. 17.3. Also, in asymptomatic patients with bilateral hilar adenopathy, the

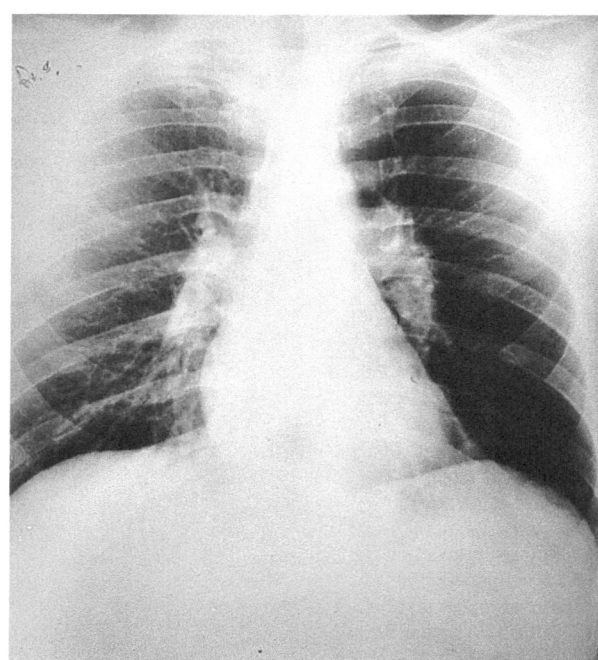

Fig. 17.3 Radiographic appearance of the typical hilar adenopathy of sarcoidosis

diagnosis is highly likely to be sarcoidosis. In a study of 100 subjects with bilateral hilar adenopathy, sarcoidosis was found in all 30 asymptomatic patients with bilateral hilar adenopathy and in 50 of 52 patients with bilateral hilar adenopathy and an absence of abnormal physical examination findings. Parenthetically, in this study, the 11 patients with neoplastic disease all exhibited telltale symptoms [2].

1. Shigemitsu H, et al. A 65-year-old woman with subcutaneous nodule and hilar adenopathy. Chest. 2008;134:1080.
2. Winterbauer RH, et al. A clinical interpretation of bilateral hilar adenopathy. Ann Intern Med. 1973;78:65.

Routine immediate lumbar imaging of patients with low back pain who have no manifestations of serious underlying disease does not improve clinical outcomes.

A systematic review and meta-analysis of six trials involving 1804 patients assessed clinical outcomes in patients receiving immediate imaging of the lumbar spine with radiography, magnetic resonance imaging, or computed tomography versus usual care without immediate imaging. They found no significant differences, whether short term or long term, in regard to pain, function, or other outcomes [1].

1. Chou R, et al. Imaging strategies for low back pain: systematic review and meta-analysis. Lancet. 2009;373:463.

Jugular venous ultrasound is a sensitive test for identifying pulmonary edema on chest x-ray in dyspneic patients with suspected heart failure [1].

The statement above is taken directly from the conclusion of a report describing a prospective study of ultrasonic assessment of jugular venous distension (US-JVD) in the context of suspected congestive heart failure in the emergency department setting. The report, published in a European journal in February 2011, showed that in detecting pulmonary edema in dyspneic patients, US-JVD had a sensitivity of 98.2 % (95 % CI, 89.2–99.9), a specificity of 42.9 % (95 % CI, 30.7–55.9), and a positive likelihood ratio 1.7 (95 % CI, 1.4–2.1) [1]. In fact, the authors liked their data so much that later that year, in an American journal, they published a *secondary analysis* with even better sensitivity, specificity, and likelihood ratio figures [2].

1. Jang T, et al. Jugular vein ultrasound and pulmonary edema in patients with suspected congestive heart failure. Eur J Emerg Med. 2011;18:41.
2. Jang T, et al. Jugular venous distension on ultrasound: sensitivity and specificity for heart failure in patients with dyspnea. Am J Emerg Med. 2011;29:965.

The designation of the esophageal pouch sign as pathognomonic for fetal esophageal atresia (EA) seems to be a plastic pearl.

Solt et al. have challenged what they describe as the sonographic finding of an esophageal pouch being pathognomonic of EA. These investigators followed six fetuses with an esophageal neck pouch associated with polyhydramnios and small or apparently absent stomachs. When examined weeks later, in all six fetuses the polyhydramnios had resolved and the stomach was normal [1].

1. Solt I, et al. The esophageal pouch sign: a benign transient finding. Prenat Diagn. 2010; 30:845.

Selected Problems Related to Laboratory and Imaging Diagnosis

Preoperative laboratory tests ordered are often unnecessary.

A survey of 1,000 consecutive patients scheduled for surgery revealed, based on testing guidelines, that more than half of them had at least one unnecessary test. The single variable that seemed to increase the likelihood of ordering unnecessary testing was completing medical training prior to 1980 [1].

1. Katz RI, et al. Survey study of anesthesiologists' and surgeons' ordering of unnecessary preoperative laboratory tests. Anes Analges. 2011;112:207.

Diagnostic phlebotomy can cause anemia in adults and even prompt the need for transfusion.

In a study of phlebotomized patients, 50 patients in intensive care settings had an average of 762.2 mL removed by phlebotomy during their stay. Of 36 patients in the study who received transfusions, 17 (47 %) had made large donations as laboratory specimens, contributing to their need for transfused blood [1].

1. Smoller BR, et al. Phlebotomy for diagnostic laboratory tests in adults. N Engl J Med. 1986; 314:1233.

Diagnostic imaging is a leading contributor to our lifetime exposure to ionizing radiation.

One reported study used utilization data to estimate cumulative exposure to radiation from imaging procedures in 952,420 subjects. During the 3-year study period, 655,613 (68.8 %) had at least one radiation-involved imaging procedure. The investigators report that 193.8 subjects per 1,000 per year received moderate effective doses of radiation, while 18.6 received high doses and 1.9 per 1,000 per year received very high doses of radiation [1]. The National Institutes of Health has responded to data such as these by requiring that vendors provide information describing the radiation exposure resulting from use of their equipment [2].

1. Fazel R, et al. Exposure to low-dose ionizing radiation from medical imaging procedures. N Engl J Med. 2009;361:849.
2. Neumann RD, et al. Tracking radiation exposure from diagnostic imaging devices at the NIH. J Am Coll Radiol. 2010;7:87.

Glossary of Statistical Terms Used in This Book

Confidence interval (CI) The probability that a result will fall between two set values. The confidence interval is often expressed as being 95 or 99 %. For example, an author describing a *95 % CI* is saying that if things are done the same way 100 times, we would expect similar results in at least 95 % of instances.

Hazard ratio (HR) According to the National Cancer Institute, the hazard ratio describes how often a particular event happens in one group compared to how often it happens in another group, measured over time. Here is an example from a study of multiple sclerosis (MS) patients (Healy, BC et al. Arch Neurol. 2009 66:7.): "At longitudinal analysis, MS in smokers progressed from relapsing-remitting to secondary progressive disease faster than in never-smokers (hazard ratio for current smokers vs. never-smokers, 2.50; 95 % confidence interval 1.42–4.41)."

Likelihood ratio (LR) The odds that a given test result would be expected in a patient with the specific disease compared to the chances that that same result would be expected in a patient without the disease in question. The LR is helpful in assessing the probability that a specific diagnostic test will provide useful information. It does so by providing a direct estimate of how much a test result will change the odds of finding a disease and incorporates both the sensitivity and specificity of the test. The likelihood ratio for a positive test result is sensitivity/ 1 − specificity. The likelihood ratio for a negative test result is 1 − sensitivity/ specificity. An LR less than 1 indicates a lower likelihood of disease, while an LR greater than 1 indicates a higher likelihood of disease. Tests with LRs less than 0.2 or greater than 5.0 tend to be the most useful clinically.

Number needed treat (NNT) The NNT is the number of persons that must be treated with a drug or that must undergo some other intervention (such as stopping smoking) in order to achieve a specific result in one individual in the study group. If a drug has an NNT of 100, then 100 persons must be treated to achieve the desired result. For example, a recent Cochrane review (Wells, et al. Cochrane Database Syst Rev. 2008;1. Art. No. CD001155.) found that for primary prevention of vertebral fractures with alendronate (Fosamax), the NNT was 50. The ideal NNT is one, and the higher the NNT, the less effective the intervention.

R.B. Taylor, *Diagnostic Principles and Applications*,
DOI 10.1007/978-1-4614-1111-6, © Springer Science+Business Media, LLC 2013

Odds ratio (OR) The odds ratio is a descriptive statistic used to assess the chance of a particular outcome, typically a disease, if a certain risk factor or event is present. For example, a study reported in JAMA (Mokdad AH, et al. JAMA. 2003;289:76) found that, compared with adults with normal weight, adults with a BMI of 40 or higher had an OR of 7.37 (95 % confidence interval [CI] 6.39–8.50) for diagnosed diabetes. Thus the odds ratio is a relative measure of risk, telling us how much more likely it is that someone who is exposed to the factor being studied will develop the disease or other outcome as compared to someone who is not exposed.

P-**value** The likelihood that a result could occur by chance is traditionally expressed as a *p*-value. The *p* stands for *probability*. The smaller the *p*-value, the less likely it is that the findings reported are the result of chance. For example, if the *p*-value is 0.05, then there is a 5 % chance that the findings occurred by chance. A *p*-value of 0.01 is even better, as described below under **statistical significance**.

Relative risk (RR) Also sometimes called the **risk ratio**. The RR describes the probability of an adverse outcome occurring during a specified time interval in a study group exposed to some sort of event versus the outcome without the exposure. For example, we might be concerned with the relative risk of stroke among persons with and without hypertension.

Relative Risk Reduction (RRR) An expression of the degree to which an intervention decreases the probability of developing a disease, complication, or other adverse outcome. For example, we might conduct a study to see what protection against stroke is afforded by various categories of antihypertensive agents.

Reliability The consistency of an assessment method. If the speedometer on my car happens to be set to read 50 miles per hour (mph) when the actual speed is 60 mph, it will reflect this error every time and thus be reliable even though it is not accurate. This will make scant difference to the traffic officer who writes the summons for speeding.

Retrospective cohort study An examination of what has already happened to a group of individuals who experienced an exposure or intervention compared with an otherwise similar group who did not experience the exposure or intervention. An example of such a study might be the record review to determine the uterine cancer risk that has already occurred in women previously exposed to hormone replacement therapy (HRT) compared to a similar group with no HRT exposure. A prospective cohort study, in contrast, would follow exposed and unexposed women into the future.

Selection bias In a cohort or case control study, selection bias occurs when, for one reason or another, study groups and control groups differ from the start. Suppose, for instance, that in a cohort study to determine the outcome of treating heart failure with a specific drug, the intervention group had far more diabetic patients than the control group. Selection bias may also be termed **allocation bias**.

Sensitivity (Sn) A measurement of the portion of items correctly detected as present. This usually has to do with tests used to detect disease. Thus a test with 100 % (also stated as 1.0) sensitivity for tuberculosis, for example, would identify all persons with the disease, and a test with a 0.5 sensitivity would detect half of those infected. Compare this term with **Specificity**, described below. A test with a high sensitivity will have few false negatives.

Specificity (Sp) A measurement of the proportions of items correctly identified as not present, often represented as the percentage of healthy people who are correctly identified as not having a particular disease. Thus a test with 100 % (or alternatively, 1.0) specificity for tuberculosis, for example, would not identify (incorrectly) anyone from the healthy group as sick. A test with a high specificity will have few false positives. For example, a study of patients with possible myocardial infarction (Mahajan N, et al. Int J Cardiol. 2006;111:442) found that in the first 24 h of a myocardial infarction, an elevated level of cardiac troponin-T has a high sensitivity (99 %) for acute myocardial infarction and a specificity of 86 %.

Statistical significance The term refers to the likelihood that a result could occur by chance, usually expressed as a *p-value*. The smaller the *p*-value, the less likely it is that the findings reported are the result of chance. If the level is 0.05, then there is a 5 % chance that the findings occurred by chance. In research terminology, a setting in which a so-called null hypothesis (see above) is often employed, the *smaller* the *p*-value, the *less* likely the null hypothesis is true, and consequently the more statistically significant the reported result is considered. Thus a *p*-value of 0.01 represents a higher level of statistical significance than a *p*-value of 0.05.

Stratification The process of separating research subjects into clinically relevant subgroups for analysis. For example, we might stratify the analysis of a drug used to treat hypertension by separately studying patients with and without elevated creatinine levels. This is one strategy for reducing confounding; another strategy would be to simply exclude patients with high creatinine levels from a study.

Systematic review A general term describing a look-back at multiple published reports on a single topic in an attempt to answer one or more focused questions relevant to the topic. Using a reproducible search strategy in bibliographic data bases and selecting all articles that meet specified criteria (e.g., sample size, randomization, or other design features) are the characteristics that make a review *systematic*, in contrast to *what's in my file drawer*.

Validity A description of the extent to which a study accurately measures what the researcher set out to measure. There are various types of validity: **Face validity** is the research "sniff test"—Do the study design and results reported seem to make sense? **Internal validity** has to do with the integrity of the research design. **External validity** is a description of the extent to which the study conclusions are generalizable to other populations. These all differ from **reliability**—the reproducibility of the actual measuring instrument or procedure, described above.

Index

A

Abdominal aortic aneurysm (AAA),
    139, 140
Abdominal bruit, 122
Abdominal distension, 167, 179
    and toxic megacolon, 179, 180
Abdominal migraine (AM), 39
Abdominal pain, 163–167, 177,
    179, 184
    and abdominal migraine, 39
    and constipation, 38, 39
    ectopic pregnancy, 226, 227
    and Henoch–Schonlein purpura, 43
    and intussusception, 38
    ovarian torsion, 218, 219
    and use of analgesics
        in acute intermittent porphyria, 167
        in acute mesenteric ischemia, 163
        in appendicitis, 165
        in pancreatitis, 164
        patient posture, 164
ABO blood groups, 176
    and pancreatic cancer, 176
Abuse
    physical, 301
    sexual, 301
Acanthosis nigricans, 279
Acoustic neuroma, 99, 100, 103
    decreased corneal reflex, 72
    nystagmus, 72
Acromioclavicular arthritis, 242
Acroparesthesia, 314
    and Fabry disease, 314
Acute cerebellar ataxia
    following varicella infection, 339
    manifestations of, 339

Acute intermittent porphyria, 167
    agitated psychosis in, 311
    peripheral neuropathy in, 311
    urine, port-wine color, 311
Acute mesenteric ischemia (AMI), 163
Acute renal failure, 194
Acute respiratory failure,
    159, 160
    and cardiogenic pulmonary edema,
        159, 160
Addison disease, 273
Adhesive capsulitis (AC), 242
Adie pupil, 82
    vs. Argyll Robertson pupil, 82
Adrenal hyperplasia, 279
Alanine aminotransferase
    (ALT), 382
Alarm symptoms, 191, 209
    dysphagia, 152
    hematuria, 152, 191
    hemoptysis, 152
    rectal bleeding, 152
Aldosteronism, 122
Alkaline phosphatase level, elevated
    in Alzheimer disease, 382
    bone related causes, 382
    hepatic related causes, 382
    spurious result, 382
Alopecia areata (AA)
    other associated diseases, 279
    and thyroid disease, 279
Alopecia syphilitica, 281
Alzheimer disease (AD), 51, 52, 71
    MRI biomarker, 52
Amenorrhea
    in adolescent athletes and dancers, 216